Butterworths International Medical Reviews

Gastroenterology 1

Foregut

Butterworths International Medical Reviews

Gastroenterology 1

Editorial Board
J. Alexander-Williams
J. H. Baron
H. J. Binder
V. S. Chadwick
W. C. Maddrey
F. G. Moody
S. F. Phillips
W. H. ReMine
R. S. Williams
K. G. Wormsley

Future volumes to include

Small Intestine

Large Bowel

Liver

Pancreatic and Biliary System

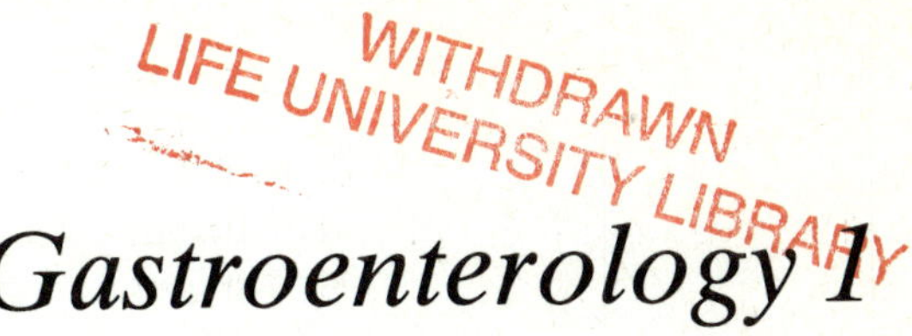

Butterworths
International
Medical
Reviews

Gastroenterology 1

Foregut

Edited by

J. H. Baron, DM, FRCP
Senior Lecturer and Consultant,
Departments of Surgery and Medicine,
Royal Postgraduate Medical School
and Hammersmith Hospital;
Consultant Physician,
St. Charles' Hospital,
London

and

Frank G. Moody, MD, FACS
Professor and Chairman,
Department of Surgery,
College of Medicine,
University of Utah,
Salt Lake City,
Utah

Butterworths
London Boston
Sydney Wellington Durban Toronto

First published 1981

©Butterworth & Co (Publishers) Ltd, 1981

British Library Cataloguing in Publication Data
Gastroenterology.
  Foregut. – (Butterworths international
  medical reviews ISSN 0260–0110)
  Vol. 1: Foregut
  1. Digestive organs – Diseases – Periodicals
  I. Baron, J. H. II. Moody, Frank G.
  616.3′305   RC801   80–42331
  ISBN 0–407–02287–2

Photoset by Butterworths Litho Preparation Department
Printed and Bound by Robert Hartnoll Ltd., Bodmin, Cornwall.

Preface

Butterworths' *Modern Trends* served a generation of clinicians and trainees, and we welcome its successor, *Butterworths International Medical Reviews*. These are neither didactic text books, nor exhaustive compendia of the whole field. Instead the coeditors (one for each hemisphere) of each book have selected about 10 important topics in their area and then chosen international experts to provide succinct critical reviews of the current state-of-the-art, to pinpoint recent advances of fruitful research, emphasizing their implication for clinical practice and also to predict future trends.

The explosive progress in gastroenterology in recent years meant that it had outgrown a single volume; it was therefore decided to divide the field into smaller components in order to give a more detailed appraisal. We were honoured to be given the exciting task of editing the first volume of the Gastroenterology series, *Foregut*, and others will follow in future years.

We decided to look in some ways at the foregut as a whole, and in other chapters we examined specific areas. Mr de Dombal has set the trend in the new approaches to assessing exactly what is the patient's complaint, in the use of information science, the concept of utility and the value of diagnosis by computer. The Helsinki group have unique prospective data on gastritis and gastric malignancy; they have given us a considered viewpoint on carcinogenesis in the foregut, with the interplay of genetic and environmental factors. Advances in physiological measurement have nowhere been more striking than in gastrointestinal motility and we have been fortunate to secure the contribution of Dr Christensen, one of the world authorities. The Hammersmith gastrointestinal endocrinology group have made major steps forward in what were once called alimentary hormones, but which, with the realization of the frequent coexistence of nerve and gut hormones, are now better entitled regulatory peptides. Upper gastrointestinal bleeding is both a common and life-threatening clinical problem, and our chapter comes from the Frankfurt group who have been in the

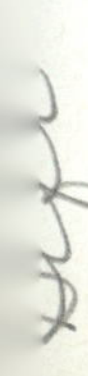

forefront of the amazing advances in diagnosis and management of alimentary haemorrhage.

In the specific organ, the oesophagus, we selected the general topic of gastroesophageal reflux and oesophagitis. The Chicago group have skillfully surveyed the surgical approaches to these disorders. Drs Maher and Woodward from the University of Florida have tackled the vexed question of the management of oesophageal strictures. We chose two complicated aspects for the stomach. The clinician is inundated continually with new drugs for gastric and duodenal ulcer and the Dallas group have provided clear guidelines for the medical therapy of peptic ulcer. The Hammersmith gastroenterologists have provided, for the first time, an authoritative analysis of the nature and management of Menetrier's disease which has been a medical mystery for a hundred years.

We are most grateful to all our contributors for their enthusiasm and wholehearted contribution in this venture, and would like to acknowledge the help and support we have received from Butterworths.

J. H. Baron
Frank G. Moody

List of contributors

T. E. Adrian, PHD,
Senior Research Officer, Department of Medicine, Royal Postgraduate Medical School, Hammersmith Hospital, London, UK

S. R. Bloom, MD, FRCP,
Reader in Medicine, Royal Postgraduate Medical School, Hammersmith Hospital, London, UK

V. S. Chadwick, MD, MSC, FRCP,
Senior Lecturer in Medicine, Royal Postgraduate Medical School, Hammersmith Hospital, London, UK

M. Classen, MD,
Professor, Abteilung für Gastroenterologie, Zentrum der Inneren Medizin, Johann Wolfgang Goethe-Universität, Frankfurt am Main, West Germany

B. T. Cooper, MD, MRCP,
Lecturer in Medicine, Royal Infirmary, Bristol, UK

James Christensen, MD,
Professor, Department of Internal Medicine and Director, Division of Gastroenterology-Hepatology, University of Iowa College of Medicine, Iowa City, Iowa, USA

Tom R. DeMeester, MD, FACS,
Professor of Thoracic and Cardiovascular Surgery, University of Chicago Department of Surgery, Chicago, Illinois, USA

F. T. de Dombal, MA, MD, FRCS,
Reader in Clinical Information Science, Department of Surgery, St James' University Hospital, Leeds, UK

Mark Feldman, MD,
Associate Professor, Department of Internal Medicine, University of Texas Health Science Center at Dallas, Southwestern Medical School, and Veterans Administration Medical Center, Dallas, Texas, USA

James W. Maher, MD,
Assistant Professor, Department of Surgery, College of Medicine, University of Mississippi, Jackson, Mississippi, USA

Gerald C. O'Sullivan, MB, MSC, FRCSI,
Fellow in Esophageal Diseases, University of Chicago Department of Surgery, Chicago, Illinois, USA

J. Phillip, MD,
Assistant Medical Director, Zentrum der Inneren Medizin, Johann Wolfgang Goethe-Universität, Frankfurt am Main, West Germany

J. M. Polak, MD, DSC,
Senior Lecturer, Department of Histochemistry, Royal Postgraduate Medical School, Hammersmith Hospital, London, UK

Lawrence R. Schiller, MD,
Assistant Professor, Department of Internal Medicine, University of Texas Health Science Center at Dallas, Southwestern Medical School, and Veterans Administration Medical Center, Dallas, Texas, USA

P. Sipponen, MD,
Head of the Department of Pathology, Jorvi Hospital, Espoo, Finland

M. Siurala, MD,
Professor, Second Department of Medicine, University of Helsinki, Helsinki, Finland

G. Smith-Laing, MRCP,
Senior Medical Registrar, Department of Gastroenterology, West Middlesex Hospital, Isleworth, UK

E. R. Woodward, MD,
Professor and Chairman, Department of Surgery, College of Medicine, University of Florida, Gainesville, Florida, USA

K. Varis, MD,
Second Department of Medicine, University of Helsinki, Helsinki, Finland

Contents

1
Esophageal strictures

James W. Maher and E. R. Woodward

History

The therapy of esophageal strictures was limited solely to attempts at dilatation until the pioneering work of Bircher in 1894 that described bypass of the stricture with an antethoracic cutaneous tube[31]. This was followed by innovative procedures utilizing subcutaneous antethoracic intestinal loops and subsequently by Torek's report in 1913 of the first successful transpleural esophagogastrectomy[27]. The advances in anesthesia that made transthoracic approaches safe, made feasible further advances such as Rienhoff's jejunal interposition[22] in 1946. This was followed in 1953 by the first intrathoracic colon interposition[23].

Modern surgery for peptic esophagitis dates from the work of Professor Phillip Allison in 1951[1]. Allison's classical description of esophagitis emphasized the role of esophagoscopy in confirming the diagnosis. He correctly attributed the esophagitis to reflux of the acid gastric contents and designed an operation to prevent further reflux. The high failure rate of his procedure has not diminished the validity of his basic concept and has led to the development of more effective antireflux procedures. These procedures now form the cornerstone of an extremely effective therapeutic strategy for the treatment of gastroesophageal reflux and its complications.

Etiology

There are numerous causes for the presence of an apparent esophageal stricture (*Table 1.1*). This chapter is limited to a discussion of strictures

Table 1.1 Etiology of apparent stricture

Intrinsic esophageal disease

Congenital esophageal disease

(1) Webs
(2) Stenosis
(3) Cysts, rests, duplications

Postinfectious esophageal disease

(1) Fungus (blastomycosis, actinomycosis)
(2) Pyogenic septicemia
(3) Tuberculosis
(4) Syphilis
(5) Diphtheria, scarlet fever
(6) Moniliasis

Post-inflammatory

(1) Endogenous corrosives
(2) Exogenous corrosives

Tumors

Miscellaneous

(1) Diffuse spasm
(2) Achalasia
(3) Plummer-Vinson syndrome
(4) Crohn's disease
(5) Penetrating injury
(6) Retained foreign body

Extrinsic compression

Vascular structures

(1) Anomalous aortic arch
(2) Aberrant right subclavian
(3) Aneurysm
(4) Cardiomegaly

Mediastinal mass

Miscellaneous

(1) Vertebral osteophyte
(2) Hepatomegaly
(3) Diaphragmatic gumma

---

secondary to intrinsic esophageal disease, their pathophysiology and treatment. Emphasis is placed on the proper treatment of strictures secondary to endogenous corrosives. The etiology of an esophageal stricture is a crucial factor in instituting proper treatment. Familiarity with the diagnostic modalities of cineradiography, esophagoscopy with esophageal biopsy, esophageal manometry, pH reflux testing and their sometimes subtle implications are important in the tailoring of therapy to the individual patient.

Congenital esophageal disease

Congenital webs are uncommon. They are thin membranes made up of mucosa and variable amounts of submucosa. Partial or complete esophageal obstruction may occur early; however, incomplete webs may present later and be confused with an acquired annular stricture or webs due to iron-deficiency anemia or trauma. Congenital webs appear to represent an abnormality in the vacuolization process and are found at all levels. Treatment usually consists of dilatation or local resection.

Congenital stenosis is also unusual and it may occur as a result of disordered development of the tracheoesophageal septum or the lateral esophageal ridges. The narrowing may be asymptomatic until the child is advanced to a solid diet. Dilatation or local resection is usually curative.

Congenital cysts, rests and duplications are generally easily enucleated or excised.

Postinfectious esophageal disease

Stenosis secondary to an infectious process usually improves with dilatation and specific medical treatment of the infection. Occasionally, however, long-standing infection will lead to severe transmural scarring necessitating resective surgery.

Endogenous corrosives

Physiology

The endogenous corrosive most commonly associated with esophageal stricture is gastric juice. Experimental studies have demonstrated an exquisite sensitivity of the esophageal mucosa to acid–pepsin solutions[20]. Gastroesophageal reflux, however, is a normal physiologic response to swallowing that can be readily demonstrated by postprandial cineradiography with barium. The regurgitated material is rapidly evacuated from the esophagus by esophageal peristalsis so that it lies in contact with esophageal mucosa for only the briefest of intervals. Gastroesophageal reflux becomes significant only when the gastric contents bathe the esophageal mucosa for a prolonged period of time. This was shown by Johnson and DeMeester whose technique of 24-hour pH monitoring demonstrated both a prolongation and an increase in the frequency of reflux episodes in patients with esophagitis[12]. This abnormal reflux may occur under a variety of circumstances, but before discussing them it is necessary to point out the details involved in maintaining normal competence.

The physiologic mechanisms involved in maintaining gastroesophageal competence is an area rife with controversies, none of which will be resolved here. Nevertheless, the most important factor appears to be the lower esophageal sphincter (LES). Resection of this area invariably results in severe prolonged reflux. Further, although substantial overlap exists with controls, patients with esophagitis usually have a decreased lower esophageal sphincter pressure. Factors previously thought to be important in maintaining competence in order of decreasing importance are listed in *Table 1.2*. These mechanical factors apparently play only minor roles in the genesis of gastroesophageal competence. Predictably, the above sentence will not be met with unanimous agreement; however, few will dispute the importance of the LES.

Since we all reflux normally, there would appear to be a secondary mechanism responsible for protection of the esophagus from prolonged contact with the gastric contents. In fact, Skinner and Booth

Table 1.2 Mechanisms of gastroesophageal competence

Lower esophageal sphincter
Phrenoesophageal ligament
Mucosal 'rosette'
Diaphragmatic 'pinchcock'
Acute angle of His
Intra-abdominal esophagus
Gastric sling fibers

showed a marked increase in the number of swallows required to restore normal intraesophageal pH in patients with esophagitis[26]. The importance of this 'acid clearing' mechanism has been supported by the previously mentioned 24-hour pH data.

Conditions that predispose one to gastroesophageal reflux are listed in *Table 1.3*. Hiatal hernia is by far the most commonly associated

Table 1.3 Factors associated with gastroesophageal reflux

Sliding hiatus hernia
Destruction of sphincter
Persistent vomiting
Indwelling nasogastric tube
Miscellaneous motor disorders

condition and in the past was nearly synonomous with the complex of symptoms we now recognize as esophagitis. There is a marked disagreement about the importance of this problem in the genesis of esophagitis and some believe that it is a result rather than a predisposing cause of the pathology[10].

Displacement of the inferior esophageal sphincter into the chest, as occurs with a hiatus hernia, exposes it to negative intrathoracic pressure. This distracting force probably has no effect on a competent lower esophageal sphincter. However, a sphincter with already borderline pressure may become grossly incompetent in this environment. While there are clearly individuals who have reflux without a hernia, 80 percent of patients with reflux will have a sliding esophageal hiatal hernia.

Gastroesophageal reflux will inevitably be produced by any procedure that destroys the lower esophageal sphincter. Excessive emesis associated with either pregnancy or pyloric stenosis can likewise lead to esophagitis as can prolonged postoperative use of a nasogastric tube.

Pathologic reflux is occasionally seen with esophageal motor disorders, the most common being scleroderma. The defect in scleroderma is characterized by aperistalsis in the lower two-thirds of the esophagus and an incompetent lower esophageal sphincter. These patients often present with severe strictures.

Pathology

Benign peptic esophageal stricture may be divided into two distinct morphologic types. The first is an annular lesion situated at or slightly above the squamocolumnar junction. it is produced by submucosal inflammation and fibrosis, and is covered by intact mucosa. The second is a longitudinal inflammatory stricture situated immediately above either herniated stomach or Barrett's heterotopic gastric mucosa. The lesion is characterized by thick fibrous scar that infiltrates the esophageal wall transmurally from an ulcerated mucosa with severe periesophageal inflammation (*Figure 1.1*). The ascending nature of the inflammation and scarring is accompanied by scar contraction in all three dimensions. This results in a lesion characterized by esophageal shortening as well as stenosis.

Esophagitis and stricture are also known to occur in non-operated achlorhydric patients and in patients who have undergone total or

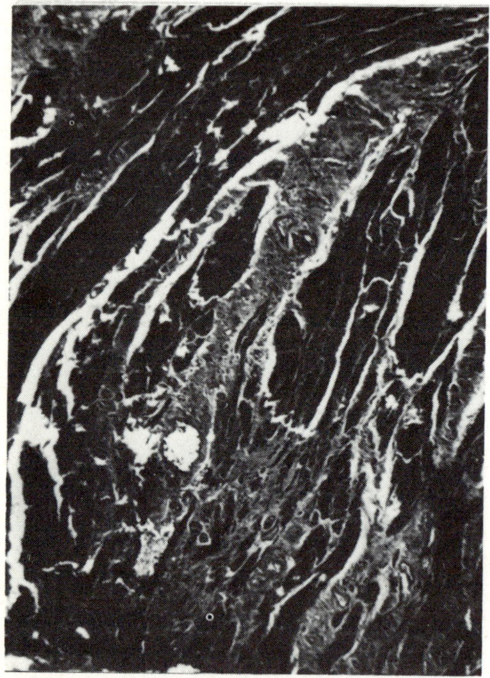

Figure 1.1 Biopsy of an esophageal stricture demonstrating transmural infiltration of muscle by fibrous tissue in a patient with reflux-induced esophageal stricture (Masson, Trichrome, original magnification × 20)

partial gastrectomy[17, 30]. This so-called 'alkaline esophagitis' is some-what of a misnomer since available evidence implicates the total duodenal content in the etiology of this condition[3].

Diagnosis

The symptoms of reflux esophagitis such as burning, regurgitation and eructation, aggravated by the recumbent position, are well known. Most patients will present with these symptoms initially, but occasionally the first symptom may be dysphagia from a far-advanced stricture. Although these symptoms are usually enough to arouse a clinician's suspicions, the diagnosis of reflux esophagitis with or without stricture cannot be made by history alone.

Barium swallow is the most common way of demonstrating gastro-esophageal reflux. Nevertheless, the high density of barium makes it suitable for only more pronounced cases of reflux. Sipping water in the Trendelberg position enhances the sensitivity of this test, but the continuous sipping of water is a powerful stimulus to sphincter relaxation. This leads to a high percentage of false positive examinations. The barium swallow remains useful for demonstrating the subtleties of local anatomy including hiatus hernia, esophageal shortening, stricture and esophageal ulcers.

Reflux may be demonstrated more reliably by pH reflux studies. In this test a miniature pH electrode is placed 2 cm above the lower esophageal sphincter which is simultaneously defined by manometry. The pH should rise promptly to 6. The patient is then instructed to perform a Valsalva maneuver and sniff vigorously three to four times. If no reflux is demonstrated 300 ml of 0.1 N-HCl is placed into the stomach through the manometric catheter and the maneuvers are repeated. The test is considered positive if pH drops to 2 or less. This test will pick up 95 percent of patients with significant reflux.

Esophageal manometry is helpful not only in ruling out the presence of a predisposing motor disorder that might complicate surgical therapy but also in predicting the results of surgery by demonstrating an increased postoperative lower esophageal sphincter pressure[5].

Esophagoscopy with biopsy remains the cornerstone of diagnostic modalities for the demonstration of reflux esophagitis and its complications. It is also useful in ruling out the presence of occult malignancy in long-standing esophageal strictures. In summary, there is no substitute for direct inspection of the afflicted area.

Treatment

There are many modes of therapy available for the treatment of esophageal strictures. Proper treatment, however, varies with the condition of the patients and the type and location of the stricture.

Dilatation and medical management

Stricture dilatation alone invariably results in recurrent reflux. This method, combined with medical therapy of the underlying gastro-esophageal reflux, has been advocated by Palmer who reported satisfactory results in 87 percent of patients. However, the pathologic types of strictures and length of follow-up are not mentioned[18].

Skinner and Belsey, in contrast, noted only 36 percent satisfactory results and a 22 percent mortality rate in patients treated in this manner[25]. We feel that this approach should now be reserved only for those patients with strict medical contraindications to surgery.

Stricture dilatation plus antireflux procedure

Annular strictures due to their limited mucosal and submucosal involvement may be adequately treated by dilatation combined with an antireflux procedure. We have combined dilatation with either a Hill posterior gastropexy or a Nissen fundoplication with excellent results in 85 percent and 100 percent of patients respectively[2, 14]. The apparent superiority of the Nissen procedure in prevention of recurrent stricture is probably related primarily to its superior effectiveness in preventing acid–peptic reflux[4]. Hill reports 85 percent good results in 86 patients followed up to six years[11]. Herrington, utilizing Nissen fundoplication and dilatation, reports similar results[9].

Hill, Hayward, and Herrington all advocate extensive intraoperative manipulations including both endoscopic dilatation with woven bougies, and retrograde transgastric dilatation or finger fracture in efforts to avoid resection or esophagofundoplasty[7, 9, 11.] In the wide spectrum between annular and transmural strictures this approach can be expected to result in a moderate degree of success when further acid–peptic injury is prevented. Dilatation of strictures in which scarring and inflammation are truly transmural, however, results in the formation of granulation tissue followed by fibroblast proliferation, collagen deposition, and recurrent stenosis secondary to contraction and cross-linking of collagen. This basic biological phenomenon of scar formation cannot be altered by an antireflux procedure. This has been well demonstrated by Skinner and Belsey who report a 37 percent failure rate of antireflux procedure and dilatation in the treatment of acquired short esophagus, a stricture which by definition is transmural[25].

The severity of a longitudinal esophageal stricture can best be judged by either pre- or intraoperative bougienage with mercury weighted dilators. The authors find preoperative dilatation under topical anesthetic most satisfactory since the force of gravity in the upright position brings considerably more weight to bear on the stricture. Forceful dilatation under general anesthesia must be approached with considerably more caution. Review of Sawyers' report on treatment of esophageal perforation at Vanderbilt revealed seven patients with iatrogenic perforation occurring at the time of attempted bougienage[24]. The authors believe that examples such as this, while almost anecdotal, provide ample evidence that not all esophageal strictures can or should be dilated.

Combined Thal-Nissen procedure

The Thal fundic patch utilizes well-established plastic reconstructive techniques to replace part of the circumference of the fibrotic esophageal wall with pliable, well-vascularized fundic tissue lined by a skin graft. The importance of the skin graft in preventing contraction of the esophageal lumen has been amply demonstrated by Thal and his associates in experimental animals[28]. The split thickness skin graft prevents re-epithelialization of the esophageal wall by granulation tissue and thus minimizes contraction of the lumen as compared to an unsurfaced patch. Initial experience with the Thal patch alone for the treatment of peptic esophageal stricture showed universally poor results because of its failure to address the underlying problem of gastroesophageal incompetence. The fundic patch was therefore combined with a complete 360° Nissen fundoplication to prevent further acid–peptic injury. The efficacy of this combination has been well documented experimentally by Jones *et al.*[13]. They demonstrated that the combined Thal-Nissen procedure effectively prevents acid–peptic reflux by augmenting lower esophageal sphincter pressure with a broad high-pressure collar of gastric fundus. They further exposed the fallacy behind the common misconception that holds that a repair must be intra-abdominal in order to be successful. The control of reflux was equally effective whether the repair was intra-abdominal or intrathoracic.

Technique

The operation is performed transpleurally through the bed of the resected seventh rib. A 42 French Hurst bougie is passed perorally to aid in identification of the level of the stricture intraoperatively and to size the lumen created by the fundic patch. The esophagus is mobilized bluntly and the stomach exposed by dividing the tendonous portion of the diaphragm radially from the hiatus. The greater curvature is

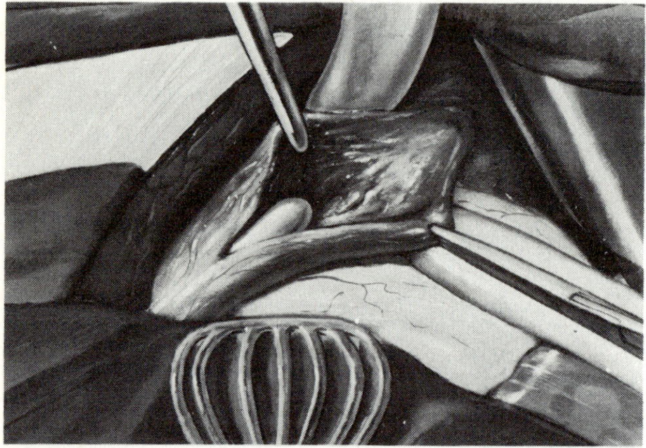

Figure 1.2 Artist rendering of the esophagotomy showing the 42 French Hurst bougie used to locate the esophageal lumen and stint the lumen during the performance of the Thal fundic patch

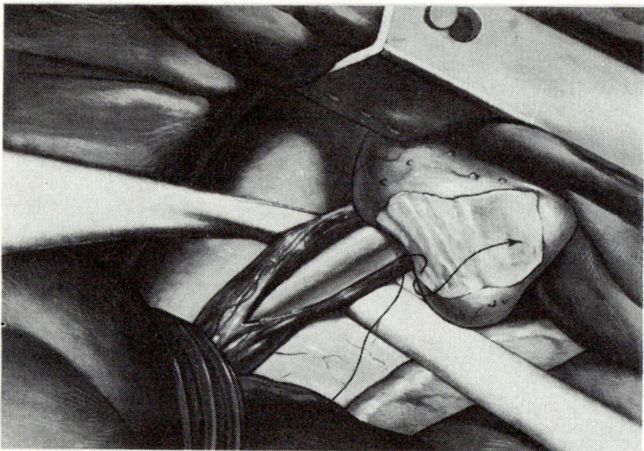

Figure 1.3 Artist rendering showing widening of the gastric inlet by transverse approximation of the full thickness of the esophageal wall to the fundus of the stomach

mobilized by dividing all short gastric branches in order to allow the fundus to prolapse easily into the chest. The stricture is then incised longitudinally from its proximal extent to the fundus (*Figure 1.2*). The dilator is passed distally into the stomach to stint the new esophageal lumen. Next, the gastric inlet is widened by transverse approximation of the posterior wall with interrupted 3–0 Dexon sutures (*Figure 1.3*). A split thickness skin graft is taken from the left shoulder and tacked

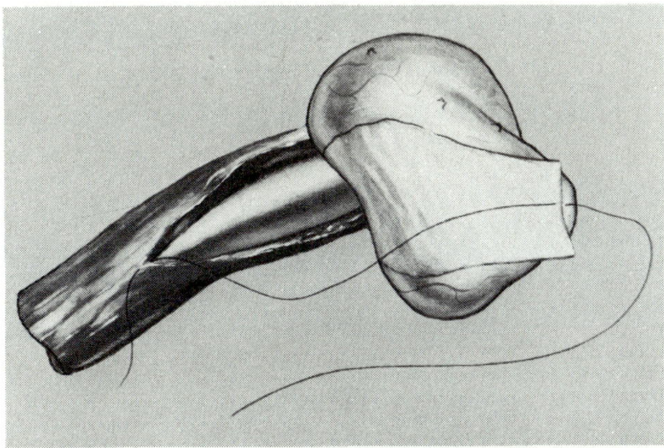

Figure 1.4 Artist rendering showing the apex stitch used to size the Thal fundic patch which is lined by a split thickness skin graft

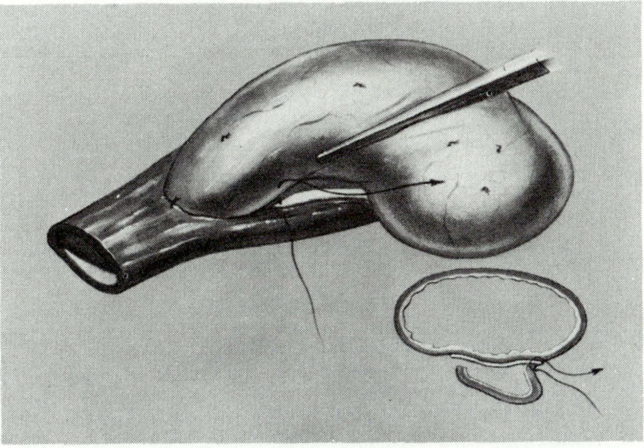

Figure 1.5 Artist rendering showing the right lateral wall of the fundic patch being constructed utilizing full thickness bites of esophagus, skin graft, and fundus. The cross-section demonstrates the degree of widening achieved by construction of the fundic patch

to the fundus following which the fundus is sutured to the defect in the anterior wall of the esophagus (*Figure 1.4, 1.5, 1.6*).

The fundoplication is then carried out by wrapping the fundus circumferentially around the esophagus and securing it on the right lateral side of the esophagus with 2–0 silk sutures to create a distal high pressure zone which prevents gastroesophageal reflux (*Figure 1.7*). The repair is left entirely in the chest. The fundus is secured circumferentially to the diaphragm with 3–0 silk sutures to prevent postoperative diaphragmatic hernia. Gastric decompression is maintained for 10 days. A chest tube is positioned near the repair with a single 4–0 chromic stitch and is not removed until an esophagogram demonstrates absence of leakage on the tenth day.

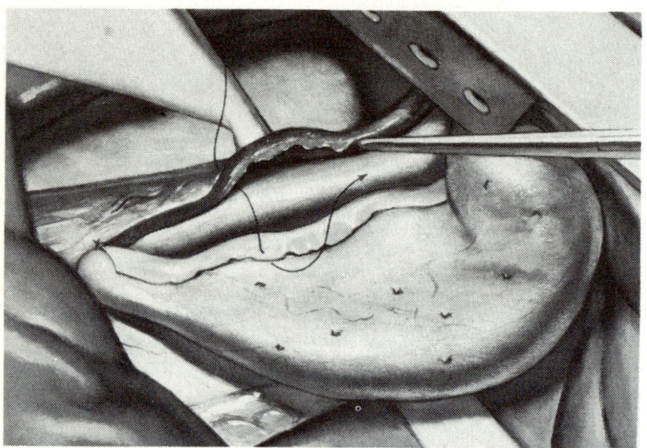

Figure 1.6 Artist rendering showing construction of the left lateral wall of the fundic patch

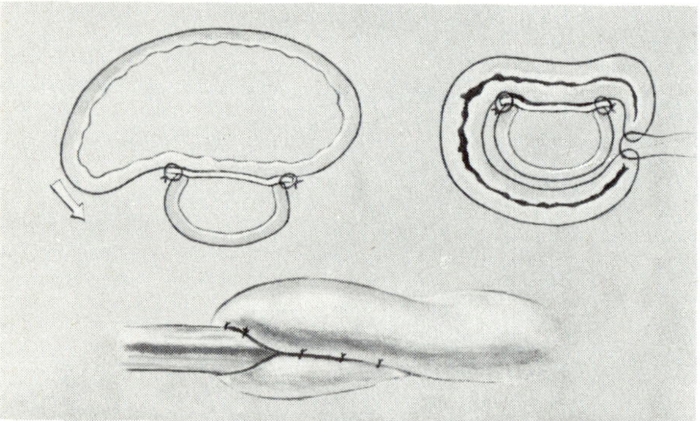

Figure 1.7 Artist rendering of the construction of the fundoplication. The cross-section demonstrates how the left side of the fundus is brought posterior to the esophagus and is used to construct a 360° fundic wrap

Patient data

Forty-nine males and 19 females underwent a combined Thal-Nissen procedure at the University of Florida Affiliated Hospitals. Age at operation ranged from 3 to 85 years with an average of 58 years (*Table 1.4*). Patients were selected on the basis of an inability to dilate them safely preoperatively using mercury-weighted bougies. In effect, this

Table 1.4 Patient data, Thal-Nissen procedure

Total number of patients	68
Males	49
Females	19
Average age (years)	58 (range 3–85)
Average length of stricture (cm)	4 (range 2–11)
Average follow-up (months)	68 (range 4–147)

criterion limits the patient population to those with longitudinal, transmural strictures of the esophagus. The average length of stricture was 4 cm; however, 33 percent of the patients had strictures that were 5 cm or longer with a maximum length of 11 cm. Two patients were later shown to have carcinoma although preoperative biopsies were negative. This emphasizes the need for intraoperative biopsy with frozen section pathologic examination. The authors have previously reported three of these patients who had scleroderma as the basis for their peptic stricture while three had achalasia with peptic esophageal stricture following an over-enthusiastic Heller procedure[16].

Preoperative evaluation in all cases included an upper gastrointestinal (GI) series and an upper GI endoscopy with biopsy. The need for esophagoscopy with biopsy cannot be over-emphasized because of the well-known propensity of these peptic strictures to harbor an occult carcinoma. Manometry is performed infrequently because of the difficulty encountered in passing the catheter assembly through these long strictures.

Follow-up

Follow-up was obtained by upper GI series, outpatient clinic visits, questionnaire, and/or telephone contact with the patient, referring physician, or next of kin if the patient had expired.

Results

Two of 68 patients were lost to follow-up, a 97 percent follow-up rate
(*Table 1.5*). There were three operation-related deaths (4 percent)
(*Table 1.5*). One patient died within 30 days of sepsis secondary to an
esophageal leak. There were two deaths in the late postoperative
period. One occurred five months postoperatively from hemorrhage

Table 1.5 Results of 68 patients undergoing Thal-Nissen procedure

	Number of patients	Percentage
Lost to follow-up	2	3
Operation-related mortality	3	4
Classification of 63 patients followed-up		
Good	44	70
Fair	13	20
Poor	3	5
Late recurrence	3	5

secondary to esophageal carcinoma which had not been detected at the
time of surgery despite multiple biopsies of the esophageal wall. The
third patient expired five weeks postoperatively from a myocardial
infarction. Three patients were demonstrated to have esophageal leaks
postoperatively. This complication was treated with drainage and
hyperalimentation. Follow-up ranged from 4 to 147 months in survi-
vors with a mean follow-up of 68 months. Twelve patients have been
followed for more than 10 years.

Results were classified as good, fair or poor. Asymptomatic patients
were considered to be good results. Patients with mild or occasional
symptoms of reflux or dysphagia were classified as fair results, and
patients who were unimproved or who required regular dilatation
were regarded as poor results.

Results are summarized in *Table 1.5*. Fifty-seven of the 63 patients
available for follow-up (90 percent) had an acceptable result while
only three (5 percent) had a poor result, as evidenced by an early
recurrence of stricture. An additional three patients (5 percent) had
late recurrence of their stricture after an initially good response period
of from 2 to 11 years. Two of the patients in the group with early
stricture required further surgery. One patient (J.K.) underwent a

jejunal interposition with good results. The other patient (C.H.) underwent a substernal colon interposition with necrosis of the interposed colon occurring on the eighth postoperative day. He is currently maintained on gastrostomy feedings. The third patient with a poor result (J.B.) suffered from achalasia with a peptic stricture that developed following a Heller myotomy performed elsewhere. He did well initially following his Thal-Nissen procedure; however, he soon required frequent dilatations to maintain an adequate lumen. He eventually underwent an esophagogastrectomy with good results.

The three patients with late stricture recurrence had good results for periods of 2, 6 and 11 years. One of the patients (H.W.) had achalasia with a peptic stricture following myotomy performed elsewhere. He did very well for six years, but he ultimately developed a recurrent stricture that required intermittent dilatation until the time of his death. Patient M.P. had scleroderma. She was asymptomatic for a period of two years. She has now had recurrence of her symptoms of dysphagia and pyrosis and requires intermittent dilatation. Patient V.C. was essentially asymptomatic for 11 years; however, she has now developed dysphagia. She has no demonstrable stricture by either endoscopy or upper GI series. Motility studies are suggestive of diffuse esophageal spasm. All other patients followed beyond 10 years had a satisfactory result.

The authors reserve the combined Thal-Nissen procedure for patients with a longitudinal, esophageal stricture that cannot be safely dilated utilizing mercury-weighted bougies. In this difficult group of patients good long-term results have been achieved in 90 percent of patients. Most of the patients with poor results suffered from severely disordered peristalsis and perhaps this group of patients would do better with an interposition procedure. The alternative to the combined Thal-Nissen procedure in patients with longitudinal strictures is a resection with either esophagogastrostomy or visceral interposition. The authors feel, therefore, that it is the morbidity and mortality of these procedures against which the results of a Thal-Nissen operation must be measured.

Stricture resection and esophagogastrectomy

Stricture resection and esophagogastrectomy is the most direct approach. Skinner and Belsey reported a 14.5 percent mortality in this group of patients with a 17 percent incidence of recurrent esophagitis[25]. Pearson, in an effort to prevent reflux, devised an 'ink well' type of anastomosis to create a high-pressure collar around the anastomosis[19]. This resulted in no mortality and a leak rate of only 6 percent. This group of patients, however, was being treated for carcinoma of the cardia and long-term follow-up was therefore not possible. Wara *et al.*[29] in contrast, reported a 25 percent rate of recurrent stricture and 87 percent recurrent esophagitis in the long-term follow-up of 17 patients who underwent 'ink well' esophagogastrostomy for benign esophageal stricture.

Reversed gastric tube

Heimlich has designed an innovative procedure combining stricture resection and a reversed gastric tube in 19 patients with benign stricture. Mortality was 5 percent with a leak rate of 11 percent and no patient developed recurrent esophagitis[8]. This procedure, however, requires a splenectomy. Furthermore, an 11 percent leak rate would be expected to result in at least some recurrent strictures and the long neo-esophageal suture line is an unnecessary step designed to create an intra-abdominal length of esophagus.

Stricture resection with jejunal interposition

Stricture resection with jejunal interposition was popularized by Merendino[15]. Results were satisfactory in his small group of patients with an 8.3 percent mortality and a similar rate of recurrent stricture. Ferrer and Bruch, however, reported a 15 percent mortality in 27 patients undergoing jejunal interposition[6]. Another 15 percent of the jejunal loops had to be discarded secondary to inadequate blood supply, but most patients with an intact loop had a satisfactory result.

Stricture resection and colon interposition

The success of colon interposition has been varied. Skinner and Belsey noted a 5 percent mortality with no late strictures or esophagitis[25]. Other investigators have reported a mortality which ranges from 7 to 20 percent with up to a 27 percent incidence of recurrent stricture[6, 21].

Late complications are unusual but colitis, colonic ulcers and perforation have been reported. Motility of the interposed colonic segment is poor, although contractions may be induced by a bolus of acid in the colon[13].

Summary

Optimum treatment of the patient with esophageal stricture requires of the operating surgeon a wide repertoire of procedures suited to the individual circumstance. Annular strictures of the esophagus can be quite satisfactorily treated by dilatation with an antireflux procedure. The Thal-Nissen procedure should be used in the patient with a longitudinal, transmural stricture which cannot be easily dilated. When used in this setting it widens the distal esophagus with a patch of well-vascularized fundus and provides extremely effective protection against gastroesophageal reflux without the high mortality associated with visceral interposition. Colonic or jejunal interposition should be reserved for those patients who either fail to respond to a combined Thal-Nissen procedure or who demonstrate sufficiently disordered peristalsis to render the esophagus an unsatisfactory conduit for the passage of food. Procedures tailored to the individual situation can be expected to produce in a high percentage of satisfactory results.

References

1 ALLISON, P. R. Reflux esophagitis, sliding hiatal hernia, and the anatomy of repair. *Surgery, Gynecology and Obstetrics*, **92**, 419–431 (1951)

2 BUSHKIN, F. L., NEUSTEIN, C. L., PARKER, T. H. and WOODWARD, E. R. Nissen fundoplication for reflux peptic esophagitis. *Annals of Surgery*, **185**, 672–677 (1977)

3 CROSS, F. S. and WANGENSTEEN, O. H. Role of bile and pancreatic juice in production of esophageal erosions and anemia. *Proceedings of the Society for Experimental Biology and Medicine*, **77**, 862–866 (1951)

4 DEMEESTER, T. R., JOHNSON, L. F. and KENT, A. H. Evaluation of current operations for the prevention of gastroesophageal reflux. *Annals of Surgery*, **180**, 511–525 (1974)

5 DIMARINO, A. J., ROSATA, E., ROSATO, F. and COHEN, S. Improvement in lower esophageal sphincter pressure following surgery for complicated gastro-esophageal reflux. *Annals of Surgery*, **181**, 239–242 (1974)

6 FERRER, J. M. and BRUCK, H. J. Jejunal and colonic interposition for non-malignant disease of the esophagus. *Annals of Surgery*, **169**, 533–543 (1965)

7 HAYWARD, J. The treatment of fibrous stricture of the oesophagus associated with hiatal hernia. *Thorax*, **16**, 45–55 (1961)

8 HEIMLICH, H. J. Esophagoplasty with reversed gastric tube. *American Journal of Surgery*, **123**, 90–92 (1972)

9 HERRINGTON, J. L., WRIGHT, R. S., EDWARDS, W. H. and SAWYERS, J. L. Conservative surgical treatment of reflux esophagitis and esophageal stricture. *Annals of Surgery*, **181**, 552–566 (1975)

10 HIEBERT, C. A. Primary incompetence of the gastric cardia. *American Journal of Surgery*, **119**, 365–371 (1970)

11 HILL, L. D., GELFAND, M. and BAUERMEISTER, D. Simplified management of reflux esophagitis with stricture. *Annals of Surgery*, **172**, 638–651 (1970)

12 JOHNSON, L. F. and DEMEESTER, T. R. Twenty-four-hour pH monitoring of the distal esophagus. A quantitative measure of gastroesophageal reflux. *The American Journal of Gastroenterology*, **62**, 325–332 (1974)

13 JONES, E. L., BOOTH, D. J., CAMERON, J. L., ZUIDEMA, G. D. and SKINNER, D. B. Functional evaluation of esophageal reconstructions. *Annals of Thoracic Surgery*, **12**, 331–346 (1971)

14 MAHER, J. W., HOLLENBECK, J. I. and WOODWARD, E. R. An analysis of recurrent esophagitis following posterior gastropexy. *Annals of Surgery*, **187**, 227–230 (1978)

15 MERENDINO, K. A. and DILLARD, D. H. The concept of sphincter substitution by an interposed jejunal segment for anatomic and physiologic abnormalities at the esophagogastric junction. With special reference to reflux esophagitis, cardiospasm and esophageal varices. *Annals of Surgery*, **142**, 486–509 (1955)

16 O'LEARY, J. P., HOLLENBECK, J. I. and WOODWARD, E. R. Surgical treatment of esophageal stricture in patients with scleroderma. *American Surgeon*, **41**, 131–135 (1975)

17 ORR, T. G. A modified technic for total gastrectomy. *Archives of Surgery*, **54**, 279–286 (1947)

18 PALMER, E. D. The hiatus hernia-esophagitis-esophageal stricture complex. *American Journal of Medicine*, **44**, 566–579 (1968)

19 PEARSON, F. G., HENDERSON, R. D. and PARRISH, R. M. An operative technique for the control of reflux following esophagogastrostomy. *Journal of Thoracic and Cardiovascular Surgery*, **58**, 668–677 (1969)

20 PLZAK, L. F., FRIED, W. and WOODWARD, E. R. Relative susceptibility of the gastrointestinal tract to experimental acute peptic ulceration. *Surgical Forum*, **7**, 389–393 (1971)

21 POSTLETHWAITE, R. W., SEALY, W. C., DILLON, M. L. and YOUNG, W. G. Colon interposition for esophageal substitution. *Annals of Thoracic Surgery*, **12**, 89–109 (1971)

22 RIENHOFF, JR., W. F. Intrathoracic esophagojejunostomy for lesions of the upper third of the esophagus. *Southern Medical Journal*, **39**, 928–940 (1946)

23 ROBERTSON, C. W., HOWE, C. W. and SMITHWICK, R. H. The use of the colon to replace the lower esophagus in man. Report of case 3½ years after operation. *Surgical Forum*, **3**, 66–71 (1953)

24 SAWYERS, J. L., LANE, C. E., FOSTER, J. H. and DANIEL, R. A. Esophageal perforation. *Annals of Thoracic Surgery*, **19**, 223–238 (1975)

25 SKINNER, D. B. and BELSEY, R. H. R. Surgical management of esophageal reflux and hiatus hernia. *Journal of Thoracic and Cardiovascular Surgery*, **53**, 33–54 (1967)

26 SKINNER, D. B. and BOOTH, D. J. Assessment of distal esophageal function in patients with hiatal and/or gastroesophageal reflux. *Annals of Surgery*, **172**, 627–637 (1970)

27 TOREK, F. The first successful case of resection of the thoracic portion of the esophagus for carcinoma. *Surgery, Gynecology and Obstetrics*, **16**, 614–617 (1913)

28 TSUKAMOTO, M. and THAL, A. P. Correction of experimental esophageal stricture with the use of skin-lined fundic patch. *Journal of Thoracic and Cardiovascular Surgery*, **52**, 682–689 (1966)

29 WARA, P., OSTER, N. J., FUNCK-JENSEN, P., ANDRESEN, J. and OTTOSEN, P. A long-term follow-up of patient's resection for benign esophageal stricture using the inkwell esophagogastrostomy. *Annals of Surgery*, **190**, 214–217 (1979)

30 WINDSOR, C. W. O. Gastro-oesophageal reflux after partial gastrectomy. *British Medical Journal*, **2**, 1233–1234 (1964)

31 YUDIN, S. S. The surgical construction of 80 cases of artificial esophagus. *Surgery, Gynecology and Obstetrics*, **78**, 561–583 (1944)

2

The surgical treatment of gastroesophageal reflux and esophagitis

Gerald C. O'Sullivan and Tom R. DeMeester

In 1951 Allison[1] clearly identified gastroesophageal reflux as the cause of symptoms such as heartburn, regurgitation, and complications such as esophagitis and stricture that were often observed to accompany hiatal hernia. Belsey[50] correctly separated the type I, or sliding hiatal, hernia from the paraesophageal, or type II, hernia. He emphasized that paraesophageal hernias should be repaired to prevent mechanical complications, but that the type I hernia was only of importance when associated with gastroesophageal reflux (GER) and its complications. Careful analysis of their clinical experience led Belsey[50] and Nissen[41], working independently, to develop the first effective operations specifically designed to control reflux. Hill[26] introduced a third antireflux operation, but has since modified it to include calibration of the cardia[27].

The use of esophageal manometry, the intraluminal esophageal pH electrode and fiberoptic endoscopy to study esophageal disease has improved the understanding of the symptomatology, pathophysiology and complications of gastroesophageal reflux, as well as the role of surgery in the management of this problem. The authors' experience indicates that the use of objective diagnostic methods, careful patient selection for surgical therapy, and the application of physiological principles to the surgical repair of the cardia gives excellent long-term results.

Gastroesophageal reflux – a diagnostic problem

A correct diagnosis provides the only rational basis for therapy, and in few other situations is this more important than in antireflux surgery.

In many patients the occurrence of GER is indicated by typical symptoms of heartburn, regurgitation and dysphagia. However, ascribing these symptoms to reflux in the absence of esophagitis may be misleading since other diseases present a similar clinical picture, e.g. achalasia, diffuse esophageal spasm, esophageal carcinoma, cholelithiasis, gastroduodenal ulceration, and coronary artery disease. Furthermore, GER may coexist with other common gastrointestinal disorders or coronary artery disease and result in a mixture of symptom complexes. On the other hand, symptoms due to regurgitation of gastrointestinal contents into the esophagus may be atypical and not attributable to GER on symptomatic grounds alone. Such symptoms are postprandial fullness, belching, angina-like chest pain, chronic cough, wheezing, hoarseness, and recurrent pneumonia. A common clinical problem is the evaluation of patients with recurrent symptoms after previous biliary, gastroduodenal, hiatal, or coronary artery bypass operations. In many of these patients, the underlying problem is GER. In these circumstances objective methods are required to determine if GER is present and to relate symptoms to reflux episodes in order to separate it from other clinical conditions.

The objective assessment of symptoms

A number of tests are available for diagnosis of GER but these vary greatly as to their reliability in indicating the presence or absence of this disease[16]. The commonly used investigative methods include roentgenographic barium studies, endoscopy, esophageal manometry and pH reflux tests.

The upper gastrointestinal tract barium studies

This can demonstrate large hiatal hernias, gross mucosal ulceration, stricture, spastic contractions, diverticula and neoplasia of the esophagus. The presence of a hiatal hernia does not necessarily indicate GER because while both conditions may coexist in the same individual, each may occur independently of the other[25]. The radiographic demonstration of reflux, i.e. the flow of barium from the stomach into the esophagus in the upright position, is a reliable indicator that reflux is present. The failure to demonstrate this, however, does not reliably indicate the absence of disease. Barium studies should be used in the preliminary stages of diagnosis, but a normal study does not exclude GER.

Endoscopy

Esophagoscopy with biopsy is essential to diagnose early esophagitis, mucosal abnormalities, or small carcinomas. More advanced esophagitis can be recognized grossly and biopsy is only necessary to exclude carcinomas masquerading as a benign stricture.

The flexible fiberoptic endoscope is the instrument of choice and permits simultaneous assessment of the stomach or duodenum. The rigid endoscope is used to assess a questionable stricture, to obtain an adequate biopsy specimen and to facilitate initial dilatation. Grade II (linear erosions) or grade III esophagitis (cobblestone esophagus) produces clear objective manifestations of disease, but there is widespread variability between endoscopists in their ability to recognize the early mucosal changes of grade I esophagitis. The accuracy of endoscopic diagnosis of grade I esophagitis can be improved by noting associated changes at the esophagogastric junction, such as protruding gastric rugae, endoscopic hiatal hernia, or a patulous cardia[29]. Biopsy is mandatory to diagnose Barrett's columnar-lined esophagus when it is suggested by a tanned velvet mucosa, esophageal ulcer, or a high stricture. Multiple biopsies are necessary to exclude carcinoma which may have a patchy distribution[36].

Esophageal manometry

The measurement of a hypotensive distal esophageal sphincter is used by many as an indicator of reflux. Initial studies of highly selected populations suggested a low esophageal sphincter pressure could distinguish asymptomatic control subjects from patients with severe symptoms[60]. Subsequent studies with large numbers of patients showed extensive overlap of the measured distal esophageal sphincter pressures in control and symptomatic subjects[16, 57]. Thus, sphincter pressure measurements have limited diagnostic usefulness. The clinical use of manometry is for the diagnosis of motor abnormalities of the body of the esophagus such as achalasia, diffuse esophageal spasm, scleroderma, the detection of disordered motility secondary to reflux, and to localize the top of the high-pressure zone prior to the accurate placement of a pH probe for reflux studies.

The acid perfusion test (Bernstein)

This test determines esophageal sensitivity to acid and implies GER[5]. When positive, it indicates that chest pain is esophageal in origin.

Many patients with esophagitis have a negative result[49] and approximately 14 percent of control subjects experience symptoms with this test[4]. While this test is helpful in relating symptoms to esophageal origin, it gives no information about the competency of the cardia and abnormal GER is assumed.

The pH withdrawal test

The pH withdrawal test was introduced by Tuttle and Grossman[57] who noted that in patients with symptoms and esophagitis, a low pH was recorded for a considerable distance above the respiratory inversion point. In contrast, asymptomatic controls had an abrupt change from an acid to a neutral pH at this level. Subsequent workers have shown that this test has a false-positive rate of 18 percent, a false-negative rate of 20 percent, and a poor correlation with symptoms[53]. Comparison of antegrade and retrograde studies revealed marked differences and suggested that retention of acid gastric mucus on the pH probe may account for the high incidence of false-positive results[56]. Consequently the measurement of the pH gradient is too imprecise to determine the reflux status of a given patient.

The standard acid reflux test (SART)

This test measures gastroesophageal reflux while the subject performs a series of maneuvers after loading the stomach with 300 ml of 0.1 M-HCl. The test gives 16 opportunities for reflux to occur during four maneuvers (deep breathing, Valsalva, Mueller and coughing) in four different positions (supine, right and left lateral decubitus and 20° head-down position). The occurrence of three or more reflux episodes (pH less than 4) during the 16 trials is considered abnormal[51]. Eighty percent of patients with severe symptoms have an abnormal SART[56], but 20 percent of asymptomatic controls also have abnormal scores[16]. These limitations are significant, but the SART is simple to perform and is sufficiently reliable when positive in all maneuvers to make it valuable in clinical practice[16].

The acid clearance test

The acid clearance test was introduced to measure the efficiency of esophageal peristalsis in clearing acid from the body of the esophagus[8]. With a pH probe 5 cm above the high pressure zone, 15 ml of

0.1 M-HCl is instilled into the esophagus 10 cm above the tip of the probe. The number of effective swallows (determined manometrically) at 30 s intervals which are necessary to elevate the esophageal pH to a value greater than 5 while lying supine are recorded. Based on results of normal controls, the requirement of 10 or more swallows to clear is considered abnormal[8]. Results of the acid clearance test have been found to correlate with the presence of endoscopically and histologically proven esophagitis and with the mean duration of reflux episodes observed with overnight pH monitoring[54]. Its limitations are that acid clearance, as measured by this technique, is a function of both dilution of esophageal contents by saliva and the efficiency of peristalsis[23].

24-hour pH monitoring of the distal esophagus

This test was refined into a practical method for detecting and studying GER[17, 28]. With an intraesophageal pH probe located 5 cm above the high-pressure zone and a reference electrode on the non-dominant forearm, the patient is monitored continuously during eating and sleeping for 24 hours without being stressed by unnatural maneuvers. Reflux of acid is defined as a drop in pH below 4 and alkaline reflux as a rise in pH to levels above 7 (between meals and during sleep)[47]. The patient is requested to write on the pH record the different body positions, the time and duration of meals, and the occurrence of symptoms so that reflux episodes may be related to these events. Competency of the cardia is evaluated by the duration of esophageal acid or alkaline exposure in both upright and recumbent positions. Reflux-induced chest pain or respiratory symptoms are determined from their relationship to the reflux episodes. The ability of the esophagus to clear the refluxed material is determined by measuring the duration of each reflux episode.

The advantage of 24-hour pH monitoring is that it combines three tests in one: a reflux, a clearance and an endogenous Bernstein test. A disadvantage of this test is that it currently must be performed in a hospital. Comparison of 24-hour pH tests with the SART or esophageal manometry has shown that it has a higher sensitivity and specificity[19].

Indications for 24-hour pH monitoring
It is the authors' opinion that 24-hour pH monitoring should be performed in all patients without esophagitis prior to an antireflux procedure in order to have objective evidence that incompetency of

the cardia is indeed present and is responsible for the patient's symptoms. Other indications for pH monitoring are:

(1) Patients with typical symptoms of GER in whom the diagnosis is in question or position of reflux needs to be identified.
(2) Patients with atypical symptoms of GER.
(3) Patients with other abdominal or thoracic diseases and symptoms suggestive of GER.
(4) Patients with dysphagia and an esophageal motility disorder thought to be secondary to GER.
(5) Pediatric or other patients who are unable to communicate their symptoms and in whom GER is suspected.
(6) Patients with previous esophageal or gastric surgery and recurrent symptoms.

The physiology of the gastroesophageal junction

Despite a great deal of investigation, the precise mechanisms that control gastroesophageal reflux are only beginning to be understood. Anatomical studies have failed to demonstrate a sphincteric muscle in humans at the gastroesophageal junction. The microdissection studies of Lieberman-Meffert[30] suggest that sphincteric function in humans may be related to the muscular architecture of the cardia (*Figure 2.1*). At this region there is an oblique gastroesophageal muscular ring due to an increase of muscle mass in the inner muscular layer. On the lesser curve side of the cardia the muscle fibers of the inner layer are orientated transversely and form semicircular muscle clasps which insert into the submucosal connective tissues. On the greater curve side of the cardia the muscle fibers form long oblique loops which run parallel to the lesser curve of stomach and encircle the distal end of the esophagus and the gastric fundus. Both the semicircular muscle clasps and the oblique fibers of the gastroesophageal ring contract in a circular manner to close the cardia. This suggests that changes in the tonicity of gastric muscle would be reflected in the lower esophageal region and the pressure differences between the distal esophageal segment and stomach would be a function of their different luminal diameters under a similar range of muscle tone. Indeed, Diamant and Akin[21] have shown in dogs that increases in distal esophageal sphincter pressure occur simultaneously with stomach contractions. The sphincter response appeared only during pressure increases in the proximal

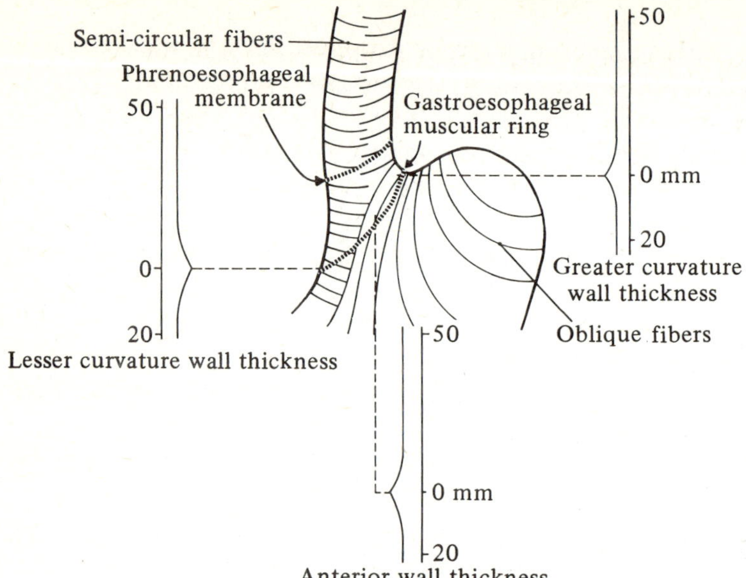

Figure 2.1 The geometric arrangement of muscle fibers in the inner muscular layer of the cardia (Reprinted by permission of the publisher from 'Muscular equivalent of the lower esophageal sphincter', by Lieberman-Meffert *et al.*, *Gastroenterology*, **76**, 31–38, 1979. Copyright © 1979 by The American Gastroenterological Association)

stomach with an approximate 8:1 ratio of sphincter to gastric pressure changes. Similarly, both the distal esophageal segment and the gastric fundus relax on deglutition[11, 31]. These factors suggest that the distal esophageal segment and gastric fundus function as a unit and have a neural or myogenic control mechanism which may differ from the rest of the esophageal or gastric muscle. The elegant experiments of Daniel on the opossum suggest that sphincter tone is purely myogenic in origin and relaxation is mediated by a neurogenic inhibitory mechanism[15].

There is a correlation between the resting pressure in the lower esophageal high-pressure zone (LEHPZ) and the incidence of GER[43]. Currently there is no explanation why the level of pressure is lower in some individuals than others. Many factors have been suggested, including neural, hormonal, myogenic and mechanical influences[40]. A neuroexcitatory mechanism for the maintenance of the basal sphincter tone has not been established in humans as truncal vagotomy has no effect on resting LEHPZ pressure[34, 35]. Pharmacological doses of cholinergic agents cause increases in the LEHPZ pressure, and anticholinergics reduce it[12], but the relevance of these observations to the normal physiological function is unknown. The influences of many hormones on this region have been investigated, but the effects noted are associated with pharmacological dosages and probably do not represent the true physiological situation. Pharmacological doses of secretin, cholecystokinin, glucagon and prostaglandins (E_1, E_2 and A), reduce LEHPZ pressure and exogenous gastrin, bombesin and motilin augment the pressure[12], but the physiological influences of these hormones have not been confirmed. Progesterone and estrogen have been shown to decrease the LEHPZ pressure[58] and are thought to be the mediators of the hypotensive LEHPZ seen in pregnancy [32,39]. It appears that under normal circumstances neither neural nor humoral factors are responsible for maintaining resting sphincter tone and the explanation for a low LEHPZ pressure in some individuals is most probably due to an abnormality of myogenic function. In support of this Biancani, Zabinski and Behar[6] have shown that the LEHPZ pressure response to stretch is reduced in patients with an incompetent cardia. This suggests that sphincter pressure depends on the length tension properties of the muscle. Reduction of the pressure may result from abnormality of the muscle length tension characteristics, as correction of this abnormality by fundoplication restores the sphincter pressure and responses to normal[6].

Despite the statistical correlation between the amplitude of pressure in the HPZ and the presence of GER on a population basis, there is now considerable evidence that other factors are as important in the control of reflux. This is based on the observation that there is a marked overlap between HPZ pressures of normal controls, non-refluxers and refluxers[16,56], and that the administration of atropine which reduced the HPZ pressure did not increase the incidence of GER in normal control subjects[52]. These findings drew attention to the presence of an intra-abdominal segment of esophagus as an additional mechanism for GER control. The anatomical dissections of Bombeck, Dillard and Nyhus[7] show a high correlation between the level of insertion of the phrenoesophageal membrane on the esophagus and the presence or absence of esophagitis. A similar correlation has been shown between the incidence of GER and the length of abdominal esophagus as determined manometrically[43]. Several reports indicate that the abdominal segment controls GER during variations of intra-abdominal pressure in a mechanical or valve-like manner[46,59]. Even in a hiatal hernia, there is a portion of distal esophagus which is exposed to the abdominal pressure due to the presence of the hernia sac which acts as a conduit to transmit the intra-abdominal pressure changes around the distal esophagus[46,59]. This results in compression of the distal esophageal segment and protection against reflux with changes of intra-abdominal pressure[59]. Shortening of the abdominal segment would therefore lead to the development of the patulous cardia, unaffected by changes of intra-abdominal pressure, and free reflux.

DeMeester *et al.*[20] developed an *in vitro* model where they were able to simulate and study individual functions of the distal esophageal segment. An important relationship between the LEHPZ pressure and the length of abdominal esophagus was shown. Competency was a function of the length of the abdominal esophagus, and as it shortened, the intrinsic pressure of the LEHPZ had to be increased exponentially to maintain control of reflux (*Figure 2.2*). This study further pointed out that a minimal length of abdominal esophagus was required to protect against changes in the intra-abdominal pressure, and a minimal pressure was required to protect against the independent changes in intragastric pressure.

A recent clinical study of 393 symptomatic patients has confirmed many of the findings of the *in vitro* model[42]. GER resulted from either a reduction in the LEHPZ pressure or the length of abdominal esophagus, or both. Conversely, competency of the cardia required

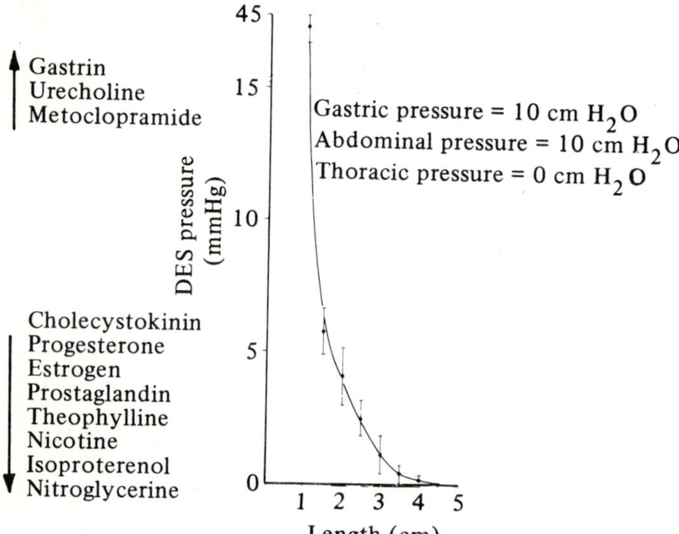

Figure 2.2 Relationship of sphincter (DES) pressure and length of abdominal esophagus to competency of the cardia. The plotted line represents the pressure necessary at a given length to obtain competence. The effects of drugs and hormones on DES pressure are indicated (From DeMeester *et al.*[20], courtesy of the Editor and Publishers, *American Journal of Surgery*)

both. The probability of GER was 90 percent when the LEHPZ pressure was less than 5 mmHg, irrespective of the length of the abdominal esophagus, and 90 percent for an abdominal segment of esophagus less than 1 cm in length, irrespective of the resting pressure. In contrast, the combination of a pressure greater than 20 mmHg and length of abdominal esophagus greater than 2 cm was associated with only an 18 percent incidence of GER. The occurrence of a low incidence of GER in the presence of adequate measurements indicates that other mechanisms are also responsible for reflux. These other mechanisms are due to the relationship of the intragastric pressure during stomach contractions and the LEHPZ pressure. A ratio of sphincter to gastric pressure of greater than one is necessary for competency and the shorter the overall sphincter length the greater the ratio required (*Figure 2.3*). The angle of entry of the esophagus

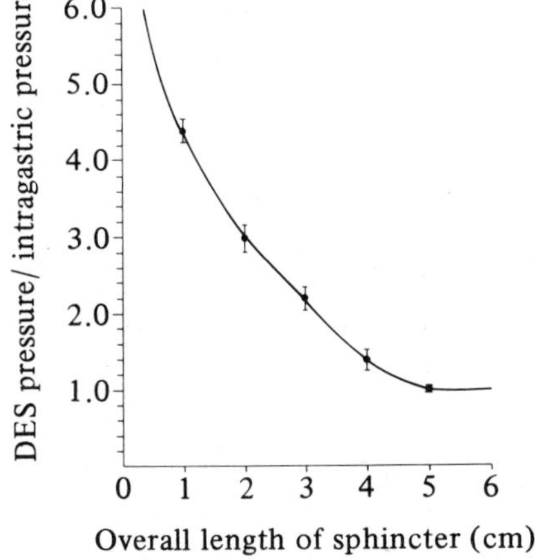

Figure 2.3 The ratio of sphincter/intragastric pressure and overall length of sphincter to competency of the cardia. The plotted line represents the pressure ratio necessary to maintain competence at a given length. For a sphincter length of 2 cm, a ratio of 3 is required

into the stomach or the angle of His has little relevance to competence[37]. The mucosal rosette formed by the esophageal mucosa in the collapsed resting state may be of some importance, but is difficult to assess. The diaphragmatic crura are also of little importance in the prevention of reflux, although correction of defects in crural anatomy form part of most antireflux operations[61].

Principles of antireflux surgery

The goal of antireflux surgery is the functional restoration of the cardia to normal. This is reflected by (1) total relief from all symptoms and complications of GER; (2) the abolition of GER as based on post-operative pH studies; (3) restoration of the patient to a normal life compatible with his age and without the necessity for postural, dietetic or medical treatment; (4) retention of the ability to swallow without discomfort and to belch or relieve gaseous distention or to vomit when necessary.

The achievement of these goals requires a complete change of the surgeon's mentality. He no longer is extirpating an organ, the function of which will be destroyed with its removal, but attempting to improve the function, by surgical manipulation, of an organ he will leave in the patient. In this situation, technique becomes paramount and will have profound effects on the organ function. No changes in technique should be made indiscriminately, but only after their effect on function has been carefully evaluated. The simple statement that the patient is symptomatically improved is not adequate in this situation.

The success of any reflux operation must be verified by sphincter manometry and intraesophageal pH monitoring to determine if the deficiency in the antireflux mechanism has been corrected and is reflected in the control of reflux. The persistence of symptoms, even if lessened, must be regarded as a failure of the procedure. The presence of symptoms during the early postoperative period may suggest another disease entity or the absence of symptoms may reflect a temporary placebo effect of surgery. The failure of a surgeon to check his results by objective methods will often give him the impression that he is achieving his goals. Patient interview alone is inadequate.

The reconstruction of a permanent and competent antireflux mechanism at the cardia requires (1) the placement of an adequate segment of the distal esophagus in the positive pressure environment of the abdomen by a method that assures its response to changes in intra-abdominal pressure; (2) that the pressure in the LEHPZ be permanently restored to a level three times resting gastric pressure; (3) that the reconstructed cardia totally relaxes on deglutition; and (4) that the resistance of the repaired valve does not exceed the peristaltic power of the body of the esophagus. The points are discussed individually below.

Response to changes in intra-abdominal pressure

The degree of competence provided by a segment of intra-abdominal esophagus in the absence of intrinsic muscle tone is a direct function of

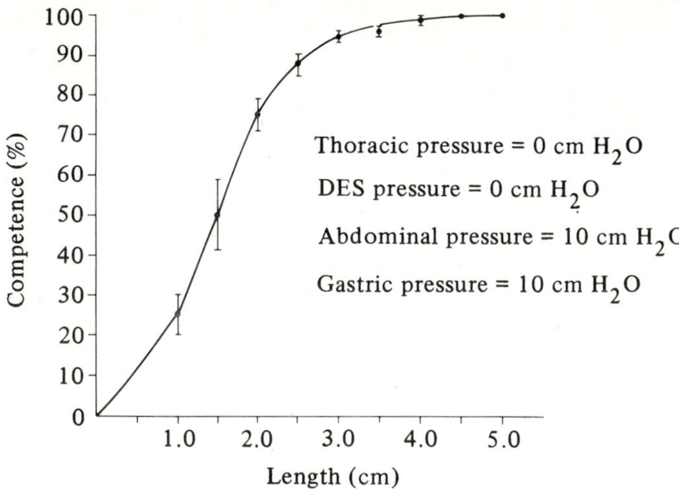

Figure 2.4 The relationship of length of abdominal esophagus (in the absence of intrinsic sphincter tone) to competency of the cardia (From DeMeester *et al.*[20], courtesy of the Editor and Publishers, *American Journal of Surgery*)

its length (*see Figure 2.4*). This is further augmented by the presence of intrinsic tone and the shorter the length the greater the tone required to maintain competency (*see Figure 2.2*). The permanent restoration of 1.5–2 cm of the abdominal esophagus in a patient with some measurable sphincter tone will maintain the competency of the cardia over various levels of intra-abdominal pressure. This is so because as the intra-abdominal pressure increases, the length of abdominal esophagus necessary for competence decreases (*Figure 2.5*). Thus the abdominal esophagus functions as a valve and assures reflux control when challenged by abdominal pressures which tend to force the cardia up into the hiatus and reduce the length of abdominal esophagus. Mobilization of the lower esophagus to assure an adequate segment below the diaphragm is, therefore, fundamental to each type of antireflux operation.

The creation of a conduit that will assure the transmission of intra-abdominal pressure changes around the abdominal esophagus is a necessary aspect of the repair. The fundoplication in the Nissen and Belsey repairs serves this purpose. In the absence of a fundic wrap, the development of periesophageal adhesions can prevent the transmission of intra-abdominal pressures to the abdominal esophagus, allowing posturally induced pressure changes in the abdominal cavity to act unequally on the stomach and abdominal esophagus and cause reflux.

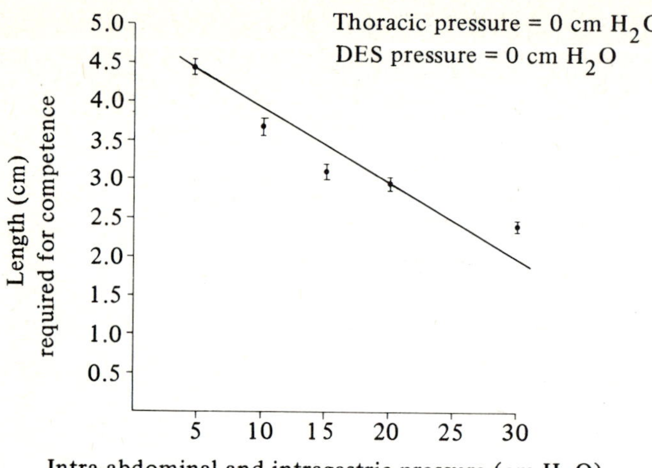

Figure 2.5 Mechanical efficiency of the intra-abdominal esophagus to counteract reflux during challenges of intra-abdominal pressure (From DeMeester *et al.*[20], courtesy of the Editor and Publishers, *American Journal of Surgery*)

Pressure in the LEHPZ

Wernly has shown that 60 percent of reflux episodes are not related to changes in intra-abdominal pressure, but are related to independent increases in the intragastric pressure which overcome the sphincter tone and cause reflux[59]. These can be due either to active contractions or to passive dilatation of the stomach. In gastric dilatation, the overall length of sphincter decreases as the neck of a balloon shortens during inflation, and a greater sphincter to gastric pressure ratio is required for competence (*see Figure 2.3*). In order to protect against reflux episodes secondary to variations in overall sphincter length, the LEHPZ must maintain a resting pressure equal to or greater than three times the resting gastric pressure. *Figure 2.6* shows that the resting sphincter pressures can be surgically augmented over the preoperative pressure values and this increase is a function of the degree of gastric wrap around the distal esophagus. The final pressure values achieved are due to the transfer of gastric muscle tone around the distal esophagus[9, 13]. This restores normal length, tension characteristics and myogenic function to the cardia[6]. The pressure augmentation appears to be permanent in that the authors have sequentially measured LEHPZ pressures after the Nissen and Belsey procedures and observed them to remain elevated 5-8 years post operation. The

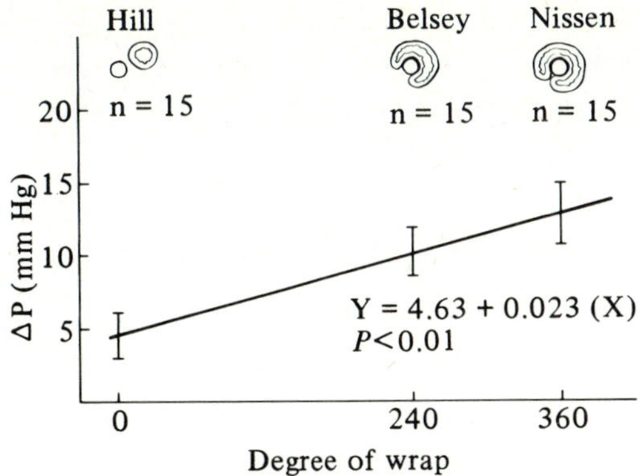

Figure 2.6 The relationship between the augmentation of HPZ pressure (ΔP) and the degree of gastric fundic wrap

fundic wrap is unique in that any change in intragastric pressure secondary to gastric contraction or dilatation will cause concomitant increases in LEHPZ pressure. Too long a wrap, however, makes belching or vomiting difficult and current evidence suggests that 1.5–2 cm in length is adequate.

Relaxation of reconstructed cardia

To facilitate normal swallowing, the ability of the high-pressure zone to relax must be present after operation. On deglutition, a vagal mediated relaxation of the distal esophagus and fundus of the stomach occurs[11, 31]. The relaxation lasts for approximately 10 s and is followed by rapid recovery to its former tonicity. To insure relaxation of the reconstructed cardia, only the fundus of the stomach should be used, since it is known to relax in concert with the esophagus. It is paramount that the innervation of the cardia be protected since inadvertent vagal damage will result in failure of relaxation.

Resistance of repaired valve

The diameter of a 360° wrap should be adequate to allow a No. 60 French bougie to pass with ease into the stomach to ensure that the relax valve will have only minimal resistance to be overcome by esophageal peristalsis. This does not seem to be a factor in the construction of a partial wrap. The choice between a total (360°) or partial (240°) wrap is influenced by the strength of the peristaltic contractions in the body of the esophagus. Esophagi having normal motility and strong peristaltic contractions do well with a 360° wrap. Where peristalsis is absent or of low amplitude, the Belsey two-thirds wrap is the procedure of choice.

Indications for operation

The indications for operation are based upon: (1) the type of hiatal hernia present; (2) the presence and pattern of GER; (3) complications of GER; (4) the response to medical therapy; and (5) the manometric evaluation of the antireflux mechanism.

The type I or sliding hiatal hernia is associated with, but is not the cause of GER, hence these patients do not require operation unless GER or its complications are present. In contrast, patients with a type II hiatal hernia (paraesophageal) or type III (paraesophageal and sliding) require operation to prevent severe mechanical complications such as incarceration, gastric bleeding, intrathoracic gastric dilatation and gangrene of the stomach. In the only prospective study performed to evaluate the fate of these patients, Belsey[50] found that six of 21 asymptomatic patients developed life-threatening complications within several years of conservative management.

In the absence of esophagitis, the presence of GER should be objectively demonstrated and related to symptoms by 24-hour pH monitoring prior to proceeding with operation. Patients who reflux only in the upright position are at a low risk to develop complications of reflux and have a generalized motility disorder of the alimentary tract. They are seldom relieved of their symptoms by operation and often develop a severe postoperative gas bloat syndrome[17].

Major complications of reflux, such as severe esophagitis, stricture, bleeding, aspiration pneumonia and reflux-induced esophageal spasm with severe chest pain, are clear indications for operation. In the latter two, 24-hour pH monitoring has proved invaluable in the assessment of these problems. Grade I esophagitis is not a sufficient indication for surgical intervention and these patients should receive a trial of medical therapy.

The failure of an adequate course of medical therapy for a period of at least six months in patients with objectively proven reflux indicates the necessity for operation. This is particularly so if there is a marked mechanical defect of the cardia indicated by a LEHPZ pressure below 5 mmHg and a length of abdominal esophagus less than 1 cm. In current surgical practice, 30 percent of patients operated for GER are in this category.

Antireflux surgery should be performed simultaneously in a patient with objectively demonstrated GER who requires operation for upper abdominal pathology such as gallstones or peptic ulceration. Failure to correct reflux will often leave these patients with postoperative symptoms that require a second operation.

Severe reflux in infancy and childhood is a particular problem that should be dealt with by early operation. Esophagitis rapidly progresses to complications in this age group and stenosis may develop in a couple of weeks[3]. Frequently the child is unable to communicate symptoms and failure to thrive, anemia and aspiration pneumonia are the only evidence that reflux is present. Once GER is objectively established as the etiology of these complaints and operation is performed, the outcome is dramatic and gratifying.

Gastroesophageal reflux associated with scleroderma or after a medical esophagomyotomy for achalasia requires early operation since reflux associated with a severe motility disorder rapidly progresses to esophagitis[3] and is frequently associated with pulmonary aspiration[45]. Furthermore, the combination of the mechanical defect of the cardia and impairment of the esophageal clearance mechanism is usually resistant to medical management. The Belsey Mark IV procedure is the operation of choice, due to the low resistance of the reconstructed valve.

Barrett's columnar-lined esophagus is usually associated with reflux and leads to stenosis and ulceration at the squamocolumnar interface[2]. Antireflux surgery can prevent the development of ulceration and future stenosis in these patients, but it is uncertain whether the Barrett's esophagus regresses after successful and objectively demonstrated control of GER[10]. As these patients are at risk for the development of an adenocarcinoma of the esophagus, they should be recalled for annual endoscopic assessment[24, 38, 55].

Incompetency of the cardia after vagotomy and gastric resection or drainage procedure allows the reflux of gastric and pancreatobiliary secretions and is associated with severe esophageal destruction and a high incidence of pulmonary aspiration[44]. Therapeutic measures which selectively control either the acid or alkaline reflux components alone usually fail; hence bile-diverting procedures are of little benefit without reconstruction of the cardia. The treatment is specific antireflux surgery, and a bile-diverting procedure if symptomatic alkaline gastritis is present.

Technique of antireflux repair

The choice between an abdominal or thoracic approach is determined by the individual assessment of each patient. A thoracic approach is indicated for (1) stricture, (2) recurrence after previous operation, (3) shortened esophagus or irreducible hiatal hernia, (4) assessment and biopsy of associated lung pathology, (5) extreme obesity, and (6) the performance of the Belsey Mark IV operation.

When a patient has had a previous hiatal hernia repair or when stricture is present, the esophagus is usually shortened or densely adherent to surrounding mediastinal structures. The thoracic approach is required to facilitate thorough mobilization of the organ in order to place the repair within the abdomen without undue tension. A peripheral incision in the diaphragm may be necessary to allow simultaneous exposure and dissection in the upper abdomen. The failure of the esophagogastric junction to drop below the diaphragm on upright barium swallow suggests shortening of the esophagus or an irreducible hiatal hernia, and in these circumstances an abdominal approach is contraindicated as the esophagus cannot be maximally mobilized. Pulmonary lesions associated with GER frequently require biopsy confirmation to exclude another etiology and the transthoracic repair will obviate the necessity for two operations. Gross obesity makes the abdominal approach difficult, whereas the thoracic approach can be performed on these patients with greater ease and less discomfort.

The Nissen procedure may be performed by either approach, but the Belsey operation can only be done by the thoracic route. In patients who undergo concomitant myotomy or where there is a severe motility disorder associated with GER, the Belsey operation is the procedure of choice. In most other circumstances, the Nissen operation can be performed transabdominally and leads to excellent symptomatic control with a very low failure rate. In situations where a fundic wrap is difficult to perform, as occurs after extensive gastric resection, the Hill operation with calibration of the cardia is an effective alternative.

The transthoracic approach

A left posterolateral thoracotomy incision is made through the sixth intercostal space or through a seventh intercostal space if a previous repair has been attempted. The esophagus is fully mobilized from the hiatus to the aortic arch with particular care to avoid injury to the vagus nerves. The superior and inferior left bronchial arteries and the esophageal branches from the descending aorta are ligated and divided. The cardia is freed from the hiatus by division of the phrenoesophageal membrane and one or more arterial branches from the inferior phrenic artery and the ascending branch of the left gastric artery. This allows the fundus and part of the body of the stomach to be drawn up through the hiatus into the thorax. The esophagus has an abundant collateral blood supply and the extensive mobilization does not predispose it to ischemic necrosis. The vascular fat pad that lies anterior to the cardia in the angle between the stomach and esophagus is excised completely (*Figure 2.7a*). This is necessary as the gastric fundus must adhere firmly to the esophagus anteriorly and the interposition of a bursa in the form of a fat pad will interfere with healing between the structures. At the start of the repair, six non-absorbable sutures of 0-silk are used to approximate the crura, but these are not tied until reconstruction of the cardia is complete (*Figure 2.7b*). In the case of a paraesophageal hernia, Teflon pledgets are used over the sutures to strengthen the closure of the hiatus.

In the Belsey procedure, a two-thirds wrap of gastric fundus is constructed over the distal 4 cm of esophagus and is held in position by two rows of non-absorbable mattress sutures (*Figure 2.7f*). Each row contains three equidistant sutures placed over a distance of 240°. The

Figure 2.7 Transthoracic approach

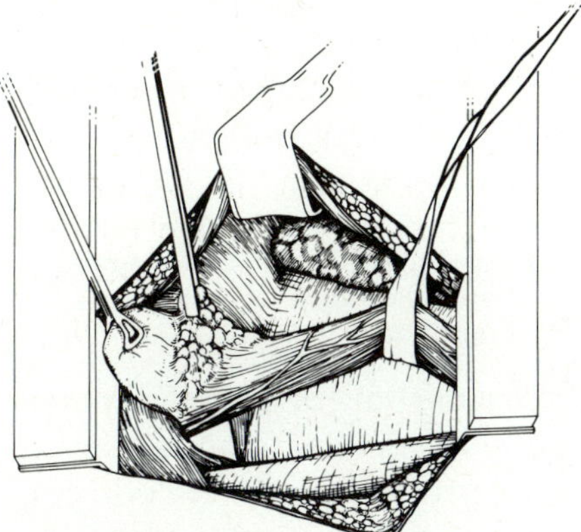

Figure 2.7a Mobilization of the esophagus and cardia with excision of the fat pad between the fundus and distal esophagus

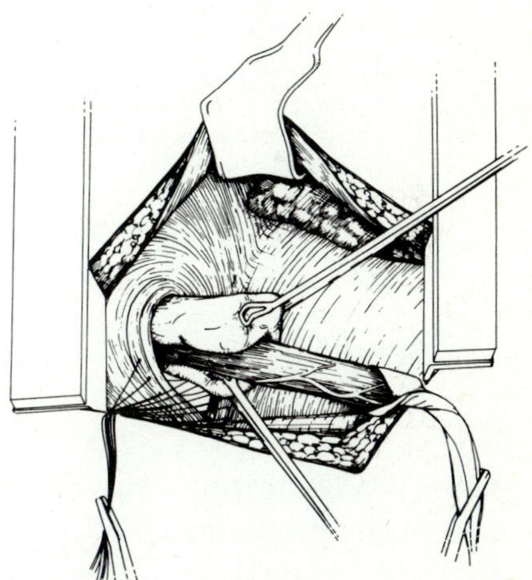

Figure 2.7b The crural sutures are inserted but are not tied until later. The fundus of the stomach is drawn up through the hiatus for construction of a fundic wrap

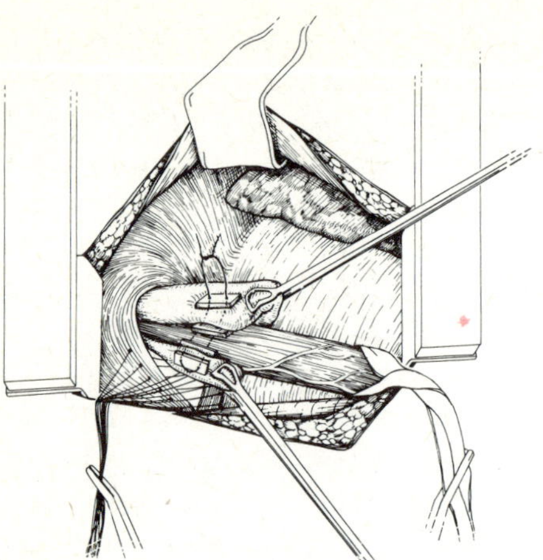

Figure 2.7c A 360° gastric fundic wrap secured with a U-stitch of 00 nonabsorbable suture reinforced with 1.5 × 0.05 Teflon pledgets

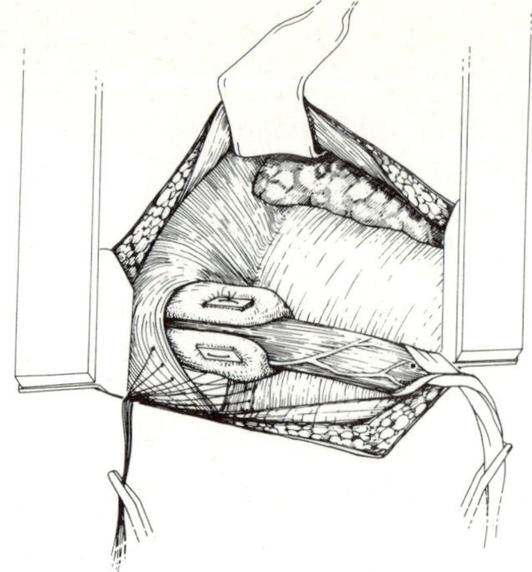

Figure 2.7d Completion of the gastric fundic wrap prior to reduction into the abdomen

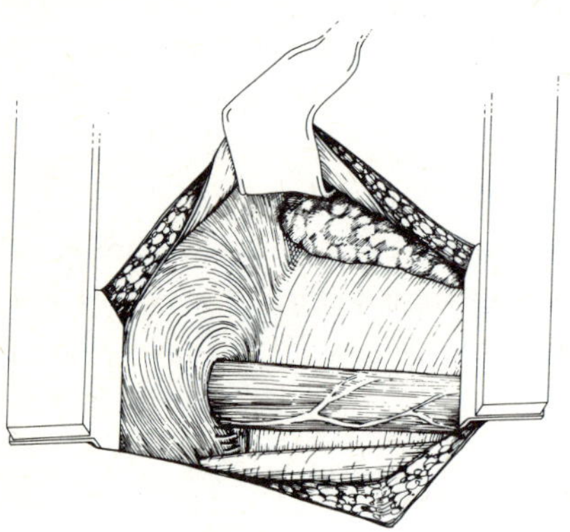

Figure 2.7e Completed transthoracic Nissen repair

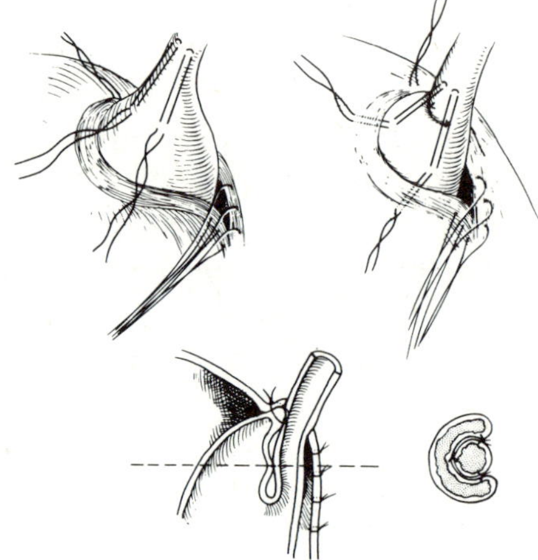

Figure 2.7f Schematic diagram of Belsey reconstruction; two rows of three equidistant 00-silk sutures are used to fashion a two-thirds gastric fundic wrap.

sutures pass through the circular seromuscular layers of the stomach and both muscle layers of the esophagus. Tissue apposition is achieved without strangulation. The second row of sutures is rethreaded on a needle and passed through the diaphragm from its abdominal to thoracic surface in order to maintain the abdominal position of the wrap after reduction of the repair. The cardia is manually placed through the hiatus into the abdomen, and when in place, it should remain there without tension on the diaphragmatic sutures. The crural sutures are then tied in a posterior to anterior direction until the hiatus allows an index finger to pass easily through it. Unused crural sutures are removed. The three transdiaphragmatic sutures are then tied.

If a Nissen fundoplication is performed transthoracically, the fundus of the stomach is wrapped totally around the distal esophagus and is held in position by one posteriorly placed non-absorbable horizontal mattress suture which passes through the wall of the stomach on both sides of the wrap and the esophagus in between. The wrap should not be longer than 1.5–2 cm and should be performed with a No. 60 French bougie within the esophagus. Accurately measured Teflon pledgets (1.5 × 0.5 cm) are used to limit the length of the wrap and reinforce the sutures as illustrated (*Figure 2.7c*). The reconstructed cardia should be manually placed in the abdomen and, as with the Belsey procedure, should remain there unsecured. Other operative details are similar to those for the Belsey procedure (*Figure 2.7d* and *2.7e*).

The transabdominal approach

The operation is performed through an upper midline abdominal incision. The esophagus is approached from the right by dividing the gastrohepatic ligament and is mobilized sufficiently to allow three to four fingers to be placed posterior to it, between the diaphragmatic hiatus and the left gastric artery (*Figure 2.8a*). Only on rare occasions is it necessary to take the left gastric artery. The crura are exposed by retracting the esophagus to the left. The right and left crura are approximated posterior to the esophagus to the extent that the tip of the surgeon's index finger can be placed easily through the esophageal hiatus (*Figure 2.8b*). For the Nissen procedure the posterior fundic wall of the stomach is pushed behind the esophagus by applying pressure on the anterior fundal wall. In the majority of circumstances, this requires interrupting the short gastric vessels in order to mobilize the fundus of the stomach. The wrap, consisting only of fundus, is held anteriorly with one non-absorbable horizontal mattress suture, incorporating both sides of the wrap and a portion of the esophageal wall in a U-stitch fashion with 1 cm of esophagus between each limb of the U. (*Figures 2.8c and 2.8d*). Accurately measured Teflon pledgets are used to limit the length of the wrap and reinforce the sutures as illustrated. From the abdominal approach it is sometimes cumbersome to perform

40

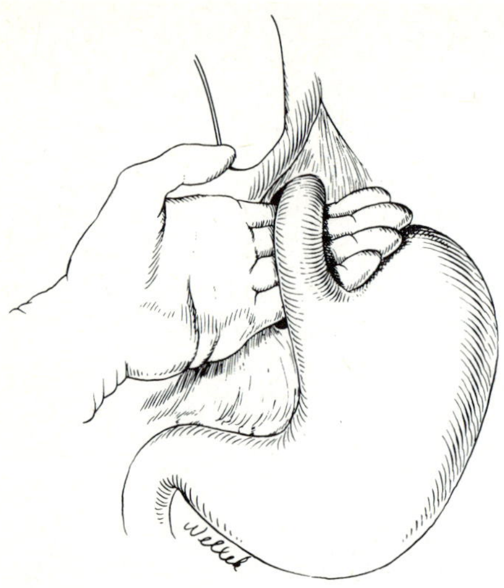

Figure 2.8a Mobilization of the esophagus and lesser curve of the stomach from the right, allowing three to four fingers to be placed posterior to it between the diaphragm and the left gastric artery

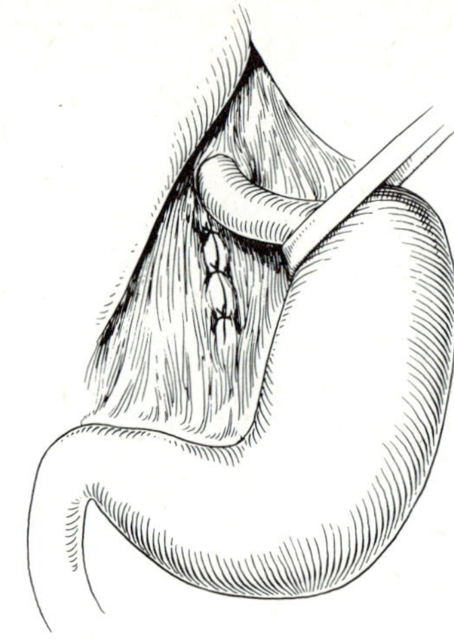

Figure 2.8b Approximation of the crura posterior to and around the esophagus

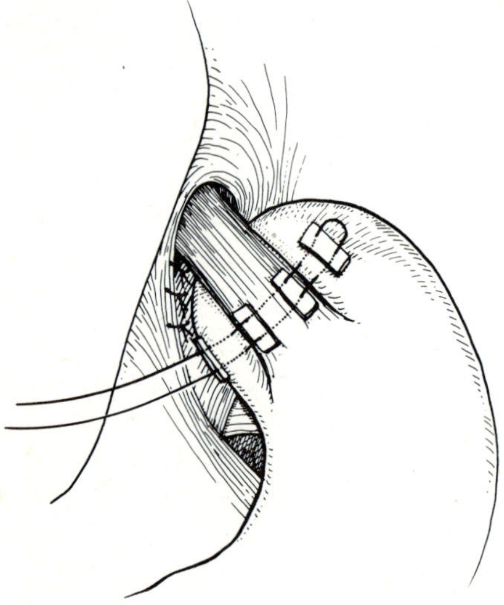

Figure 2.8c Location and placement of the U-suture and the Teflon pledgets to secure the fundic wrap in the Nissen procedure

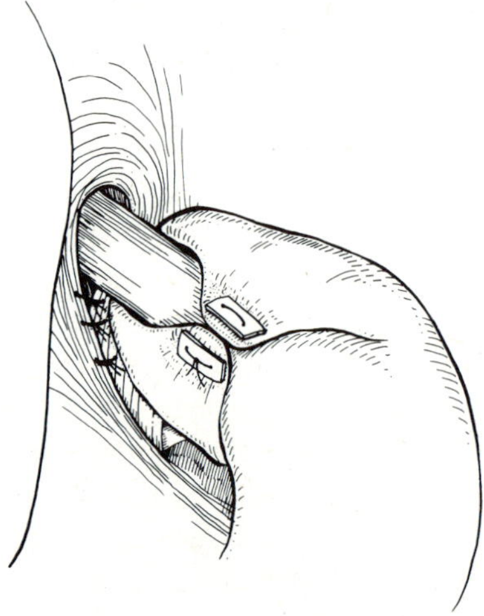

Figure 2.8d Completed Nissen fundoplication

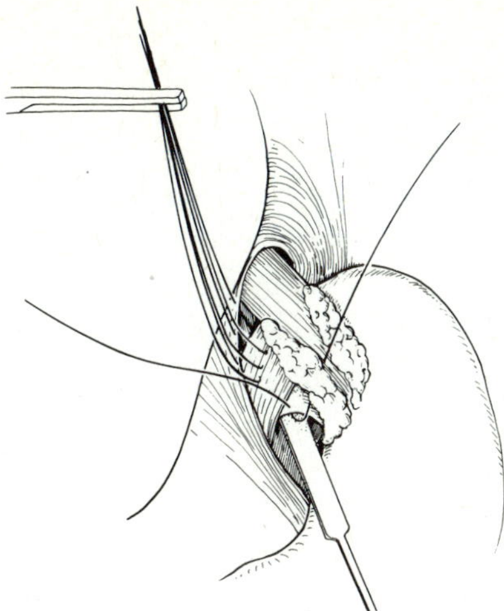

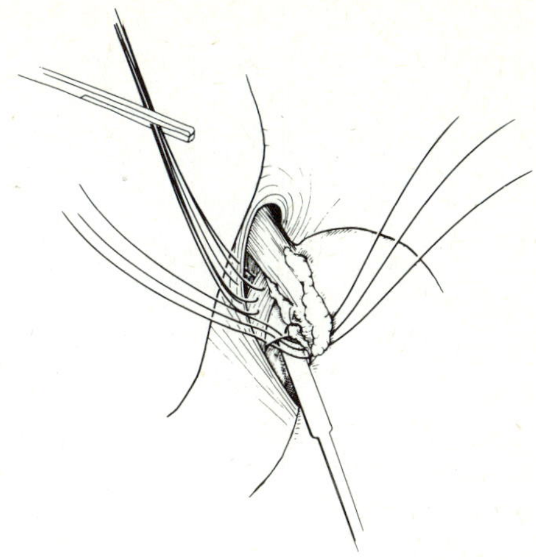

Figure 2.8e Anatomical placement of sutures through the posterior phrenoesophageal bundle, underlying stomach muscle and median arcuate ligament in the Hill esophagogastropexy

Figure 2.8f The placement of imbrication sutures for calibration of the cardia in the Hill procedure. The sutures should pass through the stomach muscle beneath both phrenoesophageal bundles and the arcuate ligament

the procedure over a No. 60 French dilator and as an alternative the wrap can be constructed over a No. 40 French dilator allowing enough room to insert a finger through the fundic tunnel adjacent to the encircled intubated esophagus.

Another transabdominal operation is the Hill posterior esophagogastropexy. Since Hill's initial description of this operation in 1960, he has modified the technique to include calibration of the cardia[27]. The distal esophagus and the cardia are mobilized as for the Nissen fundoplication. Crural sutures are placed, but are not tied until after the calibration of the cardia is complete. The leading edge of the posterior diaphragm (arcuate ligament) is identified. This can be done easily by passing a finger through the hiatus, posterior to the crura of the diaphragm on the anterior surface of the aorta. Care is taken not to injure the celiac axis. The blades of a right angle clamp are placed beneath the leading edge of the ligament from the abdominal side using the previously placed finger as a guide. A thin spatula is then used to replace the right angle clamp, and to protect the aorta and celiac vessels during passage of the sutures through this ligament. Babcock clamps are placed on the anterolateral and posteromedial phrenoesophageal bundles to visualize the anatomy. A fixation suture of 0-silk is placed through the posterior phrenoesophageal bundle and is passed through the arcuate ligament. When tied, it anchors the terminal esophagus in the abdomen (*Figure 2.8e*). The calibration of the cardia is achieved by three or four imbricating sutures (0-silk). These are placed first through the median arcuate ligament, the posteromedial portion of the cardia, again utilizing remnants of the phrenoesophageal ligament, and then similarly through the antero-lateral cardia. When these sutures are tied, approximately 180° of distal esophagus is involuted into itself (*Figure 2.8f*). The calibration sutures are tied so that a distal esophageal sphincter pressure of 50 mmHg is achieved, which indicates satisfactory narrowing of the cardia. The crural sutures are then tied so that the hiatus is narrowed to an orifice that easily accepts the tip of a finger. In doing the Hill procedure, it is necessary to monitor the DES pressure intraoperatively[27].

Assessment of results of antireflux operations

It is amazing that in an age when the physical sciences have made gigantic steps forward, the simple question as to the efficacy of one surgical procedure over another has eluded analysis. More disturbing is the realization that the methods used for objectively evaluating a surgical procedure are very meager, and most reports are based purely on the patient's symptomatic improvement and the information one can derive from a roentgenographic barium swallow. This continues to occur to the present time in spite of the knowledge that symptoms are not a reliable guide to the control of GER and that the information obtained from the barium roentgenographic swallow can be misleading.

Why is it that such a simple surgical question has eluded evaluation? One reason is that confusion exists between reports on the effect of a surgical procedure and the ability of a given surgeon to achieve the reported effect. For example, an antireflux procedure is reported to cause an elevation of the distal esophageal sphincter pressure with good control of reflux symptoms, and it is assumed that this effect can be achieved by any surgeon who so desires to perform the surgery. This assumption is erroneous. To make such a conclusion requires that a trial be undertaken to evaluate the ability of surgeons to achieve the reported effect of a procedure. This assesses the surgeon's skill and the degree of technical difficulty of the procedure, both very important when the end result of an operation is an improvement of function.

A second reason is that surgeons have shunned the development and use of diagnostic tools which can be used in the objective assessment of surgical procedures. For example, the gastroenterologist now does most of the esophagoscopy and esophageal function testing, and as a result, such procedures are no longer under control of the surgeon. This has come about through a shift in emphasis of our surgical training from disease-oriented programs to procedure-oriented programs. Only a few programs emphasize the pathophysiology of the disease and drill the trainee on all aspects of the disease from the diagnosis through the medical and surgical management of the abnormality. Today, most programs direct their attention solely to surgical procedures, and graduates of such programs find it difficult to evaluate critically a surgical procedure with existing technology.

A third reason why this simple surgical question has gone unanswered is an obstinate resistance on the part of surgeons to change technique when shown that such a change improves the result of the operation. This is potentiated by the insatiable desire of surgeons to modify a technique without knowing its effect on the results. Changes in technique are very important when the design of an operation is to improve function rather than simple extirpation of an organ.

A fourth reason is the greater difficulty in obtaining follow-up on surgical operations designed to improve function. To do so usually requires having the patient volunteer for postoperative testing, which can be difficult in today's mobile and informed consent society. This, plus economic considerations, applies pressures to the medical community which runs counter to energies expended towards answering serious questions concerning surgical problems.

A fifth reason for the failure of surgeons to answer this simple surgical question is that the pattern of patient referral has a marked effect on the ability to undertake analysis of a surgical problem. This must be dealt with if the science of surgery is to be advanced, because it alone gives rise to some of the specific problems with randomized trials of surgical procedures which are peculiar to surgery and not pertinent, for the most part, in medical trials.

The current state

The medical literature on antireflux surgery is filled with reports of clinical experience with a given antireflux operation using only symptomatic improvement and a roentgenographic barium swallow as the methods of evaluation[26, 48, 50]. Only a few of these reports are retrospective comparisons of two different procedures. More recently, there are several reports which include pre- and postoperative distal esophageal sphincter pressure along with the symptomatic and roentgenographic studies, and show that each of the antireflux procedures, Nissen[22], Belsey[33], and Hill[14], elevate the distal esophageal sphincter pressure and are therefore thought to succeed in controlling reflux. We now know that distal esophageal pressure is only one of the determinants of gastroesophageal competence and its simple measurement is not a reliable guide to the control of reflux.

Currently, there is only one published randomized trial comparing the Nissen, Hill and Belsey Mark IV antireflux procedures in the surgical literature[18]. This study was done to determine which of these procedures can be safely and effectively applied in clinical practice by a surgeon endowed with average skill. The surgical results were critically analyzed by the patient's symptomatic improvement, changes in roentgenographic barium swallow, and manometry of the esophagus and distal esophageal sphincter. In addition, control of reflux was objectively assessed by the standard acid reflux test, acid clearance test, and 24-hour esophageal pH monitoring. This study showed that the Nissen repair, over and against the Belsey Mark IV and Hill repair, done by the average surgeon, best controls gastroesophageal reflux as measured objectively with the standard acid reflux test and the 24-hour pH monitoring of the distal esophagus. The Nissen repair produced a competent cardia by increasing the resting LEHPZ pressure and the length of esophagus exposed to the positive pressure environment of the abdomen. This was accomplished at the expense of a temporary and mild postoperative dysphagia and a 50 percent chance of being unable to vomit after the repair. In order to overcome these deficiencies technical modifications of the Nissen procedure have been made and are mentioned in this report. The problem with the study is the short follow-up – one month to one year. It does, however, evaluate the degree of technical difficulty and the early results one can expect with the different procedures. It does not give any information as to the durability of a given procedure over the long term. The study was performed during a period of time when intraoperative manometry, as now advocated by Hill[27], was not available or universally done. So in essence, the Hill procedure is at a disadvantage since there have been important modifications of that procedure by its originator. Another randomized trial of the three procedures is again needed in an effort to determine the ability of a given surgeon to achieve the beneficial effects stated by their originators. The practicing surgeon owes a debt of gratitude to those surgeons who have struggled with the problems of clinical investigation in order to make antireflux procedures simple, safe, and curative with minimal side effects.

References

1 ALLISON, P. R. Reflux esophagitis, sliding hiatal hernia and the anatomy of repair. *Surgery, Gynecology and Obstetrics*, **92,** 419–431 (1951)

2 BARRETT, N. R. The lower esophagus lined by columnar epithelium. *Surgery*, **41,** 881–894 (1957)

3 BELSEY, R. H. R. and SKINNER, D. B. Management of esophageal strictures. In *Gastroesophageal Reflux and Hiatal Hernia*, edited by D. B. Skinner, R. H. R. Belsey, T. R. Hendrix and G. D. Zuidema, Chapter 14. Boston, Little, Brown and Company (1972)

4 BENZ, L. J., HOOTKIN, L. A., MARGULIES, S., DONNER, M. W., CAUTHORNE, R. T. and HENDRIX, T. R. A comparison of clinical measurements of gastroesophageal reflux. *Gastroenterology*, **62,** 1–5 (1972)

5 BERNSTEIN, L. M. and BAKER, L. A. A clinical test for esophagitis. *Gastroenterology*, **34,** 760–781 (1958)

6 BIANCANI, P., ZABINSKI, M. P. and BEHAR, J. Pressure, tension, and force of closure of the human lower esophageal sphincter and esophagus. *Journal of Clinical Investigation*, **56,** 476–483 (1975)

7 BOMBECK, C. T., DILLARD, D. H. and NYHUS, L. M. Muscular anatomy of the gastroesophageal junction and role of phrenoesophageal ligament–Autopsy study of sphincter mechanism. *Annals of Surgery*, **164,** 643–654 (1966)

8 BOOTH, D. J., KEMMERER, W. T. and SKINNER, D. B. Acid clearing from the distal esophagus. *Archives of Surgery*, **96,** 731–734 (1968)

9 BOWES, K. L. and SARNA, S. K. Effect of fundoplication on the lower esophageal sphincter. *Canadian Journal of Surgery*, **18,** 328–333 (1975)

10 BRAND, D. L., YEVISAKER, J. T., GELFAND, M. and POPE, C. E. Regression of columnar esophageal (Barrett's) epithelium after antireflux surgery. *New England Journal of Medicine*, **302**(15), 844–848 (1980)

11 CANNON, W. B., LIEB, C. W. The receptive relaxation of the stomach. *American Journal of Physiology*, **29,** 267–272 (1911)

12 CASTELL, D. O. The lower esophageal sphincter physiologic and clinical aspects. *Annals of Internal Medicine*, **83,** 290–401 (1975)

13 CONDON, R. E., KRAUS, M. A. and WALLHEIM, D. Cause of increase in 'lower esophageal sphincter' pressure after fundoplication. *Journal of Surgical Research*, **20,** 445–450 (1976)

14 CSENDES, A. and LORRAIN, A. Effect of posterior gastropexy on gastroesophageal sphincter pressure and symptomatic reflux in patients with and without hiatal hernia. *Gastroenterology*, **63,** 19–24 (1972)

15 DANIEL, E. E., CRANKSHAW, G. and SARNA, S. Myogenic control of esophageal motor function. *2nd International Symposium on the Esophagus and Gastroesophageal junction*, Vol. 2, 14–20 , Ixtapu, Mexico, Marion Laboratories (1978)

16 DEMEESTER, T. R. and JOHNSON, L. F. The evaluation of objective measurements of gastroesophageal reflux and their contribution to patient management. *Surgical Clinics of North America*, **56**, 39–53 (1976)

17 DEMEESTER, T. R., JOHNSON, L. F., JOSEPH, G. J., TOSCANO, M. S., HALL, A. W. and SKINNER, D. B. Patterns of gastroesophageal reflux in health and disease. *Annals of Surgery*, **184**, 459–470 (1976)

18 DEMEESTER, T. R., JOHNSON, L. F. and KENT, A. H. Evaluation of current operations for the prevention of gastroesophageal reflux. *Annals of Surgery*, **180**, 511–524 (1974)

19 DEMEESTER, T. R., WANG, C. I., WINANS, C. S., JOHNSON, L. F. and SKINNER, D. B. Comparison of clinical tests for the detection of gastroesophageal reflux. *European Journal of Surgical Research*, **11**, (Supplement 2) (1979)

20 DEMEESTER, T. R., WERNLY, J. A., BRYANT, G. H., LITTLE, A. G. and SKINNER, D. B. Clinical and in vitro determinants of gastroesophageal competence: a study of the principles of antireflux surgery. *American Journal of Surgery*, **137**, 39–46 (1979)

21 DIAMANT, N. E. and AKIN, A. W. Effect of gastric contractions on the lower esophageal sphincter. *Gastroenterology*, **63**, 38–44 (1972)

22 ELLIS, F. H., EL-KURD, M. F. A. and GIBB, S. P. The effect of fundoplication on the lower esophageal sphincter. *Surgery, Gynecology and Obstetrics*, **143**, 1–5 (1976)

23 HELM, J. F., RIEDAL, D. R., DODDS., W. J., HOGAN, D. G., PATEL, G. W. and ARNDORFER, R. C. Determinants of esophageal acid clearance in normal subjects. (Abstract) *81st Annual Meeting of the American Gastroenterological Association* (1980)

24 HAGGITT, R. C., TRYZELUAR. J., ELLIS, F. H. and COLCHER, H. Adenocarcinoma complicating columnar epithelial lined (Barrett's) esophagus. *American Journal of Clinical Pathology*, **70**, 1–5 (1978)

25 HIEBART, C.A. and BELSEY, R. H. R. Incompetency of the cardia without radiologic evidence of hiatus hernia. *Journal of Thoracic and Cardiovascular Surgery*, **42**, 352 (1961)

26 HILL, L. D. and TOBIAS, J. A. An effective operation for hiatal hernia: an eighth year appraisal. *Annals of Surgery*, **166**, 681–692 (1967)

27 HILL, L. D. Intraoperative measurements of lower esophageal sphincter pressures. *Journal of Thoracic and Cardiovascular Surgery*, **75**, 378–382 (1978)

28 JOHNSON, L. F. and DEMEESTER, T. R. Twenty-four-hour pH monitoring of the distal esophagus: a quantitative measure of gastroesophageal reflux. *American Journal of Gastroenterology*, **62**, 325–332 (1974)

29 JOHNSON, L. F. and DEMEESTER, T. R. Endoscopic signs of gastroesophageal reflux objectively evaluated. *Gastrointestinal Endoscopy*, **22**, 151–155 (1976)

30 LIEBERMAN–MEFFERT, D., ALLGOWER, M., SCHNEID, P. and BLUM, A. Muscular equivalent of the lower esophageal sphincter. *Gastroenterology*, **76**, 31–38 (1979)

31 LIND, J. F., DUTHIE, H. L., SCHLEGEL, J. F. and CODE, C. F. Motility of the gastric fundus. *American Journal of Physiology*, **201**, 197–202 (1961)

32 LIND, J. F., SMITH, A. M., MCIVER, D. K., COOPLAND, A. T. and CRISPIN, G. S. Heartburn in pregnancy: a manometric study. *Canadian Medical Association Journal*, **98,** 571–574 (1968)

33 LIPSHUTZ, W. H., ECKERT, R. G., GUSKINS, R. D., BLANTON, D. E. and LUKASH, W. Normal lower esophageal sphincter function after surgical treatment of gastroesophageal reflux. *New England Journal of Medicine*, **291,** 1107–1110 (1974)

34 MANN, C. V. and HARDCASTLE, J. D. The effect of vagotomy on the human gastroesophageal sphincter. *Gut*, **9,** 688–695 (1968)

35 MAZUR, J. M., SKINNER, D. B., JONES, E. L. and ZUIDEMA, G. D. Effect of transabdominal vagotomy on the human gastroesophageal high pressure zone. *Surgery*, **73,** 818–822 (1973)

36 MCDONALD, G. B., BRAND, D. L. and THORNING, D. R. Multiple adenomatous neoplasms arising in columnar lined (Barrett's) esophagus. *Gastroenterology*, **72,** 1317–1321 (1977)

37 MOOSSA, A. R., COOLEY, G. R. and SKINNER, D. B. Intraluminal and intraperitoneal pressures at the cardia: effect of hormones and surgical intervention. *Surgical Forum*, **21,** 370–372 (1973)

38 NAEF, A. P., SAVERY, M. and OZELLO, L. Columnar lined lower esophagus; an acquired lesion with malignant predisposition. Report on 140 cases of Barrett's esophagus with 12 adenocarcinomas. *Journal of Thoracic and Cardiovascular Surgery*, **70,** 826–835 (1975)

39 NAGLER, R. and SPIRO, H. M. Heartburn in late pregnancy: manometric studies of esophageal motor function. *Journal of Clinical Investigation*, **40,** 954–970 (1961)

40 NEBEL, O. T. and CASTELL, D. O. Lower esophageal sphincter changes after food ingestion. *Gastroenterology*, **63,** 778–783 (1972)

41 NISSEN, R. Gastropexy and 'fundoplication' in surgical treatment of hiatus hernia. *American Journal of Digestive Diseases*, **6,** 954–961 (1961)

42 O'SULLIVAN, G. C. and DEMEESTER, T. R. The interaction between distal esophageal sphincter pressure and length of the abdominal esophagus as determinants of gastroesophageal competance: a clinical study. *American Journal of Surgery* (In press)

43 O'SULLIVAN, G. C., DEMEESTER, T. R., SMITH, R. B., BLOUGH, R., JOHNSON, L. F. and SKINNER, D. B. The importance of the gastric wrap component in surgical restoration of the cardia. *Surgical Forum*, **31,** 136–137 (1980)

44 O'SULLIVAN, G. C., DEMEESTER, T. R., SMITH, R. B., RYAN, J. W., JOHNSON, L. F. and SKINNER, D. B. The objective evaluation of esophageal function in patients with symptoms after truncal vagotomy and gastric resection or drainage. *Archives of Surgery* (In press)

45 PELLEGRINI, C. A., DEMEESTER, T. R., JOHNSON, L. F. and SKINNER, D. B. Gastroesophageal reflux and pulmonary aspiration: incidence, functional abnormality and results of surgical therapy. *Surgery*, **86,** 110–119 (1979)

46 PELLEGRINI, C. A., DEMEESTER, T. R. and SKINNER, D. B. Response of the distal esophageal sphincter to respiratory and positional maneuvers in humans. *Surgical Forum*, **27,** 380–382 (1976)

47 PELLEGRINI, C. A., DEMEESTER, T. R., WERNLY, J. A., JOHNSON, L. F. and SKINNER, D. B. Alkaline gastroesophageal reflux. *American Journal of Surgery*, **135,** 177–183 (1978)

48 POLK, H. C., JR. and ZEPPA, R. Hiatal hernia and esophagitis: a survey of indications for operations and technique and results of fundoplication. *Annals of Surgery*, **173**, 775–781 (1971)

49 SIEGAL, C. J. and HENDRIX, T. R. Esophageal motor abnormalities induced by acid perfusion in patients with heartburn. *Journal of Clinical Investigation*, **42**, 686–695 (1963)

50 SKINNER, D. B. and BELSEY, R. H. R. Surgical management of esophageal reflux with hiatus hernia: long-term results with 1,030 cases. *Journal of Thoracic and Cardiovascular Surgery*, **53**, 33–54 (1967)

51 SKINNER, D. B. and BOOTH, D. J. Assessment of distal esophageal function in patients with hiatal hernia and/or gastroesophageal reflux. *Annals of Surgery*, **172**, 627–637 (1970)

52 SKINNER, D. B. and COMP, T. R., JR. Relation of esophageal reflux to lower esophageal sphincter pressures decreased by atropine. *Gastroenterology*, **54**, 543–551 (1968)

53 SKINNER, D. B. and DEMEESTER, T. R. Gastroesophageal reflux. *Current Problems in Surgery*, **13**, 1–62 (1976)

54 STANCIU, C. and BENNETT, J. R. Esophageal acid clearing: one factor in the production of reflux esophagitis. *Gut*, **15**, 852–857 (1974)

55 STILLMAN, A. E. and SELWYN, J. T. Primary adenocarcinoma of the esophagus arising in a columnar-lined esophagus. *American Journal of Digestive Diseases*, **20**, 577–582 (1975)

56 THURER, R. L., DEMEESTER, T. R. and JOHNSON, L. F. The distal esophageal sphincter and its relationship to gastroesophageal reflux. *Journal of Surgical Research*, **16**, 418–423 (1974)

57 TUTTLE, S. G. and GROSSMAN, M. I. Detection of gastroesophageal reflux by simultaneous measurement of intraluminal pressures and pit. *Proceedings of the Society of Experimental Biology and Medicine*, **98**, 225–227 (1958)

58 VANTHIEL, D. H., GAVALER, J. S. and STREMPLE, F. Lower esophageal sphincter pressure in women using sequential oral contraceptives. *Gastroenterology*, **71**, 232–234 (1976)

59 WERNLY, J. A., DEMEESTER, T. R., BRYANT, G. H., WANG, C. I., SMITH, R. B. and SKINNER, D. B. Intraabdominal pressure and manometric data of the distal esophageal sphincter. *Archives of Surgery*, **115**, 534–539 (1980)

60 WINANS, C. S. and HARRIS, L. D. Quantitation of lower esophageal sphincter competence. *Gastroenterology*, **52**, 773–778 (1967)

61 WOODWARD, E. R., THOMAS, H. F. and MCILHANEY, J. C. Comparison of crural repair and Nissen fundoplication in the treatment of esophageal hiatus hernia with peptic esophagitis. *Annals of Surgery*, **173**, 783–790 (1971)

3
Analysis of foregut symptoms

F. T. de Dombal

Introduction

The analysis of foregut symptoms seems to be enjoying something of a timely and appropriate revival at the present moment. Timely, because the last few decades have witnessed an increasing tendency to substitute '?dyspepsia – for barium meal' for a detailed skilful symptomatic enquiry, and appropriate, not least because the diagnostic problem posed by a patient with 'foregut' symptoms is in practice extremely common.

Other presentations, for example by Almy *et al.*[1], remind us that approximately 10 per cent of adults have recognizable digestive disease, and that approximately 15 per cent of all absences from work result from this problem. In the United States alone in 1968, nearly 74 000 persons died from diseases of the digestive system and these diseases cost in financial terms around 10 billion dollars. Foregut disease is responsible for a large proportion of these illnesses, and it is difficult to argue with the proposition that the analysis of foregut symptoms is both a common problem and an important one[16].

Moreover, in foregut disease, analysis of the symptoms assumes additional importance, since in this clinical situation physical examination is usually unhelpful, and since analysis of the symptoms is potentially extremely useful. Moynihan[30] claimed in 1905 that 90 per cent of patients with 'dyspepsia' could be accurately diagnosed simply by talking to them and listening to their symptoms. In recent years confirmatory evidence of an indirect nature has been provided to support this hypothesis by Hampton *et al.*[20] and direct evidence by Horrocks and de Dombal[21].

Long-standing aphorism is thus supported by recent evidence that 90 per cent of patients with foregut disease *can* be diagnosed simply by listening to their symptoms. But does this state of affairs come about in practice? Unfortunately, there is also rather good evidence to suggest that this is not the case. On both sides of the Atlantic, studies by Ross and Dutton[31] in the USA and the Leeds group in the UK[21], have indicated that in clinical practice only around 45–50 per cent of all adults who present *de novo* as 'dyspepsia' patients are correctly diagnosed when they are first seen in hospital. Further studies in other centres have indicated that these figures are indeed representative of clinical practice in many centres in Europe and North America.

Perhaps even more striking, these same studies have shown that one major reason for current diagnostic performance, which is far less than would appear optimal from the evidence presented, is failure on the part of the clinician both to elicit and to analyze symptomatic information from the first patient contact at all adequately. *Figure 3.1* is taken from one of these studies (Horrocks and de Dombal[22]) and illustrates the problem by studying diagnostic performance in a group of 25 patients selected at random from those presenting for their first out-patient visit to hospital with 'dyspepsia'. In practice a correct diagnosis was made at this first contact in 11 patients (44 per cent). In the remaining cases either an incorrect diagnosis was made, or no firm diagnostic prediction was possible. The reasons for this are explored in the figure.

In this particular study, the information elicited by the clinician at this first out-patient contact was recorded and given to four further clinicians of several years experience, with the results shown in *Figure 3.1*. Diagnostic accuracy of these clinicians, given the above data, ranged from 44 to 50 per cent. It is difficult to escape the conclusion that – given the information elicited – few clinicians could achieve a high diagnostic accuracy in these cases, even when pressed to make a firm diagnosis.

Crucial to the study, the same clinicians were *also* given, for the same patients, information elicited at the same out-patient contact via a detailed, structured, pre-defined interview with a non-medically qualified physician's assistant. Of course precautions were taken to 'disguise' the patients by varying the order of presentation of the data to each clinician and so on. As shown in the figure, every clinician's diagnostic accuracy was substantially higher *in the same patients*, usually between 75 and 80 per cent when presented with this type of case history. It is difficult to escape the further conclusion that in the

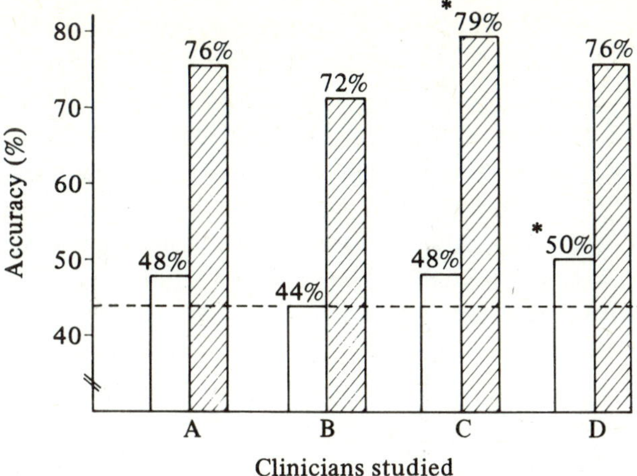

Figure 3.1 Performance of four clinicians using 'routine'
and 'paramedical' data in a series of dyspepsia cases
presenting '*de novo*' to out-patient department and seen
by two experienced clinicians.* Clinicians C + D each
recognized one patient in the relevant series, so that
analysis was restricted in these series to the remaining
cases. For details see text. □ Accuracy using conventional
data; ▨ accuracy using assistant's data; _ _ _ _ accuracy at
original clinical contact. (From Horrocks and de Dombal[22]
courtesy of the Editor and publishers, *British Medical
Journal*)

diagnosis of foregut problems, acquisition of detailed and pre-defined
data improves most clinicians' diagnostic accuracy by about 25 per
cent. It is also difficult therefore to avoid the additional conclusion
that foregut symptoms are (1) intrinsically useful, but (2) poorly
utilized in clinical practice.

The final feature which has made foregut symptoms an important
and topical clinical problem to consider here (and a much more
constructive aspect of the problem) has been the recent revival of
interest in patient symptoms *per se* and particularly the application of
information science methods to the problem of obtaining information
from patients. This has in turn been stimulated not only by technical
advances, such as the advent of the simple, cheap, powerful computer,
but by the realization that in health-care delivery, infinite demand is
currently chasing finite diminishing resource. All of a sudden, more is
not necessarily better, and this particularly applies to expensive,
time-consuming special investigations. The clinical symptom has once
again become attractive, not least because it is cheap to obtain and

can, at worst, be useful to ensure optimal scheduling of subsequent investigations. In a phrase, the humble symptom is back in fashion in the 1980s.

One beneficial effect of this has been to stimulate clinicians to take a new look at symptoms in general and foregut symptoms in particular. There have been several developments in this field in the last few years. The objective of the remainder of this contribution is not to repeat 'textbook' descriptions of foregut disease, but rather to review some of these recent developments.

Evaluation of foregut symptoms

What constitutes a 'useful' symptom? Ten or 20 years ago such a question would have been answered simply, though the grounds for so doing would have been largely anecdotal. In recent years, however, as investigation has become more complex and expensive, an increasing number of observers have begun to ask in a rather critical fashion 'how useful is the test?' What amounts almost to a new medical discipline has grown up, vitally concerned with the evaluation of innovation in medicine, and exemplified by the exploits of members of the Society for Medical Decision-Making in the United States, and the Royal College of Physicians Computer Workshop in the UK.

Much of this work has 'spilled over' into the analysis of patient symptoms. Therefore, before discussing the analysis of foregut symptoms in any detail, it may be helpful to pose an important fundamental question, namely how does one evaluate or assess the worth of any symptom in clinical medicine?

In the last decade or so several authors have addressed this problem and examined it in some detail[6, 27, 28, 41, 42]. From this work it emerges that for a symptom to be 'useful' – e.g. worthwhile in any clinical medical situation – it must fulfil three criteria:

(1) it must be pre-defined and clearly defined. All too often a symptom is so ill-defined as to be almost meaningless. An example is the word 'dyspepsia' (*see below*).
(2) as a corollary, a symptom must be capable of elicitation reproducibly. Any symptom is clearly of little use if in practice it is incapable of reproducible elicitation.
(3) the symptom must be 'useful' either in a diagnostic or therapeutic sense.

Table 3.1 Examples of useful, and also of merely interesting, symptoms in patients with foregut disease. (Taken from database of information about approximately 800 Yorkshire patients)

		Percentage of patients with disease having symptom					
Symptom	*Functional*	*Duodenal ulcer*	*Gastric ulcer*	*Cholecystitis*	*Hiatus hernia*	*Gastric cancer*	*Comment*
Pain comes on after food	44	40	42	16	64	48	Surprisingly little value
'Episodic'* pain	26	52	21	2	13	1	Valuable
Jaundice	1	1	2	20	0.1	5	Valuable when present
Nausea	63	60	65	76	54	77	Interesting but not much use

*Defined as periods of at least 3 weeks with symptoms, interspersed with periods of at least 1 month when patient is symptom-free

As regards diagnosis, Edwards[12] cogently reminds us that there is an urgent need to distinguish in diagnostic terms between information which is helpful and information which is merely interesting, and the concept of symptom 'utility' has aroused a good deal of controversy in recent years. In essence for a symptom to have a high objective utility, it should either be sensitive, i.e. present in most if not all patients with a particular disease, or specific, i.e. absence of the symptom effectively rules out a particular disease. Some examples of useful and less useful symptoms are shown in *Table 3.1* and the topic is discussed in greater detail by Lusted[28], Lindley[27] and Galen and Gambino[17].

In therapeutic terms, for example when one is assessing the results of therapy, there is by contrast a need to ensure that the assessment of a symptom does in some way reflect not only the objective status of a patient but also the subjective impression which the patient has of the disease[3, 19].

It may be worth therefore considering the value of foregut symptoms and their analysis as currently practised under these three headings – definition, reproducibility and utility; and this discussion will now follow.

Definition

The current state of the art as regards definition of foregut symptoms leaves a great deal to be desired. It is not the purpose of this presentation to reiterate a further series of detail symptom definitions but some general points need to be made on this topic.

First of all, a random survey of the literature[7] reveals that less than a quarter of presentations and publications which deal with foregut symptoms contain any definition at all of the symptoms concerned. Fully three-quarters of presentations totally ignore this important facet. Of course, this would not matter if the definitions themselves were identical around the world, but this is not the case. A more extensive survey of the literature reveals that – as regards the vague but crucial term 'dyspepsia' – over 20 different definitions exist, most of them mutually incompatible, and some of them diametrically opposed to each other.

To take just two illustrative examples of this problem, Dorland's *Medical Dictionary*[9] claims that dyspepsia is 'an impairment of the power or function of digestion' whereas French's *Differential Diagnosis*[15] states that 'dyspepsia is not at all synonymous with incapacity to digest food'. Many authorities skirt round the problem by referring to 'dyspepsia' as consisting of upper abdominal (or retrosternal) pain or discomfort, accompanied by 'symptoms referable to the upper gastrointestinal tract'.

As before, this would not matter much if 'symptoms referable to the upper gastrointestinal tract' were themselves precisely defined. Unfortunately, however, the lack of definition surrounding the term 'dyspepsia' extends to many of the symptoms which are thought to indicate foregut disease. For example, Roth[32] claims in Bockus' superb collection of essays on gastroenterology, that anorexia (loss of the desire to eat and failure to take in food) may occur even though the hunger state is present, that nausea by definition implies an imminent desire to vomit, and that reflux (or regurgitation) involves the ejection of gastric juice from the mouth. Others would dispute some or all of these assertions. The point need not be laboured, but it is a sad fact that no universally agreed set of definitions of foregut symptoms exists. In jargon perhaps more appropriate to the European Economic Community, there is an urgent need for harmonization in this area of clinical medicine.

Reproducibility

Nevertheless, as Saiger[33] and Schleff[34] remind us, mere disagreement about the definitions of symptoms may well be irrelevant. What really matters is whether the symptoms are elicited reproducibly in clinical practice and if not, whether such failure in the reproducible elicitation of each symptom is harmful in terms of clinical performance. It is worth asking therefore at this juncture whether the demonstrable lack of agreed definition as regards foregut symptoms has an effect upon the reproducibility of their elicitation in clinical practice.

Yet again, unfortunately there is some rather good evidence that this is the case. Studies both in the United States[39] and in the United Kingdom (both in Glasgow and in Leeds) have shown considerable observer variation in eliciting symptoms from patients with upper gastrointestinal problems[18, 19].

The Leeds results[18] have been particularly disquieting in this respect. During these studies a single clinician interviewed a series of patients and the interview was recorded using standardized data-sheets by three further observers. In no less than one in five of all questions, the three observers were unable to agree amongst themselves as to whether the question was asked or not, so vaguely was it phrased. In one in six of these questions which *were* agreed to have been asked, the patient's answer was so vague that the three observers could not agree as to whether the patient had said 'yes' or 'no'. Other studies more recently have confirmed these findings.

It is difficult not to conclude that the symptoms of upper gastro-intestinal disease are poorly, in the sense of non-reproducibly, elicited by clinicians in clinical practice.

Utility of symptoms

Nevertheless as remarked earlier, many workers[33, 34] would argue that what really matters is the utility of the symptoms in clinical practice. Nihilism is all very well but it must be seen to have a practical basis.

Several recent surveys have studied this problem. In particular, two aspects of the problem have been studied. First, are these symptoms *used*? Are symptoms which we generally think of as indicating 'foregut disease', e.g. nausea, anorexia, actually enquired after in routine clinical practice?

Until recently there was little data on this subject, but in the last 10 years there have been several studies which have addressed the problem: 'What do clinicians actually do when interviewing a patient apparently suffering from foregut disease?', an example being the study of Leaper *et al.*[26]. These studies have clearly indicated that many of the symptoms traditionally associated with foregut disease are *not* routinely enquired after in clinical practice. Their utility is thus diminished since it is difficult for a symptom to be useful in diagnosing the cause of a patient problem if it has not been elicited in the first place.

Another aspect of the problem which a larger number of workers have studied, involves a slightly more fundamental question. Are the data, if sought after and properly elicited, inherently useful? In other words, under what circumstances – if at all – does a particular symptom provide a reliable, useful indicator of a specific foregut disease? As recently as 1948, Friedmann bemoaned the lack of hard data in this area of medicine claiming that 'although peptic ulcer has been recognized for over 100 years and affects over 10% of the entire population, our knowledge [of the symptoms] of this disease has surprising limitations'.

Over 30 years later this lament remains uncomfortably true, for most research work in foregut disease has concentrated upon physiological or therapeutic problems and symptomatology has been the Cinderella of biomedical sciences. In recent years, however, there have been at least some studies which have attempted to look more closely and objectively at the symptoms of foregut disease as evidenced in large series of patients[4, 10, 11, 13, 23, 25, 37].

It would be both impractical and undesirable to deal in detail with the results of all these studies, particularly where they have merely confirmed textbook impressions. But it may be useful to illustrate some of this recent work by referring to misconceptions – that is to say areas of symptom study where current textbook impressions appear to be totally at variance with the observed findings in large and apparently representative series of patients.

One example may be cited which is both important and rather typical – namely the relationship between 'peptic ulcer pain' and food. In many textbooks the pain of peptic ulcer is said (1) to be extremely constant, and (2) to appear at a definite time after each meal. The time at which the pain appears is said to vary from half an hour to two hours – earlier pain being more likely to result from gastric rather than duodenal ulcer and vice versa[5, 14, 29, 38].

The findings in many large recent series are quite at variance with this classical textbook picture. Horrocks and de Dombal[23] found that less than half of all patients with peptic ulcer complained of pain related to meals in the sense that eating food aggravated the pain. Just over half of all patients studied with dyspepsia (some 360 in all) *with or without peptic ulcer* claimed that eating did *not* affect their pain and there was little difference between patients with 'functional' dyspepsia, i.e. those with negative results on X-ray and/or endoscopy, and patients whose dyspepsia was proven to be due to peptic ulceration.

Similarly Scheinok and Rinaldo[36] found that under one-third of gastric ulcer patients and less than 10 per cent of duodenal ulcer patients actually claim in practice that eating makes their symptoms worse. In another major study[13], the comparable figures for patients who claimed their pain was aggravated by eating were 24 per cent for gastric and 10 per cent for duodenal ulceration. In the more recent study of Earlam[10], out of 100 patients with radiologically proven duodenal ulcer, only 24 claimed that their pain came on at the classical time, between one-half and two hours after a meal.

It is rather difficult to escape the conclusion that, at least in Europe and the United States, the pain of peptic ulceration is not typically made worse by meals. Indeed if a stereotype patient were to be constructed with peptic ulcer, on the balance of probability and based on factual observation one would have to envisage a patient whose pain was *totally unrelated* to meals. The absence of relationship between meals and pain is therefore meaningless in terms of diagnosis and one can only wonder how long these standard but erroneous descriptions of peptic ulceration can endure in the textbooks.

Moreover, it is possible to speculate from this situation, and others where observed findings in large series of patients do not fit in at all well with textbook descriptions, that a major cause of poor current diagnostic performance in this area of medicine resides in the fact that the clinician has – at the conclusion of formal training – an inaccurate impression of the value of foregut symptoms. In other words, in practice the clinician may analyze a patient's symptoms 'correctly', but use a faulty set of reference points from which to do so, and hence still arrive (avoidably so!) at the wrong diagnosis.

New approaches to foregut symptoms

No problem can be solved until its existence is admitted, but it is also possible to argue – as pointed out previously – that unconstructive nihilism is *per se* of little practical value. For these reasons it is at least partially reassuring to report that in the last decade or so considerable quantities of work have been undertaken in an attempt to remedy the deficiences in our current approach to the problem of analyzing symptoms in foregut disease.

Definitions

First, several authors have attempted to reduce the inherent observer variation by closely defining each symptom, and carrying out observer variation studies to assess the effects of pre-defined terminology prior to each interview. Studies in this area have been carried out both in Leeds and Glasgow in the United Kingdom[18] and by Vickery[39] in the United States.

Some indication of this type of approach is set out in *Table 3.2* which extracts some 'definitions' data from the reverse side of the data sheet used in Leeds and elsewhere for paramedical workers to collect clinical data[25]. Whether the reader accepts these definitions personally is not at issue – the pragmatic point is whether in practice they have any effect in clarifying the issues and lowering observer variation in eliciting symptoms.

In fact, there is some evidence from these studies that the observer variation described previously can be reduced quite markedly by this type of careful pre-definition of symptoms before an interview is undertaken. For example, Gill *et al.*[18] showed that the observer

Table 3.2 Extract from detailed symptom definitions taken from 'worksheet' for paramedical interviewers in Leeds

---

TYPE OF PAIN

(a) *Pattern of pain*:

Continuous – pain present more or less every day since onset.

Attacks   – pain comes on for a short duration < 2 days and then ceases. Attacks may be frequent (> 1 per week) in which case put 'continuous attacks', or infrequent (< 1 per month) in which case put 'isolated attacks'.

Episodic   – pain comes on for a few weeks (need not be present 100% of the time), and this 'episode' is followed by complete remission (lasting at least 1 month), then by a further 'episode'.

If pain does not fall readily into any of these categories leave blank.

(b) *Relation to meals*:

Immediate – pain comes on regularly within 15–20 minutes after eating.

Delayed   – pain comes on regularly within 20 minutes to 2 hours after eating.

In all other cases put 'not related'. If pain comes on before meals, and is relieved by food, enter under aggravating and relieving factors.

(c) *Night pains*:

– pain must have repeatedly woken patient from sleep. If pain occurs at once on lying down, note under 'aggravating factors – posture'.

---

variation referred to previously (16–20 per cent) concerning the elicitation of foregut symptoms can be reduced to under 5 per cent by discussion and pre-definition of each symptom and subsequent work has shown that even paramedical interviewers can obtain reproducible answers to carefully pre-structured questions[8, 25].

Detailed observations

Once agreed definitions of terminology are available, the next logical step is to record the findings in a large series of patients, wherever possible representative and unselected. Studies in this domain, currently or recently carried out in the United Kingdom by Crean, Knill-Jones and their colleagues in Glasgow (unpublished observations), by Earlam and others[10, 13] in London and by the Yorkshire group in Airedale and Leeds[23] have already been discussed. Detailed observations now exist therefore in respect of several thousand patients, which provide a firm foundation for future work.

Multivariate analysis

The definition of each symptom may be crystal clear, and the clinician's analysis impeccable – but it is still unfortunately true that no *single* foregut symptom gives an absolutely reliable indication of disease on its own. Therefore if analysis of foregut symptoms is to be optimal, it is necessary to study not merely single symptoms but *groups* of symptoms. Several studies have been undertaken in this area on both sides of the Atlantic using a variety of mathematical and statistical techniques. One of the earliest surveys was that of Scheinok and Rinaldo[36] who used a variety of mathematical methods in this respect (including optimal sub-sets, discriminant analysis, and Bayes theorem).

More recently, particularly in the UK, increasing use has been made of computer-aided analysis, using a variant of Bayes theorem, to study simultaneously *all* of a patient's symptoms of foregut disease[21, 22, 24]. *Figures 3.2* and *3.3* show an illustrative example of this type of analysis, aided by a small desk-top computer in which a 'new' patient's symptoms, elicited by a non-medically qualified 'physician's assistant' are compared, using a variant of Bayes theorem, with just under 1000 similar patients, and a diagnostic prediction generated on the basis of this multiple comparison.

CLINICAL DIAGNOSIS – DYSPEPSIA

NAME	**REGISTRATION NO.**
SEX MALE	**SERIAL NO.** ⟶ GAS
AGE 58	

A. PRESENTING SYMPTOM	**F. GENERAL EXAMINATION**
B. PAIN	1. Mood. ANXIOUS 2. Colour. NORMAL 3. Temp. NORMAL 4. Pulse. 85 150/90 6. Pain during interview. NIL
1. Site at onset	
2. Site at present	
3. Duration of pain or Asstd. Symptoms. 2 MONTHS	**G. ABDOMINAL INSPECTION**
4. Cont/Ep/Ca/la. CONT. ATTACKS 5. Freq & Durn of episodes. — 6. Freq & Durn of attacks. — 7. Severity. MODERATE 8. Radiation. NIL 9. Relieving factors. VOMITING 10. Aggravating factors. NIL 11. Progress. WORSE 12. Related to meals. NIL 13. Night pains or attacks. NIL	1. Movement. NORMAL 2. Distention NIL 3. Succussion Splash. NIL 4. Lymphadenopathy. NIL
C. OTHER SYMPTOMS	**H. ABDOMINAL PALPATION**
1. Nausea. YES 2. Vomiting. YES 3. Haematemesis. NO 4. Appetite. DECREASED 5. Dysphagia. NO 6. Previous Indigestion. YES 7. Jaundice. NO 8. Bowels. NORMAL 9. Micturition. NORMAL 10. Weight. DECREASED	1. Tenderness. MILD 2. Rebound. NO 3. Guarding. NO 4. Rigidity. NO 5. Swellings. NO 6. Murphy. NEGATIVE
	I. ABDOMINAL AUSCULTATION NORMAL
D. P.M.H.	**J. RECTAL EXAMINATION** N.A.D.
1. Previous Opn. NONE 2. Drugs. NONE	**K. OTHERS** —
E. SOCIAL	Clinicians Outpatient D ? Clinicians Pre Op D GASTRIC CA. Operative & Final D GASTRIC CA. (? included Pathology).
1. Family History. NIL RELEVANT 2. Smoking/Drinking Habits. —	

Figure 3.2a Case sheet in Leeds experiments, for subsequent computer analysis

SITE OF PAIN: Mark on diagrams   SEVERITY: Self explanatory   PROGRESS: Self explanatory

AGGRAVATING FACTORS: What makes the pain worse – e.g. Nil/Movement/Food/Other (give details)

TYPE OF PAIN: Intermittent – patient has *pain-free intervals*

(when present)   Steady – pain present and constant all the time

Colicky – pain present all the time but varies rhythmically in intensity

Continuous – pain present all the time since onset

Episodic – pain that comes on for a few weeks (not all the time) and afterwards patient is free of pain for weeks or months

Cont/Attacks – attacks of pain occurring for an hour or two at frequent intervals

RELATIONS TO MEALS: Immediately after food i.e. pain comes on within 15–20 mins of eating. Delayed after food i.e. pain comes on more than 20 mins after food. Not related to meals in all other cases.

NIGHT PAINS: To be 'Yes', the pain must wake patient from sleep.

NAUSEA and VOMITING: Vomiting = regurgitation appreciable stomach content (c.f. reflux)

HAEMATEMESIS: Usually fresh blood. ('Coffee grounds' also accepted *if* witnessed by medical or nursing staff.)

APPETITE. Self explanatory. Recent change especially significant.

DYSPHAGIA: Difficulty in swallowing. REFLUX = small amount of acid/bile no nausea (c.f. vomiting)

PREV INDIGESTION: Any form of indigestion (flatulence, heartburn) prior to onset of present symptoms.

JAUNDICE: During present attack only.

RECTAL PAIN: Pain felt in rectum, with or without accompanying abdominal pain.

WEIGHT: Note whether any loss is recent, voluntary or not. Extent? Over what period?

BOWELS: Varies from person to person. We really want to know any recent change – Normal/Constipation/Diarrhoea/Alternating diarr and constip/Melaena/Pale stools/Blood/Mucus.

MICTURITION: (recent change) – Normal/Frequency/Dysuria/Dark urine.

Figure 3.2b Definitions used in interview for case sheet in *Figure 3.2a*

The results of these studies have been modestly encouraging, particularly when set alongside the previously discussed (rather poor) current clinical diagnostic performance. Thus the Leeds group[21] showed that computer-aided analysis of 212 consecutive patients, using a pre-structured interview conducted by the house surgeon at the time of admission to hospital, led to an overall accuracy of 88 per cent, as opposed to a 'conventional' diagnostic accuracy of about 55 per cent in these patients. Later these workers were able to show that the same system, used in an out-patient environment, where a further 154 patients were interviewed by a non-medically qualified physician's assistant, gave a similar overall accuracy of computer prediction when

Case ref.

Male	Nausea
Age 50–59	Vomiting
Site onset upper half	No haematemesis
Site present upper half	Decreased appetite
No radiation of pain	No dysphagia
Duration 1–3 months	Previous indigestion
Continuous attacks	No jaundice
Moderate pain	Bowels normal
Getting worse	Normal micturition
No aggravating factors	Weight decreased
Unrelated to meals	No previous operations
Relieved by vomiting	Not taking drugs
No night pains	

Diagnostic prediction

FUNCT.	D.U.	G.U.	CHOLE.	H.H.	G.CA
0.17	0.01	3.16	1.51	0.07	95.05

Figure 3.3 Computer analysis of case history obtained as *Figure 3.2* from patient with foregut symptoms

compared with final diagnosis of just over 81 per cent. More recently, these findings have been confirmed in other hospital centres[25, 43] and in General Practice[8]. These levels of accuracy are of course far higher than can be obtained from consideration of *any* single clinical feature – and whatever one feels about the use of computers, it seems reasonable to argue that for maximizing diagnostic accuracy, we need to consider several clinical features at once. Humans do this rather badly and computers do this rather well.

'New' questions and techniques

In the most recent and perhaps the most important of all current developments, various workers have begun to study the problem 'are we asking the right questions?', and to develop additional and alternative techniques for seeking a patient's opinion. One excellent example of the new thinking behind this approach is that of Edwards[12] who over the past 10 years has developed a series of flow charts and diagnostic keys particularly relevant to the diagnosis of dysphagia. An important feature of these charts and keys is that they depend not merely upon the classical series of questions suggested by tradition over the years, but upon a series of questions which result from a careful analysis of what his patients actually have reported.

Another fascinating recent trial has been carried out by Balmforth[2] who presented patients on arrival at his clinic with a series of cards, each with a stereotype of disease, such as duodenal ulcer or cholecystitis. The patients were asked to select the card most appropriate to their symptoms. Balmforth reported, interestingly, that the diagnostic accuracy of this patient prediction was as high as the diagnostic accuracy of clinical prediction.

Other authors, for example Cay *et al.*[3] and Hall *et al.*[19], have posed a further important question, namely 'does the doctor's impression of the patient's status actually tally with the patient's own subjective impression?' Such studies have shown that – as well as being open to considerable observer variation – traditional measures for estimating patient status, such as the Visick Scale[40], often fail to reflect patients' own opinions of their state of health.

More constructively, these studies have also used quite new techniques for analysing symptoms resulting from foregut disease – techniques related particularly to the problem of whether the doctor's assessment of patient symptoms actually matches what patients think. These further studies have mainly dealt with postoperative patients and attempted to relate a variety of techniques, e.g. questionnaire scores, linear analogue scores and even measures of nuisance similar to those employed at airports, to the patients' subjective impression of their status[3,7]. Clearly, even though this work has focused upon postoperative problems, it nevertheless has important implications for the analysis of foregut symptoms in terms of selection of patients for therapy.

Conclusions

We may conclude from the above evidence that something of a quiet revolution is currently taking place in respect of the analysis of foregut symptoms. Over the last 10 years the chief features of this quiet revolution have perhaps been (1) the realization that traditional methods of obtaining and analysing data from patients with foregut disease leave much to be desired, and (2) a determination to employ new techniques as well as to re-examine old ones in an attempt to improve the usage of, and enhance the value of, foregut symptoms.

Perhaps the most encouraging facet of this state of affairs is that there seems, albeit rather undramatically, for the first time to be some evidence that this attention to detail has had some benefit in terms of practical clinical performance. If these trends continue over the next few years, we may ultimately be able to agree with Moynihan's assertion when he remarked three-quarters of a century ago, that he was 'compelled to dissent very confidently' from the view that symptomatic diagnosis of dyspepsia is impossible[30].

References

1 ALMY, T. P., MENDELOFF, A. I., RICE, D., LILIENFELD, A., KLARMAN, H., RAWSON, R. and CUNNICK, W. R. Panel 1. Prevalence and significance of digestive disease. *Gastroenterology*, **68**, 1351–1371 (1975)

2 BALMFORTH, G. Data presented to Royal College of Physicians (London) Computer Workshop 1979 meeting

3 CAY, E. L., PHILIP, A. E., SMALL, W. P., NEILSON, J. and HENDERSON, M. A. Patients assessment of the result of surgery for peptic ulcer. *Lancet*, **1**, 29–30 (1975)

4 CLEATOR, I. G. M., STOLLER, J. L., NUNN, P. N., HOLUBITSKY, I. B., JOHNSTONE, F. R. C. and HARRISON, R. C. Discriminant analysis of data in ulcer and non-ulcer populations. *American Journal of Digestive Diseases*, **18**, 301–310 (1973)

5 COTTON, L. T. (Editor). *Hey Groves' Synopsis of Surgery*, 476, Bristol, Wright (1973)

6 DE DOMBAL, F. T. and GREMY, F. *Decision Making and Medical Care: Can Information Science Help?* Amsterdam, North Holland (1976)

7 DE DOMBAL, F. T. and HALL, R. In *Measuring the Efficacy of Medical Action*, edited by A. Alperovitch, F. T. de Dombal and F. Gremy. Amsterdam, North Holland (1979)

8 DE DOMBAL, F. T. and WENHAM, J. S. Early detection of gastrointestinal cancer by computer. In *Gastroenterology for Nurses*. London, Pitman (In press)

9 DORLAND'S *Illustrated Medical Dictionary*, 25th edition. Philadelphia, W. B. Saunders (1974)

10 EARLAM, R. A computerized questionnaire analysis of duodenal ulcer symptoms. *Gastroenterology*, **71**, 314–317 (1976)

11 EDWARDS, D. A. W. Flow charts, diagnostic keys and algorithms in the diagnosis of dyspepsia. *Scottish Medical Journal*, **15**, 378–385 (1970)

12 EDWARDS, D. A. W. Discriminant information in the diagnosis of dysphagia. *Journal of the Royal College of Physicians of London*, **9**, 257–264 (1975)

13 EDWARDS, F. C. and COGHILL, N. F. Clinical manifestations in patients with chronic atrophic gastritis, gastric ulcer and duodenal ulcer. *Quarterly Journal of Medicine*, **37**, 337–360 (1968)

14 ELMSLIE, R. G. and LUDBROOKE, J. *An Introduction to Surgery*, 85. London, Heinemann (1971)

15 FRENCH, H. *Index of Differential Diagnosis*, 8th edition. Bristol, Wright (1960)

16 FRIEDMAN, M. H. Peptic ulcer and functional dyspepsia in the armed forces. *Gastroenterology*, **10**, 586–606 (1948)

17 GALEN, R. S. and GAMBINO, S. R. *Beyond Normality*. New York, Wiley (1976)

18 GILL, P. W., LEAPER, D. J., GUILLOU, P. J., HORROCKS, J. C. and DE DOMBAL, F. T.. Observer variation in clinical diagnosis. *Methods of Information in Medicine*, **12**, 108–112 (1973)

19 HALL, R., HORROCKS, J. C., CLAMP, S. E. and DE DOMBAL, F. T.. Observer variation in assessment of results of surgery for peptic ulceration. *British Medical Journal*, **1**, 814–816 (1976)

20 HAMPTON, J. R., HARRISON, M. J. G., MITCHELL, J. R. A., PRICHARD, J. S. and SEYMOUR, C.. Relative contributions of history-taking, physical examination and laboratory investigation to diagnosis and management of medical outpatients. *British Medical Journal*, **2**, 486–489 (1975)

21 HORROCKS, J. C. and DE DOMBAL, F. T. Computer aided diagnosis of dyspepsia. *American Journal of Digestive Diseases*, **20**, 397–406 (1975)

22 HORROCKS, J. C. and DE DOMBAL, F. T. Diagnosis of dyspepsia using data collected by a 'physician's assistant'. *British Medical Journal*, **2**, 421–423 (1975)

23 HORROCKS, J. C. and DE DOMBAL, F. T. Clinical presentation of patients with dyspepsia. *Gut*, **19**, 19–26 (1978)

24 HORROCKS, J. C., LAMBERT, D. E., McADAM, W. A. F., MORGAN, A. G., PACSOO, C., DARNBOROUGH, A. and DE DOMBAL, F. T. Transfer of computer-aided diagnosis of dyspepsia from one geographical area to another. *Gut*, **17**, 640–644 (1976)

25 KINGSTON, R. E. and WINDSOR, C. W. O. Flatulent dyspepsia in patients with gallstones undergoing cholecystectomy. *British Journal of Surgery*, **62**, 231–233 (1975)

26 LEAPER, D. J., GILL, P. W., STANILAND, J. R., HORROCKS, J. C. and DE DOMBAL, F. T. Clinical diagnostic process; an analysis. *British Medical Journal*, **2**, 569–574 (1973)

27 LINDLEY, D. V. *Making Decisions*. London, John Wiley and Sons (1971)

28 LUSTED, L. B. *Introduction to Medical Decision Making*. Springfield, Illinois, C. C. Thomas (1968)

29 MOYER, C. A., RHOADS, J. E., ALLEN, J. G. and HARKINS, H. M. *Surgery Principles and Practice*. Philadelphia, J. P. Lippincott, 780 (1967)

30 MOYNIHAN, B. G. A. On Duodenal Ulcer. *Lancet*, **1**, 340–346 (1905)

31 ROSS, P. and DUTTON, A. M. Computer analysis of symptom complexes in patients having upper gastrointestinal examination. *American Journal of Digestive Diseases*, **17**, 248–254 (1977)

32 ROTH, J. A. L. History taking. In Bockus' *Gastroenterology*, 2nd edition, Vol. 1, Philadelphia, Saunders (1963)

33 SAIGER, G. L. Observations on the probability of error in medical diagnosis. *Annals of Internal Medicine*, **56**, 860–864 (1962)

34 SCHLEFF, T. J. Decision rules, types of error and their consequences in medical diagnosis. *Behavioural Sciences*, **8**, 97–107 (1963)

35 SCHEINOK, P. A. and RINALDO, J. A. Symptom diagnosis optimal subsets for upper abdominal pain. *Computers and Biomedical Research*, **1**, 221–236 (1967)

36 SCHEINOK, P. A. and RINALDO, J. A. Symptom diagnosis – A comparison of mathematical models related to upper abdominal pain. *Computers and Biomedical Research*, **1**, 475–489 (1968)

37 SEGAL, A. W., HEALY, M. J. R., COX, A. G., WILLIAMS, I., SLAVIN, G., SMITHIES, A. and LEVI, A. J. Diagnosis of gastric cancer. *British Medical Journal*, **2**, 669–672 (1975)

38 TAYLOR, S., COTTON, L. T. and MURRAY, J. G. *Short Textbook of Surgery*, 266. London, London University Press (1967)

39 VICKERY, D. M. Computer support of paramedical personnel: The question of quality control. *Medinfo 74*. Amsterdam, North Holland (1974)

40 VISICK, A. H. A study of the failures after gastrectomy. *Annals of the Royal College of Surgeons of England*. **3**, 266–284 (1948)

41 WARNER, H. M. *Computer Assisted Medical Decision Making*. New York, Academic Press (1979)

42 WULFF, H. R. *Rational Diagnosis and Treatment*. Oxford, Blackwell (1976)

43 ZOLTIE, N., HORROCKS, J. C. and DE DOMBAL, F. T. Computer assisted diagnosis of dyspepsia. *Methods of Information in Medicine*, **16**, 89–92 (1977)

4

Regulatory peptides of the foregut

T. E. Adrian, S. R. Bloom and J. M. Polak

Introduction

Progress in gut endocrinology has in the past few years been rapid and this may be attributed first to improvements in methods of purification, secondly to new methods of detection of these peptides in tissue and plasma by immunochemical means and finally their availability in synthetic form for physiological studies.

Although the presence of the gastrointestinal hormones gastrin and secretin was recognized at the turn of the century[17, 60], it was another sixty years before these elusive peptides were purified[80, 106]. The difficulties encountered were low tissue concentration, overlap of biological activities and proteolysis of these labile peptides. Success accompanied advances in chromatography and the recognition that small peptides are thermostable[108].

Perhaps the most exciting advance in this field has been the discovery that neural and hormonal control systems overlap and that several peptides exist both in the gut and the brain[26].

A prerequisite for studying the function of a hormone in health and disease is a sensitive and specific method for its measurement. Radioimmunoassay has provided the required sensitivity for measuring low circulating concentrations, coupled with high specificity which is essential for gut hormones where systems are integrated. Specific antibodies have also been used for the tissue localization of peptide hormones by immunocytochemistry.

In this review each of the regulatory peptides which are predominantly localized in the foregut will be considered in turn; they are listed in *Table 4.1*. An attempt will then be made to show how the integrated responses of the various circulating hormones and neuropeptides control secretion and motor activity in the foregut.

Table 4.1 Localization and probable mode of action of the regulatory foregut peptides

Peptide	Localization	Probable mode of action on gut
Gastrin	Antrum	Circulating hormone
Secretin	Duodenum and proximal jejunum	Circulating hormone
Cholecystokinin	Duodenum and proximal jejunum	Circulating hormone
Pancreatic polypeptide	Pancreas	Circulating hormone
Somatostatin	Pancreas and antrum	Local paracrine hormone
Bombesin	Stomach and small intestine	Neurotransmitter
Enkephalin	Antrum, duodenum and pancreas	Neurotransmitter
Thyrotropin-releasing hormone	Antrum, duodenum and pancreas	Neurotransmitter

The secretory actions of the stomach and pancreas will be considered independently as will gastric motility and the control of its sphincters. Because of the interrelationship between the stimulatory actions of cholecystokinin (CCK) and the inhibitory actions of pancreatic polypeptide on the gallbladder and exocrine pancreas, the latter hormone will also be considered in this chapter although it is found in the pancreas rather than the foregut.

The other circulating gastrointestinal hormones motilin, gastric inhibitory peptide, neurotensin and enteroglucagon, and the neural peptides vasoactive intestinal peptide and substance P will be considered in a subsequent volume, *Small Intestine*, as they are localized predominantly in the jejunum and ileum.

Gastrin

In 1905 Edkins reported that extracts of antral mucosa stimulated acid secretion when injected intravenously into anaesthetized cats[60]. He called the active principle gastrin and started a controversy over the existence of this substance which lasted for almost 60 years. The problem was that the extracts prepared by Edkins's method contained the gastric secretagogue histamine. In 1938 Komarov produced antral extracts which were free of histamine but retained the ability to stimulate acid[112]. Other workers, however, failed to achieve an active extract using Komarov's method. Confirmation of the existence of gastrin came in 1964 when Gregory and Tracy isolated from porcine gastric mucosa two peptides which powerfully stimulated acid secretion[80].

Chemistry

Structural analysis by Keller and his associates revealed that the two molecules isolated by Gregory and Tracy were identical 17-amino acid peptides differing only in the presence or absence of a sulphate group on the single tyrosine residue[79]. These structures were confirmed by synthesis[12]. The nonsulphated heptadecapeptide[78] was denoted gastrin I and the sulphated molecule gastrin II (*see Table 4.2*).

Table 4.2 Amino acid sequence of human big gastrin with the smaller identified forms. Tyrosine in position 29 can be unsulphated (gastrin I) or sulphated (gastrin II)

1	Glp		18	Gln		
2	Leu		19	Gly		
3	Gly		20	Pro		
4	Pro		21	Trp		
5	Gln		22	Leu		
6	Gly		23	Glu		
7	His		24	Glu		
8	Pro		25	Glu		
9	Ser		26	Glu		
10	Leu		27	Glu		G-14 } G-17
11	Val		28	Ala		
12	Ala		29	Tyr		
13	Asp		30	Gly		
14	Pro		31	Trp	G-4	
15	Ser		32	Met	(tetrin)	
16	Lys		33	Asp		
17	Lys		34	Phe-NH$_2$		

Following the discovery of gastrin Yalow and Berson reported the presence of larger molecular forms in both tissue and plasma[19, 182]. It is now well established that plasma gastrin exists in several molecular forms and that the predominant form in the fasting state is big gastrin. This larger molecular form was subsequently shown to be a 34 amino acid peptide, in which the C-terminal sequence was identical to heptadecapeptide gastrin G-17 and is thus often referred to as G-34 gastrin[81]. The N-terminal pentadecapeptide[52] of G-34 is linked to the G-17 sequence via two lysine residues which are particularly susceptible to tryptic digestion, suggesting a precursor role for G-34. Other minor forms of gastrin detectable in plasma include a large molecular form, similar in size to proinsulin (component 1), and a C-terminal tetradecapeptide (mini gastrin or G-14). Big gastrin (G-34) and mini gastrin (G-14) are found in sulphated or nonsulphated forms[154] usually in similar quantities like the little gastrins I and II.

Early structure-activity studies on gastrin revealed that the C-terminal tetrapeptide amide was biologically active, and when the amino group on the N-terminus of this peptide is blocked its potency is increased[12]. The synthetic peptide pentagastrin, in which an N-terminal blocking group (tertiary butyl oxycarbonyl) and β-alanine are linked to the C-terminal tetrapeptide amide of gastrin, has been used to investigate acid secretion for many years[173].

As the biologically active C-terminal pentapeptide of gastrin is also common to cholecystokinin it is of no surprise that the biological activities of the two hormones overlap. The important structural difference between gastrin and CCK is the position of the sulphated tyrosine residue. In gastrin the tyrosine residue is positioned next to the active pentapeptide whereas in CCK it is separated by a methionine residue[82]. This governs the relative specificity of the peptides for their target tissues[82]. Cholecystokinin-like peptides stimulate acid secretion in man with a potency an order of magnitude below gastrin. As a partial agonist, however, CCK-like peptides can act as inhibitors of the action of gastrin when the relative doses are appropriate[102]. Similarly, at high doses gastrin will stimulate pancreatic enzyme secretion and contract the gallbladder.

Distribution

Gastrin is found in highest concentration in the antral mucosa where it is located in a discrete endocrine cell type called the G cell[137]. In the gastric antrum G-17 predominates comprising more than 90 per cent of the immunoreactive gastrin. G cells are also found in the duodenum and upper jejunum in man, where substantial amounts of G-34 are localized. The concentration of gastrin in the proximal duodenum is about one-tenth of that in the pyloric antrum and concentrations fall towards the distal duodenum.

In 1975 Vanderhaegen reported the presence of gastrin-like peptide in several regions of the vertebrate brain[175]. It is now clear, however, that CCK-like peptides are present in the brain in considerable quantities and the original claim that gastrin was present had been made using cross-reacting antibodies[54]. Gastrin itself has, however, been found in the hypothalamus, pituitary and also in the vagus nerve[151, 174].

Release

The mechanisms by which plasma gastrin concentrations rise following the ingestion of food are complex, involving interaction between gastric contents bathing the microvilli on the terminal surface of the G cells and the vagus nerves. In some animals, such as the dog, vagal stimulation releases gastrin, but in man vagal activity is predominantly inhibitory[84]. Gastric distension and the presence of partially digested protein are both effectors of gastrin release. The release of gastrin is, however, strongly inhibited by low gastric pH. This negative feedback mechanism thus reduces acid secretion when gastric pH is low. Fasting concentrations of gastrin are below 10 pmol/l in young healthy adults and levels rise substantially following the ingestion of a meal. G-17 and G-34 appear to be released in parallel and although G-17 is more potent it is cleared from the circulation more rapidly than G-34. Both forms are probably important in promoting postprandial gastric secretion[176]. In a study utilizing an antibody specific for G-17 Dockray has reported that following a light meal, G-17 concentrations increased to a peak 20 minutes after feeding (G-17 mean rise 19 pmol/l) whereas G-34 concentrations peaked at 50 minutes (G-34 mean rise 27 pmol/l)[55]. From the known relative potencies of the two peptides it was concluded that G-17 accounts for about 75 per cent of the biologically active gastrin in blood after a meal even though G-34 is present in higher molar concentrations[55].

Several blood-borne stimuli can cause a release of gastrin including calcium and adrenaline, although it is unlikely that any of these would reach a high enough concentration to cause release of gastrin under normal conditions[150, 166]. Bombesin is a powerful releaser of gastrin when administered intravenously and as a local hormone it may well be involved in the physiological control of gastrin release[20].

Physiological role

Gastrin exhibits a wide range of secretory, motor and trophic actions on the gastrointestinal tract. With the exception of its role in gastric secretion, and perhaps its trophic actions, the other observed biological effects are unlikely to occur at physiological concentrations in man[177]. Thus, stimulation of acid and pepsin secretion with a concomitant increase in gastric mucosal flow, occurs at plasma gastrin levels similar to those seen after food. The other notable, and perhaps physiological action of gastrin is its trophic effect on the stomach, small intestine and pancreas. Patients with gastrinoma have marked hyperplasia of the gastric mucosa[136], an effect which can be mimicked by administration of large doses of pentagastrin to rats[45]. Conversely, antrectomy causes atrophy of the gastric mucosa, although this may be reversed by exogenous pentagastrin[100]. The profound atrophy of the stomach, small intestine and pancreas seen in starving rats can be reversed by continuous administration of pentagastrin[101]. A trophic action on gastric mucosa, therefore, appears to be important in man and a similar role may also exist in the small bowel and pancreas.

Clinical significance

Elevated serum gastrin levels accompany acid hyposecretion in patients with atrophic gastritis or gastric carcinoma and are also seen together with hypersecretion of acid in the Zollinger-Ellison syndrome. The involvement of gastrin in peptic ulcer disease is, however, less clear cut.

Raised serum gastrin concentrations are seen in the majority of patients with atrophic gastritis and are particularly high in those patients with pernicious anaemia in whom the antrum is spared by the disease process[126]. This hypergastrinaemia is secondary to the loss of the inhibitory actions of acid and can be normalized by intragastric instillation of acid[71]. Moderate elevation of gastrin levels also frequently accompanies the relative hypochlorhydria following surgical vagotomy[99, 127]. There have been some reports that postprandial hypergastrinaemia can accompany long-term H_2-receptor blockade[87] which is particularly marked in patients whose pretreatment gastrin levels were raised[15].

The measurement of plasma gastrin has proven to be extremely useful in the diagnosis of the Zollinger-Ellison syndrome or gastrinoma[97]. Patients with this rare condition have a tumour, usually located in the pancreas, which secretes gastrin and causes chronic gastric hypersecretion resulting in multiple and recurrent duodenal ulcers. Before gastrin radioimmunoassays became widely available many of these patients died from perforation or haemorrhage. The diagnosis can be made by finding an elevated fasting plasma gastrin level in a duodenal ulcer patient with elevated gastric acid secretion[97]. Renal function which should also be assessed as hypergastrinaemia is also seen in patients with renal impairment, as fragments formed from gastrin degradation are not removed from plasma[88].

The majority of gastrinomas undergo metastatic change and multiple pancreatic tumours are also common. The chances of finding a single resectable lesion have been reported[97] to be less than 1 in 5. As the tumours are slow growing, however, the prognosis can be improved considerably by treatment of the hypergastrinaemia. Before the H_2-receptor blockers became available the treatment of choice was total gastrectomy – an operation associated with a high morbidity[63]. Cimetidine has now been used with considerable success in this syndrome, first to heal the ulcer and make operation safe allowing possible tumour localization and excision as an alternative to total gastrectomy. Secondly it can be used for long-term therapy in patients in whom total gastrectomy is considered too dangerous.

In contrast to the usefulness of gastrin radioimmunoassay in the diagnosis of gastrinoma, this assay is of no value in the diagnosis of duodenal ulcer. Although duodenal ulcer disease is related to excessive gastric acid secretion[83] basal gastrin levels are in the normal range[52]. The postprandial release of gastrin is often moderately elevated in patients with duodenal ulcer but there is a large overlap with levels seen in healthy controls[52]. A small proportion of duodenal ulcer patients have hypergastrinaemia and acid hypersecretion, although no gastrin-producing tumour can be detected. In some such cases increased gastrin levels may result from antral G cell hyperplasia, a condition which can be rectified by antrectomy alone[157]. In patients with borderline normal or moderately elevated fasting plasma gastrin a secretion test may help to differentiate this condition from gastrinoma[167]. In normal subjects gastrin secretion is suppressed following intravenous pure secretin (1 u/kg) whereas patients with gastrinoma usually show a rise.

Secretin

Working from earlier observations that intraduodenal acid stimulated pancreatic juice secretion, Bayliss and Starling observed that the effect was seen even when the pancreas was totally denervated[17]. They went on to show that this effect could be mimicked by intravenous injection of crude small intestinal extracts[17] and concluded that a messenger must be released from the duodenum, to act on the exocrine pancreas via the bloodstream. They called this substance secretin. After many unsuccessful attempts to purify the peptide, Jorpes and Mutt finally succeeded in 1961 using the intestines of 10 000 pigs as starting material[106]. In 1966 the amino acid sequence of secretin was elucidated[107] and this was confirmed in the same year[30].

Chemistry

As *Table 4.3* shows secretin has considerable sequence homology with glucagon, 14 of its 27 amino acids being identical. The entire secretin molecule appears to be necessary for biological activity in contrast to gastrin where small fragments are active[108].

Table 4.3 Amino acid sequence of porcine secretin

1	2	3	4	5	6	7	8	9	10	11	12	13
His	Ser	Asp	Gly	Thr	Phe	Thr	Ser	Glu	Leu	Ser	Arg	Leu

His-Ser-Asp-Gly-Thr-Phe-Thr-Ser-Glu-Leu-Ser-Arg-Leu

14	15	16	17	18	19	20	21	22	23	24	25	26	27

Arg-Asp-Ser-Ala-Arg-Leu-Gln-Arg-Leu-Leu-Gln-Gly-Leu-ValNH$_2$

Localization

Secretin is produced by endocrine cells called the S cells which are localized in the intermediate part of the mucosa between the villous and crypt regions[144]. The highest concentrations of secretin are found in the duodenum although considerable quantities are also present in the proximal jejunum[34].

Actions

In addition to stimulation of a watery bicarbonate secretion from the exocrine pancreas, secretin has a number of other secretory effects. These include inhibition of gastric acid secretion and stimulation of hepatic bile and intestinal secretion.

Physiology

Plasma secretin concentrations rise promptly following duodenal acidification[31, 159, 179]. The pH threshold for secretin release is about 4.5 and below this the secretin release is proportional to the acid load. Physiological studies have demonstrated that duodenal pH does transiently fall below this level postprandially. These intermittent spikes of low pH appear to be accompanied by an increase in plasma secretin concentrations the magnitude of which is sufficient to stimulate bicarbonate secretion from the pancreas[86, 158] (*Figure 4.1*). Indeed

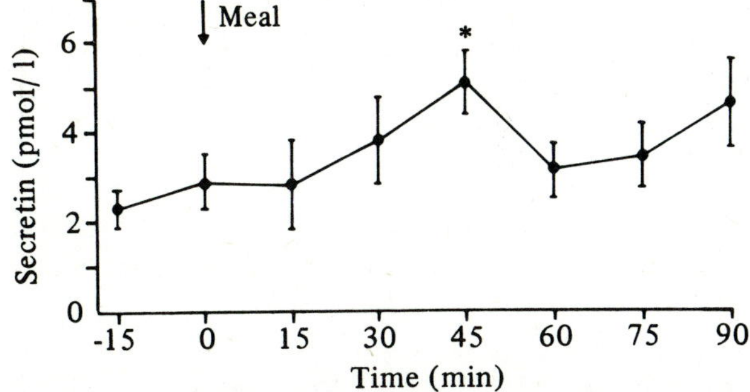

Figure 4.1 Plasma secretin concentrations during breakfast in 9 healthy subjects. *P<0.005. (From Häcki, Greenberg and Bloom[86], courtesy of the Publishers, *Gut Hormones*)

very small doses of exogenous secretin do cause significant pancreatic secretion although they have no other detectable effects. The other actions of secretin could probably, therefore, be considered as pharmacological.

Anti-secretin antiserum has been reported to strongly inhibit pancreatic exocrine secretion. This is evidence in favour of an important role for secretin in the postprandial control of bicarbonate secretion[40]. However, these findings are at variance with a previous report using similar methods where no significant effect on Lundh test meal stimulated bicarbonate was seen following secretin antiserum[110].

It is also apparent that synergism between secretin and CCK exists and, therefore, a small increase in circulating CCK levels will substantially enhance the bicarbonate response to a low dose of secretin[180]. This could be important postprandially, as in all probability is the vagus[39].

Clinical significance

Failure to neutralize acid in the duodenum could possibly give rise to the formation of peptic ulcers. It was, therefore, clearly of interest to investigate the potential role of secretin in patients with duodenal ulcers. Results from two such studies have, however, unfortunately been conflicting. In one study a group of patients awaiting gastric surgery showed a significantly reduced response to intraduodenal acid[29]. A second study of medically treated outpatients failed to demonstrate any significant difference in secretin release from healthy subjects[96]. It is possible that duodenitis in patients with the more severe ulcer disease could account for the difference. Indeed in coeliac disease, a condition characterized by small intestinal villous atrophy, the failure of secretin release is thought to be due to inflammation of the mucosa (*Figure 4.2*)[21].

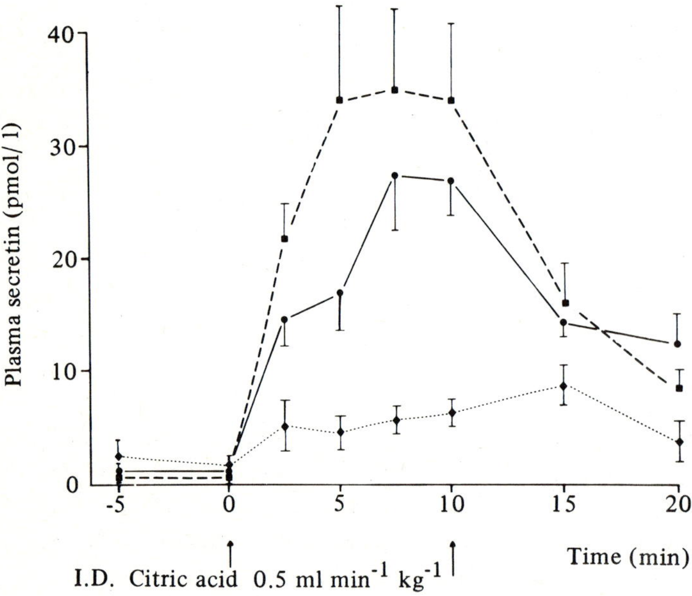

Figure 4.2 Plasma secretin response to intraduodenal citric acid in patients with active coeliac disease (♦....♦), patients treated with a gluten-free diet (■....■), and healthy controls (●—●). (From Besterman *et al.*[21], courtesy of the Editor and Publishers, *Lancet*)

Cholecystokinin

The story of cholecystokinin (CCK) goes back to 1914 when Okada, working in Starling's laboratory observed that gallbladder contraction was stimulated by duodenal acidification in the dog[138]. In 1928 Ivy and Oldberg observed that the intravenous injection of small intestinal extracts could mimic the potent effect of intraduodenal fat on gallbladder contraction[98]. In 1964 Jorpes and Mutt isolated a 33-amino acid peptide from porcine intestine which exhibited the biological activity of CCK[109]. In addition, this peptide also possessed the properties of another hormone, pancreozymin, described by Harper and Raper in 1943 as stimulating pancreatic secretion[90].

Chemistry and localization

The hormone originally isolated by Jorpes and Mutt is a basic straight chain peptide of 33 amino acids (CCK-33). During the final stages of purification the nature of a major contaminant became clear when it was shown to be a 39-amino acid peptide which contained the entire

Table 4.4 Amino acid sequence of porcine cholecystokinin variant (CCK-39) with the smaller identified forms

1	Tyr	20	Gln		
2	Ile	21	Ser		
3	Gln	22	Leu		
4	Gln	23	Asp		
5	Ala	24	Pro		
6	Arg	25	Ser		
7	Lys	26	His		
8	Ala	27	Arg		
9	Pro	28	Ile		
10	Ser	29	Ser		
11	Gly	30	Asp		CCK-33
12	Arg	31	Arg		
13	Val (CCK-33)	32	Asp		
14	Ser	33	Tyr HSO$_3$		
15	Met	34	Met		
16	Ile	35	Gly	CCK-8	
17	Lys	36	Trp		
18	Asn	37	Met (CCK-4)		
19	Leu	38	Asp (tetrin)		
		39	Phe		

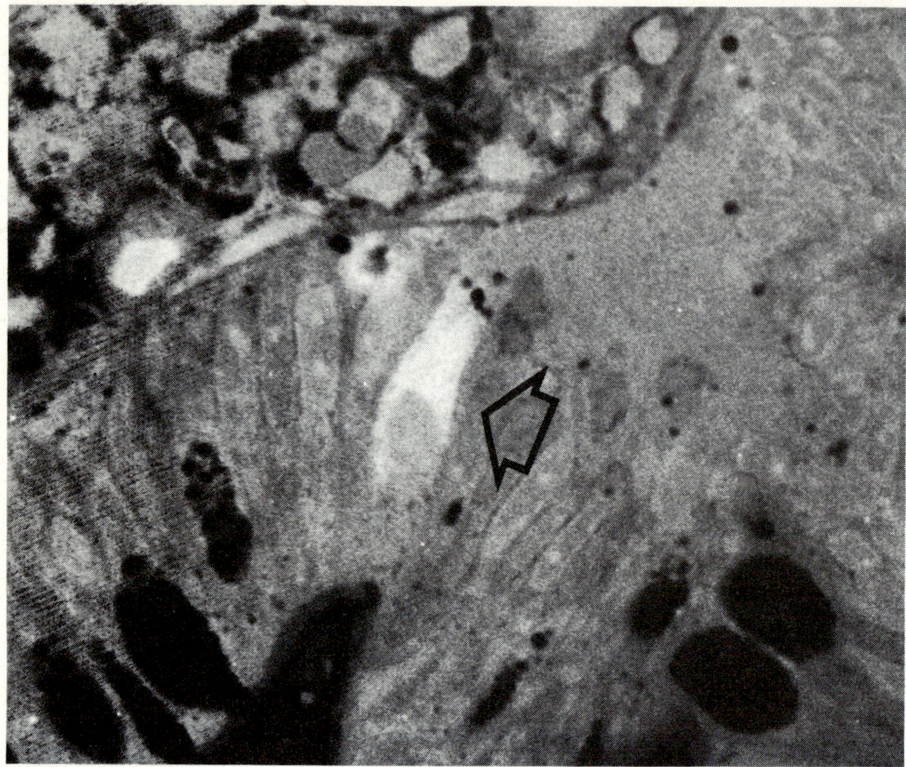

Figure 4.3 (a) Semithin (800 nm) section of human duodenum immunostained with CCK-specific antiserum showing positive cell (arrow) (×800)

sequence of CCK-33, but was extended by six amino acids in the N-terminus (*see Table 4.4*). This larger peptide has been denoted CCK variant (CCK-V or CCK-39)[134]. Investigation of the activity of fragments of CCK revealed that its biological activity resides in the C-terminal octapeptide. This fragment CCK-8, which can be produced from the larger forms by tryptic digestion, has greater potency than the parent molecules[107].

CCK is produced by an endocrine cell in the small intestinal mucosa called the I cell (*Figure 4.3*)[146]. These cells are most numerous in the duodenum and proximal jejunum, in accordance with the distribution as assessed by radioimmunoassay[23].

In 1975 Vanderhaegen described the presence of gastrin-like immunoreactivity in cerebral tissue of man and other species[175]. Dockray using different antibodies directed preferentially toward either gastrin or CCK-8 showed that much of the gastrin-like immunoreactivity in

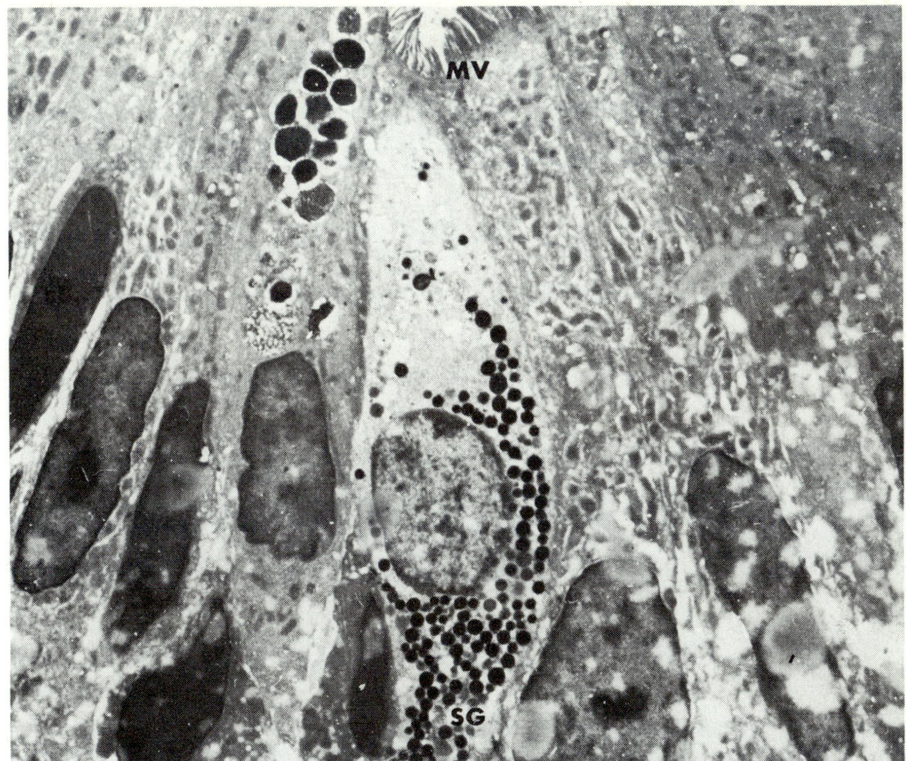

Figure 4.3 (b) The same cell identified in a serial thin (80 nm) section showing the characteristic secretory granules (MV = microvilli, SG = secretory granules) (×4000)

cerebral extracts more closely resembled CCK than gastrin[50]. The octapeptide form of CCK has now been shown to exist naturally and is indeed the most abundant form of CCK in both brain and gut[51, 152]. It is possible that CCK-33 and CCK-39 are precursor molecules. The cholecystokinins all share a common C-terminal pentapeptide with the gastrins, and as this is the biologically active fragment of both hormones it is of no surprise that gastrin shows some cholecystokinetic activity and vice versa[135]. The presence of the C-terminal tetrapeptide, common to both gastrin and cholecystokinin, in both brain and gut has recently been reported[152].

Actions

In addition to its potent actions of gallbladder contraction and stimulation of pancreatic enzyme secretion, CCK has a number of secretory and motor effects on the gastrointestinal tract[135]. Secretory effects include stimulation of the hepatic bile secretion, gastric secretion and insulin release[135]. Motor effects reported are relaxation of the sphincter of Oddi, inhibition of gastric emptying and stimulation of intestinal motor activity[135]. In addition CCK is trophic to the pancreas and is said to reduce food intake of animals[135].

Physiology

The role of cholecystokinin in the postprandial release of pancreatic enzymes and bile is assumed but as yet unproven. The control of these secretions is, in all probability, much more complex, involving other hormones such as chymodenin[1] and nerves. The vagus is almost certainly of importance in this respect[131]. Indeed the transplanted canine pancreas responds quite normally to exogenous CCK, but not to intraduodenal fat, suggesting that mechanisms other than circulating CCK are involved in the mediation of enzyme secretion[165].

The status of cholecystokinin as a circulating hormone can only be established when a specific and sensitive method is available for its measurement. Failure to fully resolve the problems in the radioimmunoassay of this peptide has led to enormous variations in the published values of its circulating concentrations. Results have often conflicted with each other and also with established physiological concepts[53]. A recent study utilizing affinity chromatography to extract and concentrate CCK-like immunoreactivity from plasma, and gel chromatography to investigate molecular forms, suggested that CCK-8 was the only form of CCK in the circulation after intraduodenal fat[115].

In addition to its potential role as a circulating hormone CCK-8 fulfils most of the requirements of a neurotransmitter in both central and peripheral neurones. It is localized and synthesized in central and peripheral neurones, it is concentrated in synaptosomal vesicles and is released by specific stimuli[153]. In addition CCK-8 is a potent activator of post-synaptic membranes[153]. Confirmation of a neurotransmitter role must, however, await the availability of a specific blocking agent.

Clinical significance

Studies on CCK release in pancreatic and gastrointestinal disease are awaited with interest. Elevated plasma CCK concentrations have been reported in patients with steatorrhoea due to coeliac disease and chronic pancreatitis but so far have not been confirmed[91, 124].

Cholecystokinin and its octapeptide analogue have considerable clinical value in cholecystography and the assessment of pancreatic exocrine function.

Pancreatic polypeptide

Human pancreatic polypeptide (PP) was first discovered as a major contaminant during the purification of human proinsulin[36, 37]. PP was shown to exhibit a variety of biological actions on the canine gastrointestinal tract[118, 120]. PP circulates in plasma and levels increase in response to feeding[7, 65, 162] and it soon became apparent that PP was a circulating hormone.

Chemistry

PP has been purified and characterized from several mammalian species and all of these molecules differ in only one to four of their 36 amino acid residues[37]. The C-terminal tyrosine amide appears to be essential for biological activity. Indeed biological activity appears to reside in the C-terminal hexapeptide, the structure of which is identical in all of the mammalian homologues available[119].

Localization

PP cells are found both in the periphery of the islets of Langerhans and scattered throughout the exocrine tissue of the pancreas[116]. Within the pancreas, concentrations are higher in the head than in the body and

Table 4.5 The amino acid sequence of human pancreatic polypeptide (PP)

1	2	3	4	5	6	7	8	9	10	11	12
Ala	Pro	Leu	Glu	Pro	Val	Tyr	Pro	Gly	Asp	Asn	Ala

13	14	15	16	17	18	19	20	21	22	23	24
Thr	Pro	Glu	Gln	Met	Ala	Gln	Tyr	Ala	Ala	Asp	Leu

25	26	27	28	29	30	31	32	33	34	35	36
Arg	Arg	Tyr	Ile	Asn	Met	Leu	Thr	Arg	Pro	Arg	Tyr-NH_2

---

tail[73]. Significant amounts of PP-like immunoreactivity are detectable in the antrum duodenum and rectum in man, but the concentration is only about 0.2 per cent of that in the pancreas. Following surgical pancreatectomy PP is undetectable in the circulation even postprandially, suggesting that the pancreas is the only source of plasma PP in man[5].

Actions

A systematic study revealed that PP has widespread actions on the canine digestive tract including both secretory and motor effects. PP stimulated basal gastric acid secretion but inhibited that stimulated by pentagastrin[120]. PP had a biphasic effect on secretin-stimulated pancreatic juice flow, first stimulating and then suppressing output[120]. Trypsin output in response to secretin and cholecystokinin was markedly reduced, and in addition PP relaxed the gallbladder and increased choledochal tone whilst having no net effect on liver bile flow[118, 120].

Physiology

Plasma PP levels have been reported to rise within three minutes of the start of a meal in man[66]. Because of its localization in the pancreas the secretion of this peptide in response to food adds an interesting facet to the already puzzling picture of the enteroinsular axis in man. The PP response is selectively initiated following the ingestion of protein and fat, although intravenous nutrients are ineffective, suggesting an indirect chemical signal[5, 6, 66]. The prompt rise of PP suggested a neural element[162] and certainly vagal stimulation is a potent mechanism, as evidenced by the dramatic rise of PP in the circulation following hypoglycaemia[5, 67]. Responses to sham feeding and gastric distension, which are thought to act neurally, are, however, at best modest inducers of PP release[67, 161, 163], whereas gut hormones, for example cholecystokinin and secretin or neurotensin, can be extremely potent releasers of PP[3, 22]. Some degree of cholinergic tone appears to be required for the release of PP, because the response of PP to all stimuli so far tested in man can be blocked by atropine, although interestingly not by vagotomy[3, 75].

Thus the PP response to food, which is biphasic, is brought about by a complex entero-PP axis probably involving both the vagus (early

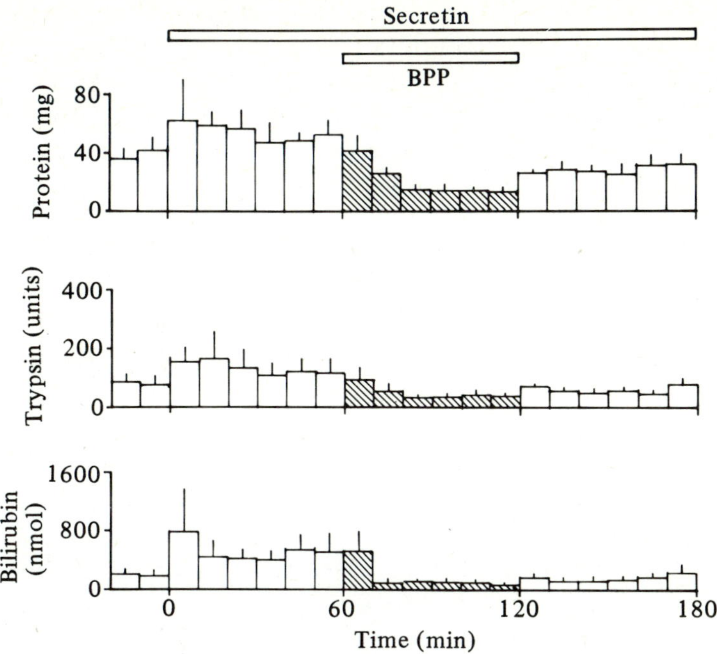

Figure 4.4 Duodenal juice bilirubin, trypsin and total protein concentrations during background secretin stimulation (0.15 pmol kg^{-1} min^{-1}) are substantially reduced during infusion of bovine polypeptide (BPP) (3 pmol kg^{-1} min^{-1}) in 5 healthy volunteers. (From Greenberg *et al.*[77], courtesy of the Editor and Publishers, *Lancet*)

response) and gastrointestinal hormones, the latter being dependent on cholinergic, but not necessarily vagal tone[3, 5].

Infusion studies in man have revealed that at plasma levels similar to those seen after food, PP inhibits pancreatic exocrine secretion, particularly of the enzymes, as well as bile output into the small intestine (*Figure 4.4*)[77]. These actions appear to be quite independent as trypsin output was similarly reduced in cholecystectomized subjects[77]. In contrast, at these and higher doses PP had no significant effect on basal or stimulated gastric secretion or emptying rate nor on circulating metabolites[8, 76]. Similar observations of the effect of PP on canine bile and pancreatic juice outputs have been reported[121, 170].

It is of interest that plasma concentrations of motilin are substantially reduced during low dose infusion of PP[8]. PP has been shown to inhibit motility of the antrum, duodenum, jejunum and colon in the dog[121] whereas, in contrast, motilin stimulates activity in these regions.

It is tempting to speculate that PP exhibits its inhibitory actions on gastrointestinal motor activity via suppression of motilin or other factors.

Clinical significance

Elevated plasma PP levels are often seen in patients wih diabetes mellitus particularly those treated with insulin[67], although PP concentrations may be quite normal in well-controlled diabetics receiving highly purified insulin[6]. Patients with pancreatic exocrine deficiency from chronic pancreatitis[49] or cystic fibrosis have low basal PP levels

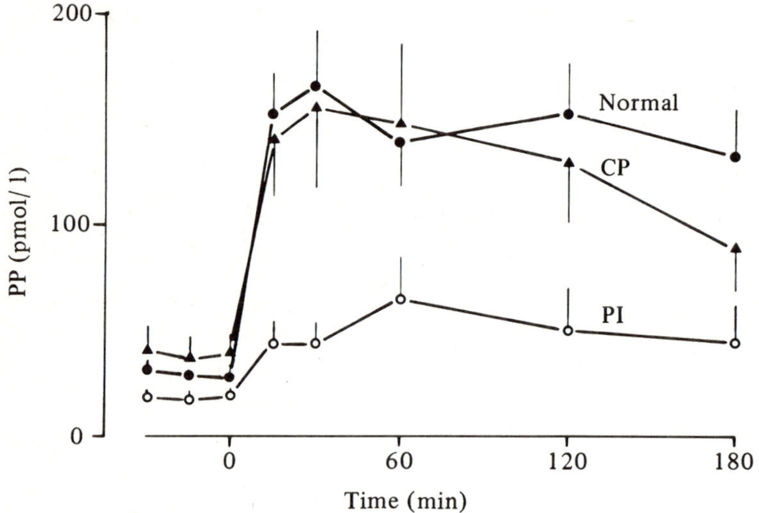

Figure 4.5 Plasma PP response to a test breakfast in patients with chronic pancreatitis with pancreatic insufficiency (PI), chronic pancreatitis without steatorrhoea (CP) and in age-matched healthy controls (normal)

and a greatly reduced postprandial response presumably reflecting the loss of PP cells from the exocrine parenchyma as well as from the islets of Langerhans (*Figure 4.5*)[4, 10].

A controversy exists regarding the association between PP and obesity. It has been reported that PP will reduce hyperphagia and resulting weight gain in genetically obese mice which subsequently become normoglycaemic[72, 129]. This observation suggested a lack of PP

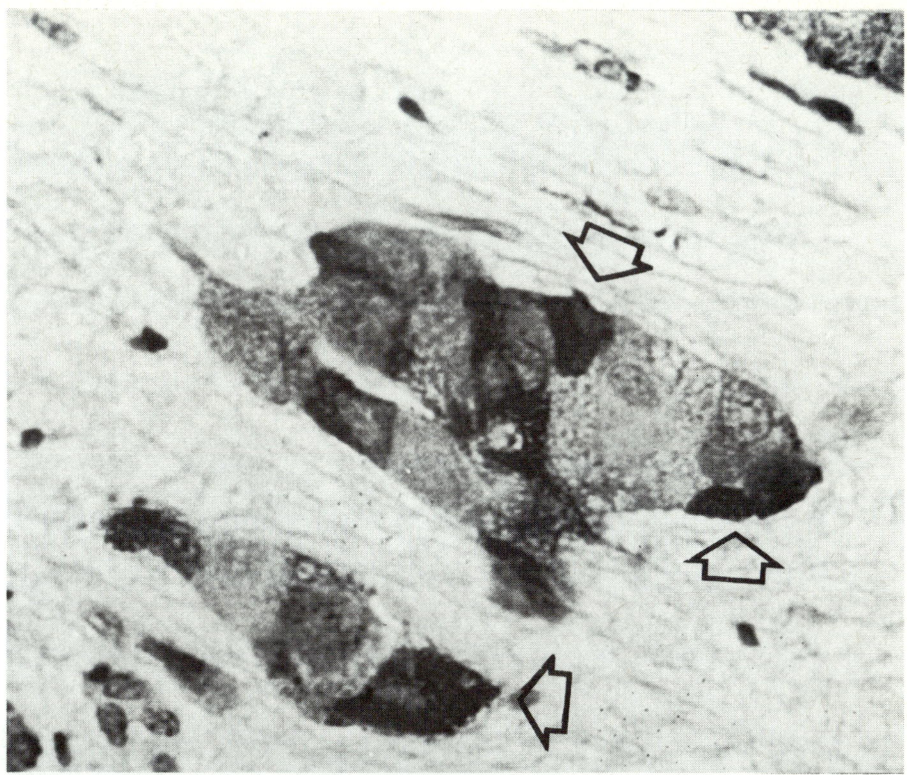

Figure 4.6 Scattered PP cells (arrows) immunostained by the peroxidase-antiperoxidase method in a gastrinoma (×450)

in obesity. Other studies have, however, indicated that both pancreatic content and plasma concentrations of PP are similar in obese mice and lean littermates[2, 74]. Low plasma PP levels have been reported in obese adult man[117], but this finding has been disputed[2, 13].

It has become apparent in recent years that pancreatic endocrine tumours are frequently composed of more than one cell type. Large numbers of PP cells are found in about half of such tumours so far investigated and tumour extracts contain high concentrations of PP (*Figure 4.6*)[2, 141]. The patients whose tumours contain PP have high-circulating concentrations which may exceed the normal postprandial response by 100-fold. These high plasma levels do not appear to be associated with any particular symptoms but may be a useful diagnostic aid.

Bombesin

Bombesin is a 14 amino acid peptide first isolated from frog skin by Esparmer and co-workers[61] (*Table 4.6*). It was shown to have powerful biological actions, including secretory and motor effects, on the mammalian gastrointestinal tract[130]. Several other active peptides

Table 4.6 Amino acid sequence of bombesin and porcine gastrin-releasing peptide (GRP)

Amphibian bombesin

1	2	3	4	5	6	7	8	9	10	11	12	13	14

Glp-Gln-Arg-Leu-Gly-Asn-Gln-Trp-Ala-Val-Gly-His-Leu-MetNH$_2$

Porcine GRP

1	2	3	4	5	6	7	8	9	10	11	12	13	14

Ala-Pro-Val-Ser-Val-Gly-Gly-Gly-Thr-Val-Leu-Ala-Lys-Met

15	16	17	18	19	20	21	22	23	24	25	26	27

Tyr-Pro-Arg-Gly-Asn-His-Trp-Ala-Val-Gly-His-Leu-MetNH$_2$

---

have been isolated from amphibian skin: caerulein, xenopsin, physaelamine, and these all have counterparts in the mammalian gastrointestinal tract, i.e. CCK, neurotensin and substance P. It was perhaps not surprising, therefore, that a bombesin-like peptide was demonstrated by immunocytochemistry in the human gastrointestinal tract[143], a finding later confirmed by radioimmunoassay[145, 178]. Bombesin-like immunoreactivity is found in considerable quantities in the stomach and upper small intestine where it is localized to fine nerve fibres (*Figure 4.7*). Recently, a gastrin-releasing peptide has been isolated from porcine intestine (*Table 4.6*). The C-terminal sequence of this material is identical to amphibian bombesin and the biological activities of the two peptides are similar[125].

Actions

In low doses bombesin stimulates gastric acid and gastrin secretion, pancreatic secretion, intestinal myoelectric activity and smooth muscle contractility, including that of the gallbladder[16, 43, 44]. Although bombesin releases gastrin and probably CCK, it also appears to have a

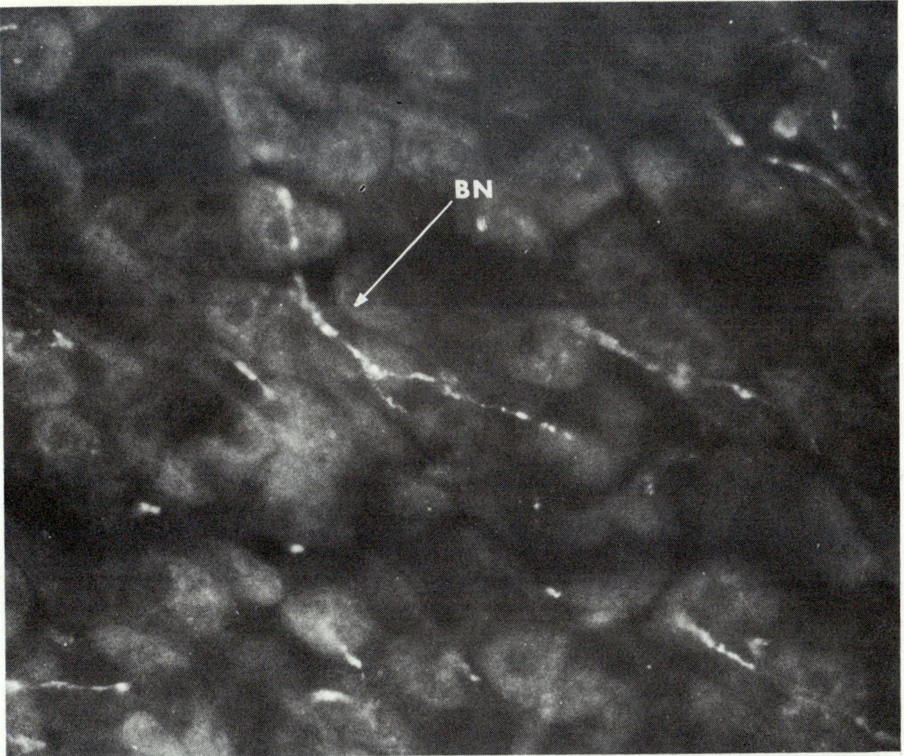

Figure 4.7 Slender and varicose bombesin nerves (BN, arrow) in rat fundic mucosa immunostained by the technique of indirect immunofluorescence (×400)

direct stimulatory effect on the gastric parietal cells and the exocrine pancreas[47]. Infusion of a liver extract into the dog duodenum causes the release of gastrin from an antral pouch, and this release cannot be blocked by antral acidification[171]. Since bombesin is the only agent known to cause a pH-independent release of gastrin, it may act locally on the G cells.

As an additional agent involved in the control of the gastric, pancreatic and biliary secretions, studies on the role of bombesin in such conditions as peptic ulcer and cholelithiasis are awaited with interest.

Somatostatin

Somatostatin was discovered during the investigation of growth hormone release by extracts of ovine hypothalamus[32]. Although the initial

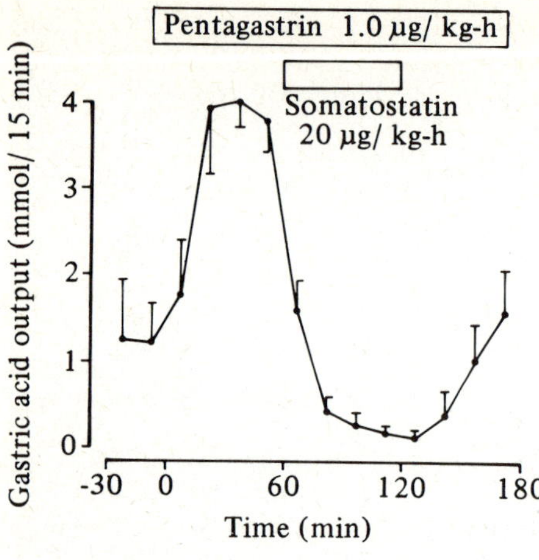

Figure 4.8 Somatostatin inhibition of gastric acid secretion, stimulated by pentagastrin in 4 dogs with gastric fistulae. (From Barros d'Sa, Bloom and Baron[15a], courtesy of the Editor and Publishers, *Lancet*)

discovery was that this peptide inhibited the release of growth hormone from the pituitary it soon became clear that its actions were more widespread. Somatostatin inhibits the release of thyrotropin (TSH) and follicle-stimulating hormone (FSH) from the pituitary. In addition, somatostatin inhibits the release of insulin and glucagon to all known stimuli as well as all of the circulating gastrointestinal hormones so far investigated[24]. As well as the inhibition of hormone release somatostatin also has other direct effects inhibiting gastric, pancreatic, small intestinal and biliary secretions and altering gastrointestinal motor activity patterns (*Figure 4.8*)[24, 25, 48, 172].

In addition to its localization in the hypothalamus, somatostatin was found to be present throughout the central nervous system and the gut with particularly high concentrations in the gastric antrum and the islets of Langerhans of the pancreas. In the gut somatostatin is localized to a discrete endocrine cell type denoted the D cells by ultrastructural classification[147]. In addition to the cyclic tetradecapeptide initially isolated (*Table 4.7*), larger molecular forms of somatostatin have been reported and a 28-amino acid peptide with an identical C-terminal sequence has recently been purified from hog

Table 4.7 Amino acid sequence of ovine somatostatin

1	2	3	4	5	6	7	8	9	10	11	12	13	14
Ala	Gly	Cys	Lys	Asn	Phe	Phe	Trp	Lys	Thr	Phe	Thr	Ser	Cys

Cys3—S–S—Cys14

intestine[149]. This big somatostatin is possibly a precursor form of the 14-amino acid peptide.

The discovery of the widespread distribution and actions of somatostatin led to the search for analogues with selective potency and longer duration of actions. Several analogues have been synthesized which have selective actions in rat[33]. $DTrp^8DCys^{14}$ somatostatin inhibits glucagon and growth hormone, but is less potent on insulin release. In contrast $DesAsp^5DTrp^8DSer^{13}$ is a potent inhibitor of insulin release, but is relatively ineffective at suppressing glucagon. Studies in man, however, have failed to demonstrate selective potency of these somatostatin analogues[9]. The octapeptide analogue, $DesAA^{1,2,4,5,12,13}DTrp^8$ somatostatin, has been shown to suppress the release of insulin, glucagon, growth hormone and gastrin for several hours following a single subcutaneous injection[122]. When infused intravenously, however, this analogue is slightly less potent than the parent molecule and is cleared from the circulation just as rapidly[9]. The increased duration of action is, therefore, probably due to slow uptake from the site of injection, a consequence of its hydrophobic structure.

Physiology

There is considerable controversy as to whether somatostatin normally acts via the circulation. Its widespread actions, which are all seen at similar doses would suggest that if somatostatin was a circulating hormone all actions would be seen simultaneously. There is a lack of agreement between different groups on the plasma concentrations of this peptide and on whether these levels change following physiological stimuli such as food. The concentrations reported using some radioimmunoassays seem inordinately high for a peptide which is so potent. The presence of large forms of somatostatin-like immunoreactivity in the plasma which are detected by these assays further complicate the picture as it is not known whether these substances are biologically active. It has been suggested that the peripheral somatostatin-like immunoreactivity measured by such assay reflects biologically irrelevant somatostatin, which is not abolished by liver passage[14].

It is perhaps more likely that somatostatin is a locally acting substance, a member of the paracrine system. Thus the D cells may exert a controlling influence on gastrin release in the antrum and on islet hormone release in the pancreas.

Clinical significance

Somatostatin-containing cells are frequently found in pancreatic endocrine tumours[27] and recently there have been a few reports of cases where a pancreatic tumour is composed entirely of D cells, a somatostatinoma[70]. These patients have several symptoms which could be attributed to the known biological effects of the peptide including diabetes mellitus, cholelithiasis, hypochlorhydria and steatorrhoea. Relative antral D cell deficiency has been suggested as a possible causative factor in peptic ulcer disease[142]. Histological evidence also suggests that the number of D cells in the pancreas is reduced in nesidioblastosis. A loss of this local inhibitory factor could be responsible for the hypersecretion of insulin seen in this condition[140]. The somatostatin content of the diabetic pancreas has also been reported to be abnormal.

Enkephalins

The enkephalins, which are found in the gut as well in as the central nervous system, are the smallest members of the family of peptides with opiate-like activity, the endorphins[95]. The two enkephalins are 5-amino acid peptides which differ only by the amino acid at the C-terminal end; this may be leucine leu-enkephalin or methionine met-enkephalin[95] (*Table 4.8*). Although the enkephalins were found

Table 4.8 The enkephalins

Tyr-Gly-Gly-Phe-Met
Tyr-Gly-Gly-Phe-Leu

---

first in the brain they were subsequently found in the gut, the highest concentrations being in the gastric antrum, duodenum and pancreas[148]. Enkephalin-like immunoreactivity can be demonstrated in fine nerve fibres in the gut wall although the cell bodies for these nerves are rarely seen. Enkephalin fibres can even be demonstrated immunocytochemically in cultures of Auerbach's plexus[160]. The physiological role of enkephalins in the gut is still unknown although some clue as to the extent of their actions comes from the well-known powerful effects of morphia, such as reduction of secretions and inhibition of motility. Enkephalin infusion studies in dogs have indeed revealed pronounced effects on gastrointestinal motility with a reduction in gastric emptying and inhibition of intestinal contractions[113]. The effects on secretions are, however, more controversial, because enkephalin has been reported to augment gastric secretion, an effect which could be reversed by naloxone[113]. Like morphine, enkephalin inhibits pancreatic secretions[113].

Thyrothropin-releasing hormone

Thyrothropin-releasing hormone (TRH pyroglutamyl-histidyl prolinamide) was the first hypothalamic releasing agent to be isolated and characterized. This has recently been demonstrated in the rodent gastrointestinal tract by radioimmunoassay[132]. TRH has recently been shown to exhibit several actions on the human gut including inhibition of gastric acid secretion and motility, and also reduction in glucose and xylose absorption[56, 57, 58, 133]. It would, thus, appear that in the gut TRH has somatostatin-like actions. The elucidation of its physiological importance is awaited with interest.

Interactions of regulatory peptides in the foregut

Effects of gastrointestinal hormones on the pyloric and lower oesophageal sphincter

Circulating gastrointestinal hormones may be involved in the control of the lower oesophageal sphincter (LES) and the pylorus; however, their physiological role is uncertain. Several peptides can be shown to effect the pressures of these sphincters, but there is little evidence that these effects are physiological. Resting LES pressure is suppressed by intragastric instillation of acid suggesting that it may be dependent on endogenous gastrin[35]. The possibility remains that gastrin may exert some background influence on the maintenance of LES pressure[69]. Glucagon, secretin and cholecystokinin antagonize the effect of gastrin on the LES but are probably not important physiologically. Infusions of motilin in man have been reported to cause a dose-dependent increase in LES pressure[59], and in addition duodenal acidification in man causes a rise in pressure concomitant with the plasma motilin rise in some[59], but not in other[92] studies. CCK, secretin and motilin have been shown to increase pyloric pressure and although gastrin has no effect on basal pressure it does antagonize the pressure increase following instillation of hydrochloric acid[64, 169]. The physiological control mechanisms for the sphincters are as yet ill understood.

Effects of hormones on gastric emptying

Several peptides including gastrin, secretin and cholecystokinin (CCK) delay the rate of gastric emptying in man[38]. Of these, however, only the effect of CCK may be considered to be physiological[46]. Motilin, a peptide with potent effects on the stomach, enhances the emptying rate of a solid meal in man at doses which are within the physiological range[42]. The effects of somatostatin on gastric evacuation are complex. At low doses the peptide speeds the rate of emptying[123], whereas at high doses somatostatin appears to be inhibitory[28].

Hormone interaction in the control of acid secretion

Gastric acid secretion is a complex physiological process involving the interactions of several hormonal and neural factors. Classically, gastric secretion was divided into the interdigestive and digestive states and the latter was further subdivided into the cephalic, gastric and intestinal phases of stimulation. The cephalic phase was thought to be neural, and hormones were implicated as being responsible for the gastric and intestinal phases. It is now evident that all three phases of postprandial acid secretion are influenced by the same hormonal and neural factors which potentiate each other. The parietal cells are exposed to a variety of stimulators and inhibitors delivered by endocrine, paracrine and neurocrine pathways (*Figure 4.9*).

There are at least three secretagogues present in the stomach which are physiologically important in the control of acid secretion: gastrin, histamine and acetylcholine. These substances all demonstrate a high degree of interaction and interdependence. Both anticholinergics and H_2 receptor antagonists block acid secretion induced by histamine, gastrin or cholinergic stimulation[85, 114, 164]. Similarly antrectomy decreases the acid response to food and to histamine[18, 114].

Vagal influence on gastrin and acid secretion is complex and show species differences. For example, in the dog vagal stimulation increases gastrin levels and stimulates acid secretion; in man its effects are much less marked. Sham feeding in man causes little or no change in gastrin levels although it stimulates acid secretion quite potently, an effect which is not blocked by antrectomy[111]. Vagal stimulation of gastrin release, appears to be noncholinergic and may perhaps be mediated by bombesin[156]. There is increasing evidence that the vagus also causes inhibition of acid and gastrin release particularly in man and the name 'vagogastrone' has been coined for the hormone mediating these effects. Vasoactive intestinal peptide (VIP) is released by vagal stimuli[62], and potently inhibits acid secretion and could therefore fit the role of the hypothetical vagogastrone.

Gastrin is released by the presence of partially digested proteins in the stomach[155] as well as by neural influences. Although gastrin is clearly the principle mediator of protein-stimulated acid secretion, amino acids may also influence the oxyntic cells directly[155]. Acid in the stomach inhibits the release of gastrin, and indeed peptic digest may stimulate gastrin release by buffering the secreted acid and raising intragastric pH as well as by their direct influence on the G cell. Distension also stimulates acid secretion, an effect partly mediated by gastrin release.

Entero-oxyntin is the name given to the small intestinal hormone postulated as stimulating acid secretion in man in response to amino acids. Gastrin from the duodenum may be partly responsible for this effect, but bombesin or the gastrin-releasing peptide recently isolated from porcine intestine is probably more important[125, 171]. Cholecysto-kinin is a partial agonist for the gastrin receptor but is unlikely to be involved in everyday control of acid secretion.

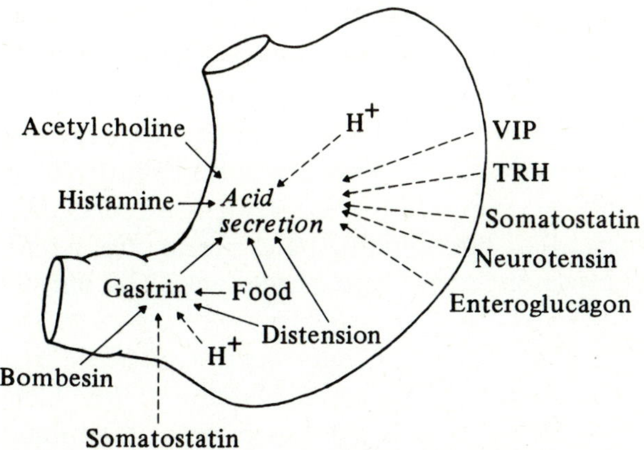

Figure 4.9 Some of the factors which may influence gastric acid secretion, demonstrating a complex inter-action of endocrine, neurocrine and paracrine control

Enkephalins are known to be present in the stomach and duodenum and have been shown to stimulate acid secretion. However, their physiological role is unknown[113].

Gastric secretion is inhibited by acid in the stomach or duodenum and inhibitory effects are also seen with fat, or hypertonic solutions in the small intestine and following hyperglycaemia[103, 181]. The antral inhibition of acid secretion has been attributed to 'antral chalone' and 'gastrone' although clearly somatostatin, present locally in high concentations, may well be involved. Secretin, glucagon and gastric inhibitory peptide (GIP) can all cause inhibition of acid secretion[103] although at doses which could be considered to be unphysiological. It is of interest that the effect of this group of peptides might be mediated by the release of antral somatostatin[41]. The physiological mechanism of the inhibition of gastrin secretion by duodenal fat or acid is as yet unknown.

Interaction of hormones on exocrine pancreatic secretion

Early experiments with pure preparations of secretin and cholecystokinin revealed that these peptides potentiated the action of each other on the exocrine pancreas[180]. Although when infused alone CCK causes little or no increase in pancreatic juice volume or bicarbonate output, it can cause a four-fold increase in that induced by secretin. Enzyme output stimulated by CCK can likewise be potentiated by the addition of secretin. Such interdependence is undoubtedly of importance in the postprandial control of pancreatic exocrine secretions particularly as the rise of secretin after food is small and intermittent[86, 158]. In addition to these hormonal interactions, vagal influence appears also to be of importance in the postprandial secretion of pancreatic juice. Pancreatic bicarbonate output stimulated by secretin is enhanced by 2-deoxyglucose and inhibited by atropine[39]. In addition, the transplanted canine pancreas responds normally to exogenous CCK but not to food[165].

There are several other peptides which may have a physiological role in the control of the exocrine pancreas (*Figure 4.10*). Chymodenin, a peptide isolated from hog duodenal mucosa, stimulates chymotrypsinogen output with little effect on other pancreatic enzymes[1]. Vasoactive intestinal peptide (VIP) stimulates bicarbonate secretion in man and can be demonstrated in neural fibres of the

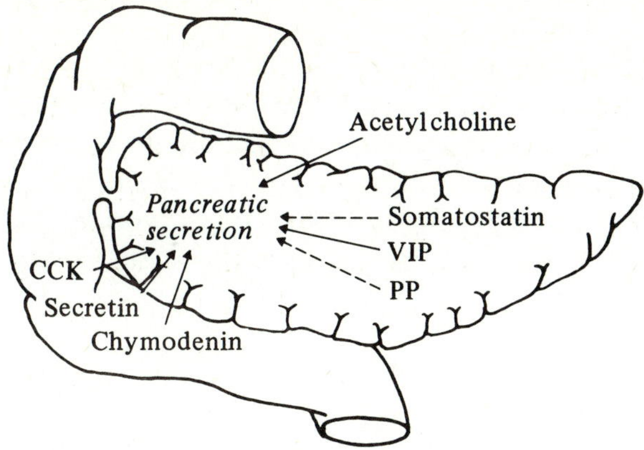

Figure 4.10 Some of the factors which may influence
pancreatic exocrine secretion of bicarbonate and
digestive enzymes

pancreas. At plasma levels similar to those seen postprandially,
pancreatic polypeptide inhibits pancreatic exocrine secretion, particularly of enzymes in both man[77] and dog[170]. Somatostatin has widespread inhibitory actions on the gastrointestinal tract and pancreatic
secretion is no exception[68, 89]. Release of secretin and cholecystokinin
is also suppressed by somatostatin. Like morphine, the enkephalins
inhibit pancreatic secretion and this may be of physiological importance.

Interaction of hormones on bile output

Several gastrointestinal hormones have been reported to stimulate bile
secretion including glucagon[104], secretin[104], vasoactive intestinal
peptide[128], cholecystokinin[105] and gastrin[105]. Secretin and VIP are very
potent choleretic agents and are possibly involved in postprandial bile
secretion[104, 128]. Both somatostatin and substance P have been reported to inhibit spontaneous bile secretion[93, 94].

Secretin potentiates the action of cholecystokinin on gallbladder
muscle although alone it has no effect[168]. Recent experiments have
revealed that motilin causes gallbladder contraction in the pig[11], whilst
PP, VIP and somatostatin all relax the gallbladder in a dose-related
manner[11, 77, 119, 139].

Conclusion

A decade ago gastrin, secretin and cholecystokinin were the known gut hormones. The list of regulatory peptides of the gut has now grown and with it our knowledge of the release and biological effects of these substances. We are slowly becoming aware, however, of the complex interactions between these endocrine, neurocrine and paracrine systems in the regulation of the secretory and motor processes of the foregut.

References

1 ADELSON, J. W. and ROTHAM, S. S. Chymodenin, a duodenal peptide: specific stimulation of chymotrypsin secretion. *American Journal of Physiology*, **229**, 1680–1686 (1975)

2 ADRIAN, T. E. Pancreatic polypeptide. *Journal of Clinical Pathology*, **33** Supplement 8, 43–50 (1980)

3 ADRIAN, T. E., BESTERMAN, H. S. and BLOOM, S. R. Importance of cholinergic tone in the release of pancreatic polypeptide by gut hormones in man. *Life Science*, **24**, 1989–1994 (1979)

4 ADRIAN, T. E., BESTERMAN, H. S., MALLINSON, C. N., GARALOTIS, C. and BLOOM, S. R. Impaired pancreatic polypeptide release in chronic pancreatitis with steatorrhoea. *Gut*, **20**, 98–101 (1976)

5 ADRIAN, T. E., BLOOM, S. R., BESTERMAN, H. S., BARNES, A. J., COOKE, T. J. C., RUSSELL, R. C. G. and FABER, R. G. Mechanism of pancreatic polypeptide release in man. *Lancet*, **1**, 161–163 (1977)

6 ADRIAN, T. E., BLOOM, S. R., BESTERMAN, H. S. and BRYANT, M. G. PP – Physiology and pathology. In *Gut Hormones*, edited by S. R. Bloom, 254–260 Edinburgh, Churchill Livingstone (1978)

7 ADRIAN, T. E., BLOOM, S. R., BRYANT, M. G., POLAK, J. M., HEITZ, PH. and BARNES, A. J. Distribution and release of human pancreatic polypeptide *Gut*, **17**, 940 –944 (1976)

8 ADRIAN, T. E., GREENBERG, G. R., CHRISTOFIDES, N. D., ALBERTI, K. G. M. M. and BLOOM, S. R. Effects of pancreatic polypeptide on motilin and circulating metabolites in man. *European Journal of Clinical Investigation*, **10**, 235–240 (1980)

9 ADRIAN, T. E., LONG, R. G., BARNES, A. J., BLOOM, S. R., BROWN, M. R., VALE, W. and RIVIER, J. The effect of analogues of somatostatin on growth hormone, pancreatic and gut hormones in man. *Journal of Endocrinology*, **85**, 41 (1980)

10 ADRIAN, T. E., MCKIERNAN, J., JOHNSTONE, D. I., HILLER, E. J., VYAS, H., SARSON, D. L. and BLOOM, S. R. Pancreatic and gut hormone abnormalities in cystic fibrosis. *Gastroenterology*, **79**, 460–465 (1980)

11 ADRIAN, T. E., MITCHENERE, P., CHRISTOFIDES, N. D. and BLOOM, S. R. Effect of motilin and other hormonal peptides on gallbladder pressure in the pig. *Regulatory Peptides*, **1**, Supplement 1 (1980)

12 ANDERSON, J. C., BARTON, M. A., GREGORY, R. A., HARDY, P. M., KENNER, G. W., MACLEOD, J. K., PRESTON, J., SHEPPARD, R. C. and MORLEY, J. S. Synthesis of gastrin. *Nature*, **204**, 933–934 (1964)

13 ANDREWS, W. J., O'HARE, M. M. T., BUCHANAN, K. D. and CORNELL, A. M. Eating, exercise and pancreatic polypeptide in obestity. *Clinical Science*, **57**, 7pp. (1979)

14 ARNOLD, R. and LANKISCH, P. G. Somatostatin and the gastrointestinal tract. *Clinicis in Gastroenterology*, **9**, 733–753 (1980)

15 BARBEZAT, G. O. and GROSSMAN, M. I. Intestinal secretion: stimulation by peptides. *Science*, **174**, 422–423 (1979)

15a BARROS D'SA, A. A. J., BLOOM, S. R. and BARON, J. H. Direct inhibition of gastric acid by growth-hormone release-inhibiting hormone in dogs. *Lancet*, **1**, 886–887 (1975)

16 BASSO, N., GIRI, S., IMPROCCA, G., LEZOCHE, E., MELCHIORRI, P., PERCOCO, M. and SPERANZA, V. External pancreatic secretion after bombesin infusion in man. *Gut*, **16**, 994–998 (1975)

17 BAYLISS, W. M. and STARLING, E. H. The mechanism of pancreatic secretion. *Journal of Physiology* (*London*), **28**, 325–353 (1902)

18 BERGEGARDH, S., BROMAN, G., KNUTSON, U., PALMER, L. and OLBE, L. Gastric acid responses to graded iv infusions of pentagastrin and histolog in peptic ulcer patients before and after antrum-bulb resection. *Scandinavian Journal of Gastroenterology*, **11**, 337–346 (1976)

19 BERSON, S. A. and YALOW, R. S. Nature of immunoreactive gastrin extracted from tissue of the gastrointestinal tract. *Gastroenterology*, **60**, 215–222 (1971)

20 BETTACCINI, G. Active peptides of non-mammalian origin. *Pharmacology Review*, **28**, 127–177 (1976)

21 BESTERMAN, H. S., BLOOM, S. R., SARSON, D. L., BLACKBURN, A. M., JOHNSTON, D. I., PATEL, H. R., STEWART, J. S., MODIGLIANI, R., GUERIN, S. and MALLISON, C. N. Gut hormone profile in coeliac disease. *Lancet*, **1**, 785–788 (1978)

22 BLACKBURN, A. M., FLETCHER, D. R., CHRISTOFIDES, N. D., FITZPATRICK, M. L., ADRIAN, T. E. and BLOOM, S. R. Neurotensin infusion in man and its effect on gastric function. *Gastroenterology*, **78**, 1142 (1980)

23 BLOOM, S. R. Hormones of the gastrointestinal tract. *British Medical Bulletin*, **30**, 62–67 (1974)

24 BLOOM, S. R. Somatostatin and the gut. *Gastroenterology*, **75**, 145–147 (1978)

25 BLOOM, S. R., MORTIMER, C. H., THORNER, M. O., BESSER, G. M., HALL, R., GOMEZ-PAN, A., ROY, V. M., RUSSELL, R. C. G., COY, D. H., KASTIN, A. J. and SCHALLY, A. V. Inhibition of gastrin and gastric acid secretion by growth-hormone release-inhibiting hormone. *Lancet 2*, 1106–1109 (1974)

26 BLOOM, S. R. and POLAK, J. M. Neuropeptides in the gut and other peripheral tissues. In *Brain Peptides: A New Endocrinology*, edited by A. M. Gotto, D. J. Peck and A. E. Boyd. Amsterdam, Elsevier Biomedical Press, 103–107 (1979)

27 BLOOM, S. R., POLAK, J. M. and WEST, A. M. Somatostatin content of pancreatic endocrine tumours. *Metabolism*, **27**, Supplement 1, 1235–1238 (1978)

28 BLOOM, S. R., RALPHS, D. N., BESSER, G. M., HALL, R., COY, D. H., KASTIN, A. J. and SCHALLY, A. V. Effect of somatostatin on motilin levels and gastric emptying. *Gut*, **16**, 834 (1976) (Abstract)

29 BLOOM, S. R. and WARD, A. S. Failure of secretin release in patients with duodenal ulcer. *British Medical Journal*, **1**, 126–127 (1975)

30 BODANSKY, M., ONDETTI, M. A., LEVINE, S. D., MARAJAN, V. L., VON SALTZA, J. T., WILLIAMS, N. J. and SABO, E. T. Synthesis of a heptacosapeptide amide with the hormonal activity of secretin. *Chemical Industry*, **42**, 1757–1758 (1966)

31 BODEN, G., WILSON, R. M., ESSA-KOUMAR, N. and OWEN, O. E. Effects of a protein meal, intraduodenal HC1, and oleic acid on portal and peripheral venous secretin and on pancreatic bicarbonate secretion.*Gut*, **19**, 277–283 (1978)

32 BRAZEAU, P. and GUILLEMIN, R. Somatostatin: newcomer from the hypothalamus. *New England Journal of Medicine*, **290**, 963–964 (1974)

33 BROWN, M., RIVIER, J. and VALE, W. Somatostatin: analogs with selected biological activities. *Science*, **196**, 1467–1469 (1977)

34 BRYANT, M. G. and BLOOM, S. R. Distribution of the gut hormones in the primate intestinal tract. *Gut*, **20**, 653–659 (1979)

35 CASTELL, D. O, and HARRIS, L. D. Hormonal control of gastroesophageal sphincter strength. *New England Journal of Medicine*, **282**, 886–890 (1970)

36 CHANCE, R. E. Discussion of presentations. *Diabetes*, **21**, Supplement 2, 536 (1972)

37 CHANCE, R. E. and JONES, W. E. Polypeptides from bovine, ovine, human and porcine pancreas. *United States Patent Office*, **842**(3), 063 (1974)

38 CHEY, W. Y., HITANANT, S. M., HENDRICKS, J. and LORBER, S. H. Effect of secretin and cholecystokinin on gastric emptying and gastric secretion in man. *Gastroenterology*, **58**, 820–827 (1970)

39 CHEY, W. Y., KIM, M. S. and LEE, K. Y. Influence of the vagus nerve on release and action of secretin in dog. *Journal of Physiology* (*London*), **293**, 435–446 (1979)

40 CHEY, W. Y., KIM, M. S., LEE, K. Y. and CHANG, T. Effect of rabbit antisecretin serum on postprandial pancreatic secretion in dogs. *Gastroenterology*, **77**, 1268–1275 (1979)

41 CHIBA, T., TAMINATO, T., KADOWAKI, S., ABE, H., CHIHARI, K., SEINO, Y., MATSUKURA, S. and FUJITA, T. Effects of glucagon secretin and vasoactive intestinal polypeptide on gastric somatostatin and gastrin release from isolated perfused rat stomach. *Gastroenterology*, **79**, 67–71 (1980)

42 CHRISTOFIDES, N. D., MODLIN, I. M., FITZPATRICK, M. L. and BLOOM, S. R. Effect of Motilin on the rate of gastric emptying and gut hormone release during breakfast. *Gastroenterology*, **76**, 903–907 (1979)

43 CORAZZIARI, E., TORSOLI, A., DELLE FAVE, G. E., MELCHIORRI, P. and HABIB FORTUNEE, I. Effects of bombesin on the mechanical activity of the human duodenum and jejunum. *Rendiconti di Gastroenterologia*, **6**, 55–59 (1974)

44 CORAZZIARI, E., TORSOLI, A., MELCHIORRI, P. and DELLE FAVE, G. F. Effect of bombesin on human gallbladder emptying. *Rendiconti di Gastroenterologia*, **6**, 52–54 (1974)

45 CREAN, G. P., MARSHALL, M. W. and RAMSEY, R. D. E. Parietal cell hyperplasia induced by the administration of pentagastrin to rats. *Gastroenterology*, **57**, 147–155 (1969)

46 DEBAS, H. T., FAROOQ and GROSSMAN, M. I. Inhibition of gastric emptying is a physiological action of cholecystokinin. *Gastroenterology*, **68**, 1211–1217 (1975)

47 DESCHODT-LANCKMAN, M., ROBBERECHT, P., DE NEEF, PH., LAMMENS, M. and CHRISTOPHE, J. In vitro action of bombesin and bombesin-like peptides on amylase secretion, calcium and adenylate cyclase activity in the rat pancreas: a comparison with other secretagogues. *Journal of Clinical Investigation*, **58**, 891–898 (1976)

48 DHARMSATHAPHORN, K., SHERWIN, R. S. and DOBBINS, J. W. Somatostatin inhibits fluid secretion in the rat jejunum. *Gastroenterology*, **78**, 1554–1558 (1980)

49 DI MAGNO, E. P., GO, W. L. W. and SUMMERSKILL, W. H. J. Relations between pancreatic enzyme outputs and malabsorption in severe pancreatic insufficiency. *New England Journal of Medicine*, **288**, 813–815 (1973)

50 DOCKRAY, G. J. Immunochemical evidence of cholecystokinin-like peptides in brain. *Nature*, **264**, 568–570 (1976)

51 DOCKRAY, G. J. Immunoreactive component resembling cholecystokinin octapeptide in intestine. *Nature*, **270**, 359–361 (1977)

52 DOCKRAY, G. J. Gastrin overview. In *Gut Hormones*, edited by S. R. Bloom, 129–139. Edinburgh, Churchill Livingstone (1978)

53 DOCKRAY, G. J. Gastrointestinal hormones II Gastrin, Cholecystokinin and Secretin. In *Hormones in Blood*, 3rd Edn, edited by C. H. Gray and V. H. T. James, 357–382. London, Academic (1979)

54 DOCKRAY, G. J., GREGORY, R. A., HUTCHISON, J. B., HARRIS, J. I. and RUNSWICK, M. J. Isolation, structure and biological activity of two cholecystokinin octapeptides from sheep brain. *Nature*, **273**, 711–713 (1978)

55 DOCKRAY, G. J. and TAYLOR I. L. Heptadecapeptide gastrin: measurement in blood by specific radioimmunoassay. *Gastroenterology*, **71**, 971–977 (1976)

56 DOLVA, L. O., HANSSEN, K. F. and BERSTAD, A. Actions of thyrotropin-releasing hormone on the gastrointestinal function in man II: inhibition of pentagastrin-stimulated acid secretion. *Scandinavian Journal of Gastroenterology*, **14**, 33–34 (1979)

57 DOLVA, L. O., HANSSEN, K. E. and FREY, H. M. M. Actions of thryrotropin-releasing hormone on gastrointestinal function in man I: inhibition of glucose and xylose absorption from the gut. *Scandinavian Journal of Gastroenterology*, **13**, 599–604 (1978)

58 DOLVA, L. O. and STADAAS, J. O. Actions of thyrotropin-releasing hormone on gastrointestinal function in man III: inhibition of gastric motility in response to distension. *Scandinavian Journal of Gastroenterology*, **14**, 419–423 (1979)

59 DOMSCHKE, W., LUX, G., MITZNEGG, P., ROSCH, W., DOMSCHKE, S., BLOOM, S. R., WUMSCH, E. and DEMLING, L. Relationship of plasma motilin response to lower oesophageal sphincter pressure in man. *Scandinavian Journal of Gastroenterology*, **11**, Supplement 39, 81–84 (1976)

60 EDKINS, J. S. The chemical mechanism of gastrin release. *Journal of Physiology*, (*London*), **34**, 133–144 (1906)

61 ESPARMER, V. and MELCHIORRI, P. Active polypeptides of the amphibian skin and their synthetic analogues. *Pure and Applied Chemistry*, **35**, 463–494 (1973)

62 FAHRENKRUG, J., SCHAFFALITZKY DE MUCKADELL, O. B. and HOLST, J. J. Nervous release of VIP. In *Gut Hormones*, edited by S. R. Bloom, 488–491. Edinburgh, Churchill Livingstone (1978)

63 FANG, M., GINSBERG, A. L., GLASSMAN, L., MCCARTHY, D. M., COHEN, P., GEELHOED, G. W. and DOBBINS, W. O. Zollinger-Ellison syndrome with diarrhoea as the predominant clinical feature. *Gastroenterology*, **76**, 378–387 (1979)

64 FISHER, R. S., LIPSHUTZ, W. and COHEN, S. Hormonal regulation of the human pyloric sphincter. *Journal of Clinical Investigation*, **52**, 1289–1296

65 FLOYD, J. C., FAJANS, S. S. and PEK, S. Regulation in healthy subjects of the secretion of human pancreatic polypeptide, a newly recognized pancreatic islet polypeptide. *Recent Progress in Hormone Research*, **32**, 146–158 (1976)

66 FLOYD, J. C., FAJANS, S. S. and PEK, S. Physiological regulation of plasma levels of PP in man. In *Gut Hormones*, edited by S. R. Bloom, 247–253. Edinburgh, Churchill Livingstone (1978)

67 FLOYD, J. C., FAJAN,S S., PEK, S. and CHANCE, R. E. A newly recognized pancreatic polypeptide; plasma levels in health and disease. *Recent Progress in Hormone Research*, **33**, 519–570 (1977)

68 FOLSH, U. R., LANKISCH, P. G. and CREUTZFELDT, W. Effect of somatostatin on basal and stimulated pancreatic secretion in the rat. *Digestion*, **17**, 194–203 (1978)

69 FREELAND, G. R., HIGGS, R. H., CASTELL, D. O. and MCGUIGAN, J. E. Lower oesophageal sphincter and gastric acid response to intravenous infusions of synthetic human gastrin I heptadecapeptide. *Gastroenterology*, **71**, 570–574 (1975)

70 GANDA, O. P., WEIR, R. C., SOELDNER, J. S., LEGG, M. A., CHICK, W. L., PATEL, Y. C., EBEID, A. M., GABBAY, K. H. and REICHLIN, S. 'Somatostatinoma': a somatostatin-containing tumour of the endocrine pancreas. *New England Journal of Medicine*, **296**, 963–967 (1977)

71 GANGULI, P. C., CULLEN, D. R. and IRVINE, W. J. Radioimmunoassay of plasma gastrin in pernicious anaemia, achlorhydria without pernicious anaemia, hypochlorhydria and in controls. *Lancet*, **1**, 155–158 (1971)

72 GATES, R. and LAZARUS, N. The ability of pancreatic polypeptides (APP and BPP) to return to normal the hyperglycaemia, hyperinsulinaemia and weight gain of New Zealand obese mice. *Hormone Research*, **8**, 189–202 (1977)

73 GERSELL, D. J., GINGERICH, R. L. and GREIDER, M. H. Regional distribution and concentration of pancreatic polypeptide in the human and canine pancreas. *Diabetes*, **28**, 11–15 (1979)

74 GINGERICH, R. L., GERSELL, D. J., GREIDER, M. H., FINKS, E. H. and LACY, P. E. Elevated levels of pancreatic polypeptide in obese hyperglycaemic mice. *Metabolism*, **27**, 1526–1532 (1978)

75 GLASSER, B., VINIK, A. I., SIVE, A. A. and FLOYD, J. C. Plasma human pancreatic polypeptide responses to administered secretin: effects of surgical vagotomy, cholinergic blockage and chronic pancreatitis. *Journal of Clinical Endocrinology*, **50**, 1094–1099 (1980)

76 GREENBERG, G. R., MCCLOY, R. F., ADRIAN, T. E., BARON, J. H. and BLOOM, S. R. Effect of bovine pancreatic polypeptide on gastric acid and pepsin output in man. *Acta Hepato-Gastroenterologica*, **25**, 384–387 (1978)

77 GREENBERG, G. R., MCCLOY, R. F., ADRIAN, T. E., CHADWICK, V. S., BARON, J. H. and BLOOM, S. R. Inhibition of pancreas and gallbladder by pancreatic polypeptide. *Lancet*, **2**, 1280–1282 (1978)

78 GREGORY, R. A. Gastrin – the natural history of a peptide hormone. *Harvey Lecture*, **64**, 121–155 (1968)

79 GREGORY, H., HARDY, P. M., JONES, D. S. KENNER, G. W. and SHEPPHARD, R. C. Structure of gastrin. *Nature*, **204**, 931–933 (1964)

80 GREGORY, R. A. and TRACY, H. J. The constitution and properties of two gastrins extracted from hog antral mucosa. *Gut*, **5**, 103–117 (1964)

81 GREGORY, R. A. and TRACY, H. J. The chemistry of the gastrins: some recent advances. In *Gastrointestinal Hormones*, edited by J. C. Thompson, 13–24. Austin, University of Texas Press (1975)

82 GROSSMAN, M. I. Gastrointestinal hormones. In *Peptide Hormones*, edited by J. A. Parsons, 105–106. London, MacMillan Press (1976)

83 GROSSMAN, M. I. Abnormalities of acid secretion in patients with duodenal ulcer. *Gastroenterology*, **75**, 524–526 (1978)

84 GROSSMAN, M. I. Vagal stimulation and inhibition of acid secretion and gastrin release: which aspects are cholinergic? In *Gastrins and the Vagus*, edited by J. F. Rehfeld and E. Amdrup, 105–114. New York, Academic Press (1979)

85 GROSSMAN, M. I. and KONTRUEK, S. J. Inhibition of acid secretion by metiamide, a histamine antagonist acting on H_2-receptors. *Gastroenterology*, **66**, 517–521

86 HÄCKI, W. H., GREENBERG, G. R. and BLOOM, S. R. Role of secretin in man I. In *Gut Hormones*, edited by S. R. Bloom, 182–192. Edinburgh, Churchill Livingstone (1978)

87 HAKANSON, R., HEDENBRO, J. and LIEDBERG, G. Activation of histidine decarboxylase by H_2-receptor blockade, mechanism of action. *British Journal of Pharmacology*, **53**, 127–130 (1975)

88 HALLGREN, R., KARLSSON, F. A. and LUNDQVIST, G. Serum level of immunoreactive gastrin: influence of kidney function. *Gut*, **19**, 207–213 (1978)

89 HANSSEN, L. E., HANSSEN, K. F. and MYREN, J. Inhibition of secretin release and pancreatic bicarbonate secretion by somatostatin infusion in man. *Scandinavian Journal of Gastroenterology*, **12**, 381–394 (1977)

90 HARPER, A. A. and RAPER, H. S. Pancreozymin, a stimulant of the secretion of pancreatic enzymes in extracts of the small intestine. *Journal of Physiology*, (*London*), **102**, 115–125 (1943)

91 HARVEY, R. G., DOWSETT, L., HARTOG, M. and READ, A. E. A radioimmunoassay for cholecystokinin pancreozymin. *Lancet*, **2**, 826–828 (1973)

92 HELLEMANS, J., VANTRAPPEN, G. and BLOOM, S. R. Endogenous motilin and the LES pressure. *Scandinavian Journal of Gastroenterology* **11**, (Supplement 39), 67–73 (1973)

93 HOLM, I., THULIN, L. and HELLGREN, M. Anticholinergic effect of substance P on anaesthetised dogs. *Acta Physiologica Scandinavica*, **102**, 274–280 (1978)

94 HOLM, I., THULIN, L., SAMNEGARD, H., EFENDIC, S. and TYDEN, G., Anticholinergic effect of somatostatin in anaesthetised dogs. *Acta Physiologica Scandinavica*, **104**, 241–243 (1979)

95 HUGHES, J., SMITH, T. W., KOSTERLITZ, H. W., FOTHERGILL, L. A., MORGAN, B. A. and MORRIS, H. R. Identification of the two related peptides from the brain with potent opiate agonist activity. *Nature*, **258**, 577–579 (1975)

96 ISENBERG, J. I., CANO, R. and BLOOM, S. R. Effect of graded amounts of acid instilled into the duodenum on pancreatic bicarbonate secretion and plasma secretin in duodenal ulcer patients and normal subjects. *Gastroenterology*, **72**, 6–8 (1977)

97 ISENBERG, J. I., WALSH, J. H. and GROSSMAN, M. I. Zollinger-Ellison syndrome. *Gastroenterology*, **65**, 140–165 (1973)

98 IVY, A. C. and OLDBERG, E. A hormone mechanism for gallbladder contraction and evacuation. *American Journal of Physiology*, **86**, 599–613 (1928)

99 JAFFE, B. M., CLENDINNEN, B. G., CLARKE, R. J. and WILLIAMS, J. A. Effect of selective and proximal gastric vagotomy on serum gastrin. *Gastroenterology*, **66**, 944–953 (1974)

100 JOHNSON, L. R. Gut hormones on growth of gastrointestinal mucosa. In *Endocrinology of the Gut*, edited by W. Y. Chey and E. P. Brooks, 163–177. Thorofare, New Jersey, Charles B. Slack Inc. (1974)

101 JOHNSON, L. R., CASTRO, G. A., LICHTENBERGER, L. M. COPELAND, E.N. and DUDRICK, S. J. The significance of the trophic action of gastrin. *Gastroenterology*, **66**, 718 (1974)

102 JOHNSON, L. R. and GROSSMAN, M. I. Intestinal hormones as inhibitors of gastric secretion. *Gastroenterology*, **60**, 120–144 (1971)

103 JOHNSON, L. R. and GROSSMAN, M. L. Intestinal hormones as inhibitors of gastric secretion. *Gastroenterology*, **60**, 120–144 (1972)

104 JONES, R. S., GEIST, R. E. and HALL, A. D. The choleretic effects of glucagon and secretin in the dog. *Gastroenterology*, **60**, 64–68 (1971)

105 JONES, R. S. and GROSSMAN, M. I. Choleretic effects of cholecystokinin, gastrin II and caerulein in the dog. *American Journal of Physiology*, **219**, 1014–1018 (1970)

106 JORPES, E. and MUTT, V. On the biological activity and amino acid composition of secretin. *Acta Chemica Scandinavica*, **15**, 1790–1791 (1961)

107 JORPES, J. E. and MUTT, V. On the biological assay of secretin. The reference standard. *Acta Physiologica Scandinavica*, **66**, 316–325 (1966)

108 JORPES, J. E. and MUTT, V. Secretin, cholecystokinin (CCK). In *Secretin, Cholecystokinin, Pancreozymin and Gastrin*, edited by J. E. Jorpes and J. Mutt, 1–144. Berlin, Springer Verlag (1973)

109 JORPES, J. E., MUTT, V. and TOCZKO, K. Further purification of cholecystokinin and pancreozymin. *Acta Chemica Scandinavica*, **18**, 2408–2410 (1964)

110 KAYASSEH, L., GYR, K., GIRARD, J., MEYER, F., RITTMAN, W. W. and STALDER, G. A. Immunological blocking of endogenous secretin and exocrine pancreatic secretion in dog. *European Journal of Clinical Investigation*, **8**, 326–329 (1978)

111 KNUTSON, U., OLBE, L. and GANGULI, P. C. Gastric acid and plasma gastrin responses to sham feeding in duodenal ulcer patients before and after resection of antrum and duodenal bulb. *Scandinavian Journal of Gastroenterology*, **95**, 351–356 (1974)

112 KOMAROV, S. A. Gastrin. *Proceedings of the Society for Experimental Biology and Medicine*, **38**, 514–516 (1938)

113 KONTUREK, S. J., PAWLIK, W., TASLER, J., THOR, P., WALUS, K., KROL, R., JAWOREK, J. and SCHALLY, A. V. The effects of enkephalin on the gastrointestinal tract. In *Gut Hormones*, edited by S. R. Bloom, 507–512. Edinburgh, Churchill Livingstone (1978)

114 KONTUREK, S. J., WYSOCKI, A. and OLEKSY, J. Effect of medical and surgical vagotomy on gastric response to graded doses of pentagastrin and histamine. *Gastroenterology*, **54**, 392–400 (1968)

115 LAMERS, C. B., VALENZUELA, J. E. and WALSH, J. H. Demonstration of cholecystokinin (CCK) 8-like immunoreactivity in the circulation of man after intraduodenal fat. *Gut*, **20**, A925 (1979)

116 LARSSON, L.-I., SUNDLER, F. and HAKANSON, R. Pancreatic polypeptide. A postulated new hormone: identification of its cellular storage site by light and electron microscopic immunocyto-chemistry. *Diabetologia*, **12**, 211–226 (1976)

117 LASSMAN, V., VAGUE, P., VIALETTES, B. and SIMON, M.-C. Low plasma levels of pancreatic polypeptide in obesity. *Diabetes*, **29**, 428–430 (1980)

118 LIN, T.-M. and CHANCE, R. E. Gastrointestinal actions of a new bovine pancreatic polypeptide (BPP). In *Endocrinology of the Gut*, edited by W. Y. Chey and F. P. Brooks, 143–145. Thorofare, New Jersey; Charles B. Slack Inc. (1974)

119 LIN, T.-M. and CHANCE, R. E. Spectrum of gastrointestinal actions of bovine PP. In *Gut Hormones*, edited by S.R. Bloom, 242–246. Edinburgh, Churchill Livingstone (1978)

120 LIN, T.-M., EVANS, D. C., CHANCE, R. E. and SPRAY, G. F. Bovine pancreatic peptide action on gastric and pancreatic secretion in dogs. *American Journal of Physiology*, **1**, E311–E315 (1977)

121 LIN, T.-M., EVANS, D. C., SHAAR, C. J. and CHANCE, R. E. Physiological versus pharmacological actions of bovine pancreatic polypeptide (BPP) on the pancreas, stomach, gallbladder choledochal sphincter and intestine of dogs. In *Gut Peptides*, edited by A. Miyoshi and M. I. Grossman, 175–181. Amsterdam, Elsevier (1980)

122 LONG, R. G., BARNES, A. J., ADRIAN, T. E., MALLINSON, C. N., BROWN, M. R. VALE, W., RIVIER, J. E., CHRISTOFIDES, N. D. and BLOOM, S. R. Suppression of pancreatic endocrine tumour secretion by long-acting somatostatin. *Lancet*, **2**, 764–767 (1979)

123 LONG, R. G., CHRISTOFIDES, N. D., FITZPATRICK, M. L., MCGREGOR, G. P. and BLOOM, S. R. Effects of motilin and somatostatin on gastric emptying and glucose tolerance. *Gastroenterology*, **78**, 1210 (1980)

124 LOW-BEER, T. S., HARVEY, R. F., DAVIES, E. R. and READ, A. E. Abnormalities of serum cholecystokinin and gallbladder emptying in coeliac disease. *New England Journal of Medicine*, **292**, 961–963 (1975)

125 MCDONALD, T. J., JORNVALL, H., NILSSON, C., VAGNE, M., GHATEI, M. A., BLOOM, S. R. and MUTT, V. Characterisation of a gastrin-releasing peptide from porcine non-antral gastric tissue. *Biochemical and Biophysical Research Communications*, **90**, 227–233 (1979)

126 MCGUIGAN, J. E. and TRUDEAU, W. L. Serum gastrin in concentrations in pernicious anaemia. *New England Journal of Medicine*, **282**, 358–361 (1970)

127 MCGUIGAN, J. E. and TRUDEAU, W. L. Serum gastrin levels before and after vagatomy and pyloroplasty or vagotomy and antrectomy. *New England Journal of Medicine*, **286**, 184–188 (1972)

128 MAKHLOUF, G. M., SAID, S. I. and YAU, W. M. Interplay of vasoactive intestinal peptide (VIP) and synthetic VIP fragments with secretin, octapeptide of cholecystokinin (Octa CCK) on pancreatic and biliary secretion. *Gastroenterology*, **66**, 737 (1971)

129 MALAISSE-LAGAE, F., CARPENTIER, J.-L., PATEL, Y. C., MALAISSE, W. J. and ORCI, L. Pancreatic polypeptide: a possible role in the regulation of food intake in the mouse. *Experientia*, **33**, 915–917 (1977)

130 MELCHIORRI, P. Bombesin and bombesin-like peptides of amphibian skin. In *Gut Hormones* edited by S. R. Bloom, 534–540. Edinburgh, Churchill Livingstone (1978)

131 MELLANBY, J. M. The mechanism of pancreatic digestion – the function of secretion. *Journal of Physiology (London)*, **60**, 85–91

132 MORLEY, J. E., GARVIN, T. J., PEKARY, A. E. and HERSHMANN, J. M. Thyrotropin-releasing hormone in the gastrointestinal tract *Biochemical and Biophysical Research Communications*, **79**, 314–318 (1977)

133 MORLEY, J. E., STEINBACH, J. H., FELDMAN, E. J. and SOLOMON, T. E. The effects of thyrotropin-releasing hormone (TRH) on the gastrointestinal tract. *Life Sciences*, **24**, 1059–1065 (1979)

134 MUTT, V. Further investigation on intestinal hormonal polypeptides. *Clinical Endocrinology*, **5**, Supplement, 183–197 (1976)

135 MUTT, V. Cholecystokinin: isolation, structure and functions. In *Gastrointestinal Hormones*, edited by G. B. Jerzy Glass, 169–221. New York, Raven Press (1980)

136 NEUBERGER, P. H., LEWIN, M. and BONFILS, S. Parietal and chief cell populations in four cases of Zollinger-Ellison syndrome. *Gastroenterology*, **63**, 937–942 (1972)

137 NILSSON, G., YALOW, R. S. and BERSON, S. A. Distribution of gastrin in the gastrointestinal tract of human, dog, cat and hog. In *Frontiers of Gastrointestinal Hormone Research*, 95–101. Stockholm, Almquist & Wiksell (1973)

138 OKADA, S. On the secretion of bile. *Journal of Physiology (London)*, **49**, 457–482 (1914)

139 PIPER, P. J., SAID, S. I. and VANE, J. R. Effects on smooth muscle preparation of vasoactive peptides from intestine and lung. *Nature*, **225**, 1144–1146 (1970)

140 POLAK, J. M., AYNSLEY-GREEN, A., BLOOM, S. R. and WIGGLESWORTH, J. S. Nesidioblastosis is a cause of sudden neonatal death. *Scandinavian Journal of Gastroenterology*, **13**, Supplement 49, 143 (1978)

141 POLAK, J. M., BLOOM, S. R., ADRIAN, T. E., HEITZ, P. H., BRYANT, M. G. and PEARSE, A. G. E. Pancreatic polypeptide in insulinomas, gastrinomas, VIPomas and glucagonomas. *Lancet*, **1**, 328–330 (1976)

142 POLAK, J. M., BLOOM, S. R., BISHOP, A. E. and MCCROSSAN, M. V. D cell pathology in duodenal ulcers and achlorhydria. *Metabolism*, **27**, Supplement, 1239–1242 (1978)

143 POLAK, J. M., BLOOM, S. R., HOBBS, S. and SOLCIA, E. Distribution of a bombesin-like peptide in human gastrointestinal tract. *Lancet*, **1**, 1109–1110 (1976)

144 POLAK, J. M., COULLING, I., BLOOM, S. R. and PEARSE, A. G. E. Immunofluorescent localisation of secretin in human intestinal mucosa. *Scandinavian Journal of Gastroenterology*, **6**, 739–744 (1971)

145 POLAK, J. M., GHATEI, M. A., WHARTON, J., BISHOP, A. E., BLOOM, S. R. SOLICIA, E., BROWN, M. R. and PEARSE, A. G. E. Bombesin-like immunoreactivity in the gastrointestinal tract, lung and central nervous system. *Scandinavian Journal of Gastroenterology*, **13**, Supplement 49, 148 (1978)

146 POLAK, J. M., PEARSE, A. G. E., BLOOM, S. R., BUCHAN, A. M., RAYFORD, P. L. and THOMPSON, J. C. Identification of cholecystokinin-secreting cells. *Lancet*, **2**, 1016–1018 (1975)

147 POLAK, J. M., PEARSE, A. G. E., GRIMELIUS, L., BLOOM, S. R. and ARIMURA, A. Growth hormone-releasing-inhibiting hormone in gastrointestinal and pancreatic D cells. *Lancet*, **1**, 1220–1222 (1975)

148 POLAK, J. M., SULLIVAN, S. N., BLOOM, S. R., FACER, P. and PEARSE, A. G. E. Enkephalin-like immunoreactivity in the human gastrointestinal tract. *Lancet*, **I**, 972–974 (1977)

149 PRADAYROL, L., JORNVALL, H., MUTT, V. and RIBET, A. N-terminally extended somatostatin: the primary structure of somatostatin-28. *FEBs Letters*, **109**, 55–58 (1980)

150 REEDER, D. D., BECKER, H. D. and THOMPSON, J. C. Effect of intravenously administered calcium on serum gastrin and gastric secretion in man. *Surgery, Gynecology and Obstetrics*, **138**, 847–851 (1974)

151 REHFELD, J. F. Localisation of gastrin to neuro- and adenohypophysis. *Nature*, **271**, 771–772 (1978)

152 REHFELD, J. F. Immunochemical studies on cholecystokinin: II Distribution and molecular heterogeneity in the central nervous system and small intestine of man and hog. *Journal of Biological Chemistry*, **253**, 4022–4030 (1978)

153 REHFELD, J. F., GOLTERMANN, N., LARSSON, L.-I., EMSON, P. M. and LEE, C. M. Gastrin and cholecystokinin in central and peripheral neurons. *Federation Proceedings*, **38**, 2325–2329 (1979)

154 REHFELD, J. F., STADIL, F. and VIKELSOE, J. Immunoreactive gastrin components in human serum. *Gut*, **15**, 102–111 (1974)

155 RICHARDSON, C. T., WALSH, J. H., HICKS, M. I. and FORDTRAN, J. S. Studies on the mechanism of food-stimulated gastric acid secretin in normal human subjects. *Journal of Clinical Investigation*, **58**, 623–631 (1976)

156 ROLAND, M., BERSTAD, A. and LIAVAG, I. Effect of carbocholine and urecholine on pentagastrin-stimulated gastric secretion in healthy subjects. *Scandinavian Journal of Gastroenterology*, **10**, 357–362

157 RUSSELL, R. C. G., BLOOM, S. R., DAVIES, W. A., POLAK, J. M. and REED, P. I. Hypergastrinaemia in a peptic ulcer patient with antral gastrin cell hyperplasia. *British Medical Journal*, **4**, 441 (1975)

158 SCHAFFALITZKY DE MUCKADELL, O. B. and FAHRENKRUG, J. Role of secretin in Man III. In *Gut Hormones*, edited by S. R. Bloom, 197–200. Edinburgh, Churchill Livingstone (1978)

159 SCHAFFALITZKY DE MUCKADELL, O. B., FAHRENKRUG, J. and RUNE, S. J. Physiological significance of secretin in the pancreatic bicarbonate secretion: I. Responsiveness of the secretin-releasing system in the upper duodenum. *Scandinavian Journal of Gastroenterology*, **14**, 79–83 (1979)

160 SCHULTZBERG, M., DREYFUS, C. F., GERSHON., M. D., HOKFELT, T., ELDE, R. P., NILSSON, G., SAID, S. and GOLDSTEIN, M. VIP-, enkephalin-, substance P-, and somatostatin-like immunoreactivity in neuron intrinsic to the intestine: immunohistochemical evidence from organotypic tissue. *Brain Research*, **155**, 239–248 (1978)

161 SCHWARTZ, T. W., GROTZINGER, U., SCHOON, I.-M. and OLBE, L. Vagovagal stimulation of pancreatic polypeptide secretion by graded distension of the gastric antrum in man. *Digestion*, **19**, 307–314 (1979)

162 SCHWARTZ, T. W., STADIL, F., CHANCE, R. E., REHFELD, J. F., LARSSON, L.-T. and MOON, N. Pancreatic polypeptide response to food in duodenal ulcer patients before and after vagotomy. *Lancet*, **1**, 1102–1105 (1976)

163 SCHWARTZ, T. W., STENQUIST, B. and OLBE, L. Cephalic phase of pancreatic polypeptide secretion studied by sham feeding in man. *Scandinavian Journal of Gastroenterology*, **14**, 313–320 (1979)

164 SOLL., A. H. and GROSSMAN, M. I. Cellular mechanisms in acid secretion, *Annual Review of Medicine*, **28**, 495–507 (1978)

165 SOLOMON, T. E. and GROSSMAN, M. I. Response of transplanted pancreas to intestinal stimulants in dogs. Effect of atropine and vagotomy and comparison to intact pancreas. *American Journal of Physiology*, **236**, E186–E190 (1979)

166 STADIL, F. and REHFELD, J. F. Release of gastrin by epinephrine in man. *Gastroenterology*, **65**, 210–215 (1973)

167 STAGE, J. G., STADIL, F., REHFELD, J. F., FAHRENKRUG, J., SCHAFFALITZKY DE MUCKADELL, O. B. Secretin and the Zollinger–Ellison syndrome: reliability of secretin tests and the pathogenetic role of secretin. *Scandinavian Journal of Gastroenterology*, **13**, 501–511 (1978)

168 STENING, G. F. and GROSSMAN, M. I. Potentiation of cholecystokinetic action of cholecystokinin (CCK) by secretin. *Clinical Research*, **17**, 528 (1969)

169 STRUNZ, U., DOMSCHKE, W. and DOMSCHKE, S., MITZNELG, P., WÜNSCH, E., JAEGER, E. and DEMLING, L. Potentiation between 13-Nle-Motilin and acetycholine on rabbit pyloric muscle in vitro. *Scandinavian Journal of Gastroenterology*, **12**, (Supplement 39), 29–35 (1976)

170 TAYLOR, I. L., SOLOMON, T. E., WALSH, J. H. and GROSSMAN, M. I. Pancreatic polypeptide Metabolism and effect on pancreatic secretion in dogs. *Gastroenterology*, **76**, 524–528 (1979)

171 THOMPSON, M. R., DEBAS, H. T., WALSH, J. H. and GROSSMAN, M. I. Release of antral gastrin by infusion of liver extract into the small intestine of dogs. *Gut*, **17**, 393 (1976)

172 THOR, P., KROL, R., KONTUREK, S. J., COY, D. H. and SCHALLY, A. V. Effect of somatostatin on myoelectrical activity of small bowel. *American Journal of Physiology*, **235**, E249–E254 (1978)

173 TRACY, H. J. and GREGORY, R. A. Physiological properties of a series of synthetic peptides structurally related to gastrin I. *Nature*, **204**, 935–938 (1964)

174 UVNAS-WALLENSTEN, K., REHFELD, J. F., LARSSON, L.-I. and UVNAS, A. S. Heptadecapeptide gastrin in the vagal nerve. *Proceedings of the National Academy of Sciences of the USA*, **74**, 5705–5711 (1977)

175 VANDERHAEGEN, J. J., SIGNEAU, J. C. and GEPTS, W. New peptide in the vertebrate CNS reacting with antigastrin antibodies. *Nature*, **257**, 604–605 (1975)

176 WALSH, J. H. A new look at peptic ulcer. Pathogenesis of duodenal ulcer. *Annals of Internal Medicine*, **84**, 59–61 (1976)

177 WALSH, J. H. and GROSSMAN, M. I. Gastrin. *New England Journal of Medicine*, **292**, 1324–1332 (1975)

178 WALSH, J. H. and HOLMQUIST, A. I. Radioimmunoassay of bombesin peptides: identification of bombesin-like immunoreactivity in vertebrate gut extracts. *Gastroenterology*, **70**, 948 (1976)

179 WARD, A. S. and BLOOM, S. R. The role of secretin in the inhibition of gastric secretion by intraduodenal acid. *Gut*, **15**, 889–897 (1974)

180 WORMSLEY, K. G. A comparison of the response to secretin, pancreozymin and a combination of these hormones in man. *Scandinavian Journal of Gastroenterology*, **4**, 413–417 (1969)

181 WORMSLEY, K. G. Response to duodenal acidication in man II. Effects on the gastric response to pentagastrin. *Scandinavian Journal of Gastroenterology*, **5**, 207–215 (1970)

182 YALOW, R. S. and BENSON, S. A. Size and charge distinctions between endogenous human plasma gastrin in peripheral blood and heptadecapeptide gastrins. *Gastroenterology*, **58**, 609–615 (1970)

5

Management of upper gastrointestinal haemorrhage

M. Classen, J. Phillip and G. Smith-Laing

Bleeding in the upper gastrointestinal tract is a serious challenge to the physician. The problem is so common as to be a daily occurrence – municipal hospitals admit just as many patients with bleeding in the upper alimentary system as patients with pneumonia or congestive cardiac failure. Prognosis depends on accurate and rapid identification of the source of the haemorrhage, and at the present time, endoscopy represents the optimal diagnostic and, in some cases, the decisive therapeutic procedure. An energetic diagnostic approach[71] in these cases not only helps the physician to make rational decisions about treatment, but at the same time can also be therapeutically effective. Despite apparent advances in the recognition and management of upper gastrointestinal haemorrhage, a number of problems still remain, such as defining the degree of severity of bleeding, the optimal time for endoscopy and the choice of suitable treatment.

Diagnostic methods

Endoscopy

Almost 30 years ago, Palmer[69] advocated an aggressive diagnostic work-up at the earliest possible moment in patients with acute upper gastrointestinal bleeding, since he was of the opinion that effective therapy was possible only when the exact location of the bleeding point was known. Owing to the rapid acceptance of fibre-optic endoscopy, emergency endoscopy is now the 'standard diagnostic approach' in case of acute bleeding, and some authors[66, 89] even claim that failure to perform endoscopy in patients with massive gastrointestinal haemorrhage must be considered unethical.

On the basis of individual observations, impressions, opinions and professions of faith, the usefulness of emergency endoscopy would appear to be without question; prospective controlled studies, however, in contrast to the numerous retrospective studies already carried out, make a favourable influence on the mortality rate of acute bleeding appear doubtful[2, 46, 65, 92]. However, now that to an ever-increasing extent attempts are being made to treat an endoscopically verified bleeding at the same time as the diagnostic examination, many critical objections to emergency diagnostic endoscopy are no longer applicable.

Emergency endoscopy is carried out as soon as the patient's vital signs have been stabilized. If resuscitation is unsuccessful, endoscopy should be performed in the operating theatre or an intensive care unit. To verify that haemorrhage is upper gastrointestinal in origin, a thin nasogastric tube may be passed prior to endoscopy. Studies by Luk, Bynum and Hendrix[52] suggest that if blood is found in the gastric aspirate, the source of bleeding will be found in the upper gastrointestinal tract in 93 per cent of the cases, while in patients with no blood in the aspirate, the bleeding point will be found in the large bowel in 60 per cent of the cases. The diagnostic and therapeutic value of ice-water lavage is controversial[35]. Most sources of bleeding in the duodenum, antrum, on the lesser curvature of the stomach and in the oesophagus, can usually be identified without previous irrigation. In addition, there is a danger of causing additional bleeding with the large-bore gastric tube, so that the actual bleeding source may not be identified accurately. Despite all the advantages offered by emergency endoscopy, the increased risk of complications accompanying endoscopy under emergency conditions, must not be forgotten[76, 103]. The authors have observed renewed bleeding from oesophageal varices during endoscopy which in several cases, appeared to be caused by retroversion of the endoscope or 'J manoeuvre'[86].

Radiology

Barium studies

The single contrast barium meal demonstrates the source of haemorrhage in about 50 per cent of patients compared with 86 per cent using endoscopy[61]. In a minority of cases the same authors found that a barium meal provided information not obtained by endoscopy so that an accurate diagnosis was made in 91 per cent of patients by combining emergency endoscopy with a barium meal. The superiority of endoscopy over the barium meal has been confirmed in other prospective studies[28].

The double contrast barium meal is a more time-consuming technique than the single contrast meal. Greater radiological detail is obtained but not always an increased diagnostic yield. A diagnosis is made in 70 per cent of patients rising to almost 80 per cent if the investigation is carried out within 24 hours of haemorrhage. Stigmata of recent bleeding such as clot or a protruding artery in the base of an ulcer are seen in about half the patients[31].

The urgency with which radiology is performed after a bleed influences the diagnostic yield. Ideally, studies should be performed within 24 hours of the haemorrhage, although if performed very early blood clot or continuing bleeding may obscure detail. After 48 hours the diagnostic yield of barium studies declines rapidly and will not affect the emergency management of the patient.

The nature of the bleeding lesion also influences the diagnostic accuracy of barium studies. Mass lesions such as carcinoma of the stomach, chronic peptic ulceration and large varices, are usually seen on a barium meal. Acute gastric and duodenal ulcers which are shallow and not accompanied by scarring are more difficult to visualize and diagnostic accuracy depends more on the skill of the radiologist. Mucosal lesions such as gastritis or Mallory-Weiss tears and small varices (usually confused with normal oesophageal mucosal folds) are frequently not demonstrated at all by barium radiology. In addition the demonstration of a *potential* source of haemorrhage on the barium meal does not necessarily mean that this *is* the source of bleeding and in this particular endoscopy is far superior to barium radiology.

Diagnostic angiography

Angiography is an invasive procedure and should not be undertaken lightly. When bleeding has stopped endoscopy and barium studies are indicated rather than angiography. If haemorrhage is massive and the patient unresponsive to resuscitation, emergency operation is usually indicated unless varices are the source of bleeding or the patient is considered too ill for surgery (cf. therapeutic angiography, p. 125).

Diagnostic angiography is indicated in the following circumstances: (1) bleeding is severe and diagnostic angiography is to be performed prior to the embolization or selective infusion of vasopressin; (2) upper gastrointestinal endoscopy has failed to reveal the source of haemorrhage and there is persistent bleeding; (3) there is chronic gastrointestinal blood loss and endoscopy and barium studies have failed to reveal its source[41]; (4) the source of bleeding is likely to be an arteriovenous malformation as in patients with Osler-Weber-Rendu syndrome[64].

Sources of haemorrhage Active arterial bleeding at the rate of 0.5 ml/ min or more is usually detected by extravasation of contrast material during angiography. All arteries that might be the source of bleeding should be selectively catheterized and adequately opacified (*Figure 5.1*). The stomach is filled with air prior to injection of contrast to extenuate the vascular pattern and care taken to include all areas of interest, including the lower oesophagus, on the films. If a bleeding

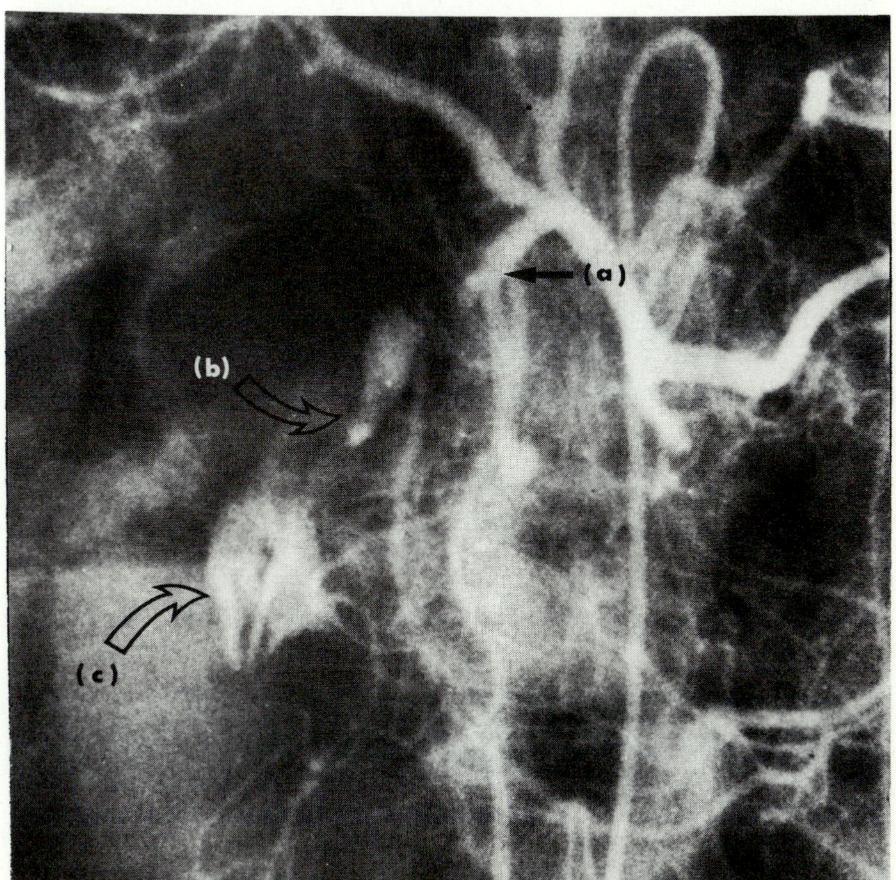

Figure 5.1 Coeliac axis injection demonstrates gastroduodenal artery (*a*) with extravasation of contrast into the duodenal bulb (*b*) and the first portion of the duodenum (*c*) (courtesy of Dr R. Dick, Royal Free Hospital)

site is not demonstrated by selective injections an aortogram should be performed in case bleeding is from an anomalous artery, or very rarely an aortoenteric fistula. Occasionally bleeding is intermittent and several injections may have to be made into the same artery before extravasation of contrast is seen[102].

Gastro-oesophageal varices are opacified during the venous phase of superior mesenteric and splenic artery injections. Opacification of the splenic and portal veins is often poor due to dilution of contrast within the venous system, particularly if there is massive splenomegaly and varices may not be visualized at all. Compared with percutaneous transhepatic portography, coeliac axis angiography is extremely poor at delineating the portal venous anatomy and the former allows measurement of portal pressure and therapeutic embolization of varices[99, 100].

Causes of failure to detect bleedings The most common cause of failure to detect arterial bleeding is that haemorrhage has ceased. In such cases the catheter may be left *in situ* for 24 hours as bleeding frequently recurs. Catheter patency is maintained by constant infusion of dextrose using a syringe pump.

Other common causes of failure to detect the site of haemorrhage are: (1) the rate of bleeding is less than 0.5 ml/min; (2) bleeding is venous in origin or occurs from small surface vessels. Extravasation of contrast medium in such circumstances may be indistinguishable from a normal mucosal blush; (3) bleeding has stopped temporarily due to low blood pressure and may recur after resuscitation measures; (4) there are technical problems with angiography. The appropriate artery may not be catheterized due to an anomalous origin or unfavourable anatomy; the area of haemorrhage may not be included on the films; insufficient contrast medium may have been injected or insufficient delayed films taken (particularly when varices are the source of haemorrhage).

Complications of angiography Arterial catheterization may lead to complications at the site of puncture including haemorrhage and haematoma formation, sepsis, arterial thrombosis, lower limb embolization, false aneurysm formation and arterial laceration. There may also be adverse reactions to contrast medium such an acute anaphylaxis or renal failure[3, 106] which may prove fatal. The chances of renal failure are increased by the presence of pre-existing hepatic or renal disease.

Bleeding sources in the upper gastrointestinal tract

The incidence of bleeding sources varies considerably. The causes for this are only partially known. Geographical reasons such as, for example, infectious diseases, schistosomiasis, religious bans on drink, or widespread alcoholism in the case material of certain hospitals, the public advertising of analgesics, etc., may be partially responsible for these differences[47].

Table 5.1 Major diagnoses in patients with upper gastrointestinal bleeding (per cent)

Hospital and reference (year)	Number of patients	Varices	Ulcer	Cancer	Mucosal lesions*	Miscellaneous	Unknown
Radcliffe, Oxford[94] (1953–67)	2149	2	45	2	0	25	26
St Thomas, London[18] (1973)	208	3	58	2	18	4	15
East Orange, NJ, Veterans Adm.[70] (1969)	1400	19	43	0	34	6	7
Portland, OR, Veterans Adm.[44] (1973)	100	16	47	2	30	4	1
Erlangen, GFR Dep. Med.[87] (1980)	1319	14	47	4	30	1	4
Europ. Emerg. Endosc. Study[77]† (1980)	638	12	52	4	26	6	15

*Esophagitis, gastritis, erosions, Mallory-Weiss tear.
†Multiple findings in 15 per cent.

The significance of ethyl alcohol in the development of bleeding in the upper gastrointestinal tract is largely underestimated. In the two American series (*Table 5.1*) alcohol abuse was probably responsible for bleedings in 50 per cent of those subjected to endoscopy.

The sources of severe bleeding in the upper gastrointestinal tract are well known. Since the introduction of endoscopy as the primary diagnostic method, not only more, but also 'new' lesions have been discovered as the source of bleeding. Thus, for example, today the superficial mucosal lesions of the stomach (erosions, Mallory-Weiss tears), formerly seen only by the pathologist[29], are frequently recognized as a source of bleeding. This also applies to oesophagitis, in particular to monilial oesophagitis in the elderly.

Emergency situations are, in the first instance, triggered by oesophageal varices and stress-induced lesions. About one-half of the patients presenting with oesophageal varices die from the first bleeding episode[105].

Acute gastric mucosal lesions are frequently described in the literature as haemorrhagic gastritis, erosive gastritis, stress lesions or stress ulcers. It would seem preferable, irrespective of aetiology and pathogenesis, to apply to them the descriptive term 'erosion' or, in the case of Mallory-Weiss tears, 'linear erosion'. Nor does the use of personal names (Curling, Cushing) in the case of ulcers following head injuries or burns, do anything to improve intercommunication. It is sufficient to say that there is an ulcer in a certain region and that it is the definitive or presumptive source of the bleeding. An estimate or accurate measurement of the size of the ulcer can be of importance for the observation of the course of healing[16].

The source of bleeding is considered to have been identified when signs of a recent or a previous haemorrhage are found in a lesion. These include a vascular stump in the floor of an ulcer, a coating of fibrin discoloured by haematin in the ulcer crater and, of course, active bleeding. If, following haematemesis, a lesion is found in the upper gastrointestinal tract, but without any unequivocal signs of haemorrhage, it is the probable source of the bleeding. In the case of melaena, however, this assumption is not necessarily valid, since melaena may also be caused by an additional lesion in the small bowel or proximal colon. Unequivocal signs of bleeding are less frequently observed the greater the interval between the start of the bleeding episode and endoscopy – probably because acute lesions heal rapidly[1]. The discovery of one lesion must not cause the endoscopist to forego a full careful inspection of the oesophagus, stomach and duodenum. Multiple lesions, such as duodenal ulcer and gastric erosions, are found simultaneously in 28 per cent to 46 per cent of the cases presenting with gastrointestinal haemorrhage.

Bleeding due to rare sources of upper gastrointestinal haemorrhage are found predominantly at gastroenterological centres. Tumours, in particular early carcinoma of the stomach, coagulopathies ruptured aneurysms, vascular anomalies, pancreatic pseudocysts, haemobilia after trauma and hepatic cysts may all be diagnosed.

Management of upper gastrointestinal haemorrhage

General measures

Slight bleeding does not require either intensive care or treatment. The nature of the lesion involved appears to be important. Bleeding from ulcers tends to recur, while bleeding erosions as a rule heal rapidly and completely. Blood transfusion becomes necessary only when the haemoglobin drops below 8 g/dl.

Massive bleeding causes shock, exsanguination and, in the case of oesophageal varices may lead to hepatic coma. The definition of what constitutes severe bleeding presents problems, since blood loss cannot be measured with great accuracy. Severe haemorrhage may be assumed when an estimated 1500 ml of blood, or 25 per cent of the total blood volume is lost in a matter of hours; when systolic and diastolic blood pressures drop or there is postural hypotension, the pulse rate rises to above 100/min; pallor and sweating occur, the haematocrit rises and oliguria develops. Ideally, the appropriate measures taken to prevent or eliminate the complications of a massive haemorrhage should be carried out by gastroenterologists with intensive care experience. The diagnosis and treatment follow a standard routine. Oesophagogastroduodenoscopy can be carried out in the intensive care unit. Initially haemorrhagic shock is corrected by the infusion of plasma substitutes and, if possible, fresh blood. The infusion of coagulation factors for the treatment of coagulopathies is effective, but expensive. Parameters such as erythrocyte count, haemoglobin, haematocrit, clotting parameters, electrolytes, blood gases, urea and urine output, and also central venous pressure, are constantly monitored and, where necessary, corrected.

A nasogastric tube is passed to remove blood and gastric contents, and to permit irrigation of the stomach with ice-water and antacids. Cooling of the gastric mucosa appears to have no haemostatic effect. The nasogastric tube can give rise to pressure ulcers and oesophagitis if left in position too long.

One of the most important of the physician's tasks is to look after the mental well-being of the patient who, after a massive bleeding episode, is in a state of high anxiety. Decisions on surgical treatment, depend upon the age, condition and associated pathology of the patient, and also on the nature, severity, and localization of the bleeding site, and should be made jointly with the surgeon.

Special conservative therapy

Oesophageal varices

The immediate life-threatening dangers are exsanguination, shock and hepatic coma. Therapy using vasopressin will be discussed later (*see* p. 126). For local control of bleeding, Sengstaken-Blakemore and Linton-Nachlas tubes are employed. The haemostatic effect appears to be greater with the Sengstaken-Blakemore tube[11, 108].

Only in the case of fundic varices may the Linton-Nachlas tube be of advantage. The main complications of balloon tamponade are obstruction of the larynx, aspiration of saliva with subsequent pneumonia, and perforation of the oesophagus. Because of the danger of pressure ulcers developing, balloon tubes must not remain inflated *in situ* for longer than 48 hours.

Hepatic coma is prevented by magnesium sulphate enemas, nonabsorbable antibiotics (Neomycin, Paromomycin), lactulose and maintenance of normal electrolyte balance.

Ulcers

In the conservative treatment of bleeding ulcers, differentiation is made between stress ulcers occurring acutely during the course of other severe diseases (postoperative, trauma), and bleeding from chronic ulcers. For the prophylaxis and therapy of bleeding erosions, the administration of high doses of antacids seems to have a favourable effect[39, 59, 98].

In contrast, a randomized study showed that cimetidine did not prevent the occurrence of acute stress ulcers[80]. In contrast to earlier publications[60] reports of the failure of cimetidine to control peptic ulcer are now becoming more common. In a controlled study, Pichard, Sonderson and South[78] noted rebleeding in 8 out of 17 patients with duodenal and gastric ulcers treated with cimetidine and in 8 out of 23 patients treated with placebo. Hoare *et al.*[40] found that cimetidine had no effect on the rebleeding rate in patients with bleeding duodenal ulcers, whereas it was effective in bleeding gastric ulcers.

Initial reports on the encouraging results of somatostatin in the management of bleeding ulcers[10, 58] have recently been confirmed by Kayasseh *et al.*[45] in a randomized controlled study.

The persisting problem associated with medical control of bleeding is the danger of failing to judge the correct time for operation in those patients in whom surgical treatment is necessary despite initial control by medical therapy.

Endoscopic treatment of bleeding

Sclerotherapy

Of the causes of gastrointestinal upper bleeding, oesophageal varices have the poorest prognosis. The liver disease which is usually the underlying cause of these varices, is incurable, so that therapy can only be palliative, with the aim of preventing or reducing the incidence of fatal variceal bleeding. In patients with good hepatic function elective shunt surgery carries a justifiable risk and may secure lengthy bleed-free intervals. The risk of therapy, however, must be acceptable, even in the presence of decompensated cirrhosis of the liver or during active bleeding. Endoscopic sclerotherapy would appear to meet this criterion to a large degree[115]. Transoesophageal variceal sclerosis in the bleed-free interval, was introduced into the treatment of oesophageal varices in 1939 by Crafoord and Frenckner[19]. In 1956 Wodak[114] started to practise sclerotherapy by injecting sclerosants close to the varices. Since 1963, Denck[20] has been using this technique with success for the treatment of actively bleeding varices.

Paravascular sclerotherapy The principle of the method proposed by Wodak[114] does not involve injection of the sclerosant into the varices themselves, but into the submucosa, with the aim of causing a thickening of the latter, and thus a displacement of the varices away from the luminal surface. Ideally, the varices are then retained as blood-conducting channels, merely being shifted into deeper layers of the oesophageal wall[21]. In the lower third of the oesophagus, where more than 90 per cent of bleeding varices are located, the varices are subepithelial (*Figure 5.2*). If these varices can be enclosed within fibrous tissue, they can no longer rupture and bleed.

The sole indication for the use of rigid oesophagoscopes is massive active bleeding, since the source of bleeding may be more readily compressed with the rigid tube.

The technique of paravascular variceal sclerotherapy is as follows. As a rule, treatment is carried out using a standard gastroscope (Olympus GIF D 3, Q, ACMI-F8) employing commercially available long, flexible needles. Fibre endoscopes provided with several large-bore suction channels have the advantage of permitting simultaneous aspiration of blood in cases with massive haemorrhage.

The patient is placed in the left-lateral position with the trunk elevated to avoid aspiration. An antifoaming agent (dimethyl polysilo-

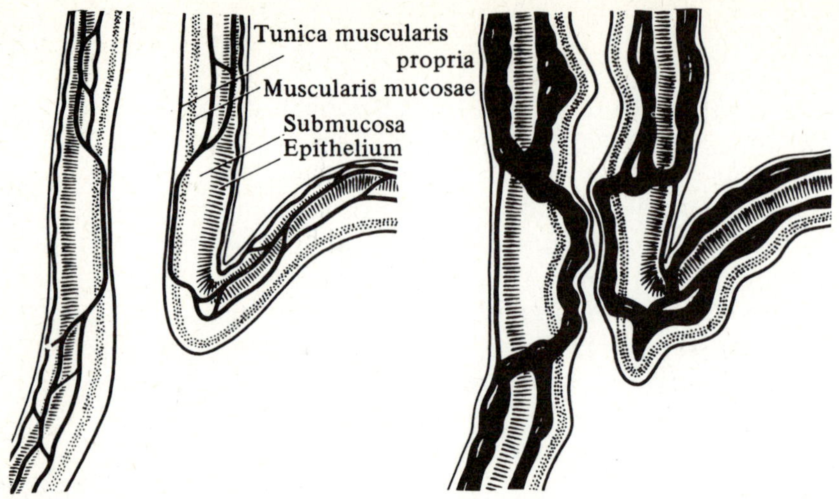

Figure 5.2 Subepithelial location of (*left*) normal veins and (*right*) oesophageal varices in the lower part of the oesophagus (From Stelzner and Lierse[104], courtesy of the Editor and Publishers, *Langenbecks Archiv für klinische Chirurgie*)

xane) and 5000 units of heparin/250 ml are added to the irrigating fluid instilled through the endoscope. This prevents foam obscuring vision and any blood that collects can be aspirated out of the stomach, uncoagulated, at the end of the procedure. The sclerosant injected by English and South African workers is ethanolamine[107], while in Germany preference is given to a 0.5 per cent or 1 per cent solution of polydocanol (Äthoxysclerol)[75, 107].

Thirty to 60 ml of sclerosant is injected in increments of 1–2 ml into the submucosa, strictly adjacent to (not into) the varices, from caudal to cranial, in two to four endoscopic procedures spaced about a week apart. A uniform swelling of the entire mucosa in the distal part of the oesophagus occurs (*Figure 5.3*). If active bleeding is encountered, submucosal 'depots' of sclerosant are injected immediately above the haemorrhage to the right and left of the varix. This frequently results in immediate cessation of bleeding. Otherwise, further quantities of sclerosant are injected. Endoscopy and, if required, repeat sclerotherapy, are carried out after 3 months and thereafter at 6-monthly intervals. When a repeat injection is made into already fibrotic tissue, or if highly concentrated sclerosant is employed, there is a risk of ulceration developing, which may heal only slowly.

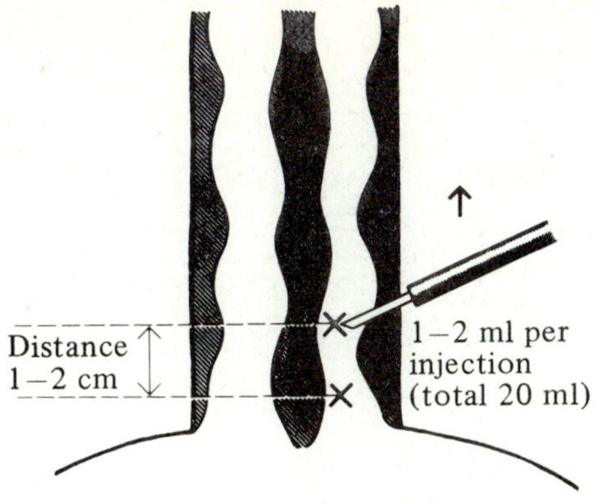

Figure 5.3 Technique of paravascular variceal sclerotherapy (From Soehendra[101], courtesy of the Publishers, *Operative Endoskopie 1979*, edited by L. Demling and W. Rösch)

Occasional accidental puncture of a varix can scarcely be avoided, but bleeding can be prevented by immediate compression of the varix using the tip of the endoscope.

Intravascular sclerotherapy In addition to the paravascular injection technique preferred by most authors, direct sclerosis of the oesophageal varices can also be induced by the intravascular application of the sclerosant. The technique is represented in *Figure 5.4*.

The removal of the sclerosant from the site of the injection by the blood, is prevented by compression with the tip of the endoscope and a special injection technique. The perivascular tissue is also infiltrated during the procedure by advancing the needle somewhat deeper and then slowly withdrawing it while injecting the sclerosant[101].

Williams and Dawson[113] have described a technique using a flexible gastroscope (GIF Q) employing a specially designed flexible plastic sheath provided with a slot through which the varix bulges into the

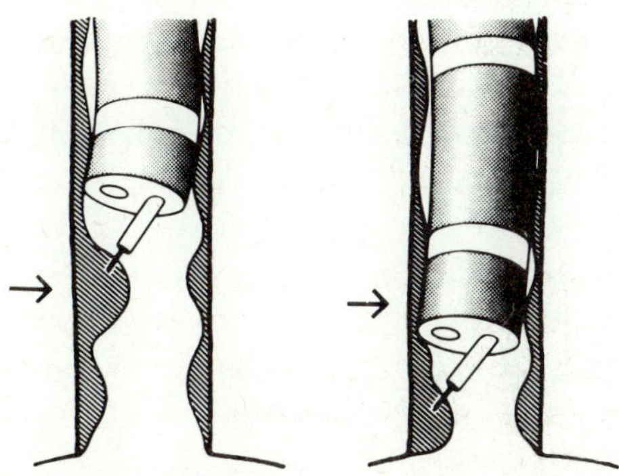

Figure 5.4 Technique of intravascular sclerotherapy (From Soehendra[101], courtesy of the Publishers, *Operative Endoskopie 1979*, edited by L. Demling and W. Rösch)

Table 5.2 Indications for endoscopic variceal sclerotherapy

Absolute indications

(1) Emergency therapy of bleeding impossible to control by conservative
    means
(2) Contraindications to elective shunt surgery
    (a) decompensated active hepatic cirrhosis
    (b) anatomical reasons
    (c) myelofibrosis
(3) Infants and children up to the age of 10 years

Relative indications

(1) Elective shunt operation intended
(2) Prophylactic
(3) Shunt operation refused by patient

lumen in a manner similar to that seen during proctoscopic sclerotherapy of haemorrhoids.

Indications for endoscopic variceal sclerotherapy The results described
in the literature suggests that sclerotherapy of oesophageal varices is
the therapy of choice for variceal bleeding that does not respond to
conservative measures.

It appears to be the equal, or superior, of all the other alternative
procedures, even when an elective shunt operation is not possible.
Because of the danger of hepatic encephalopathy after shunt surgery,
sclerotherapy is also to be preferred when portal hypertension presents in patients with myelofibrosis. In infants and children with
bleeding oesophageal varices, too, fibrosclerotherapy should also be
given preference initially, since the danger of shunt thrombosis
developing is increased in children[74]. Indications for sclerotherapy in
the treatment of oesophageal varices during and after a bleeding
episode are summarized in *Table 5.2*.

Complications The most important complications of sclerotherapy are
necrosis of the oesophageal wall with mediastinitis and/or pyothorax
(2–3 per cent), haemorrhage from gastric varices (2.5 per cent), large
pleural effusions (2 per cent) and stenosis of the oesophagus (2.5 per
cent)[15, 74].

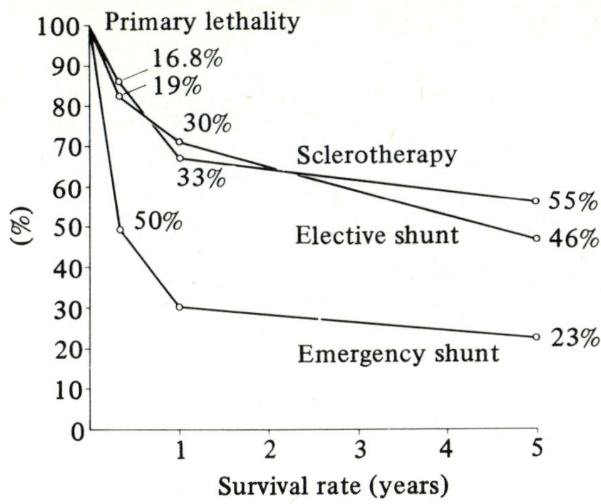

Figure 5.5 Therapeutic results in bleeding
oesophageal varices (1958–78) (From Denck and
Olbert[21], courtesy of the Publishers, *Operative Endoskopie 1979*, edited by L. Demling and W. Rösch)

Results and prognosis The results published to date are difficult to
compare directly, since the individual investigators employed different
techniques. Denck and Olbert[21] and Paquet, Albrecht and Kliems [74],
each of whom has treated more than 850 patients, have the largest case
material at the present time.

In 293 patients presenting with bleeding that did not respond to
conservative measures, Paquet, Albrecht and Kliems[74] successfully
employed sclerotherapy to arrest bleeding in 92 per cent. The 5-year
survival rate of all 858 treated patients was about 50 per cent, and is
comparable with the results obtained by Denck[21] (*Figure 5.5*). In a
prospective study carried out by Terblanche[107], the success rate in
medically uncontrollable bleeding was also 92 per cent, the mortality
rate following sclerotherapy being 18 per cent.

Laser photocoagulation

'Laser' is an acronym for *l*ight *a*mplification by *s*timulated *e*mission of
*r*adiation, and was, in principle, predicted by Einstein more than 50
years ago.

The principle of photocoagulation with laser beam is the absorption
and conversion of light energy into heat with an associated increase in
the temperature of the tissue, resulting in coagulation. For the medical

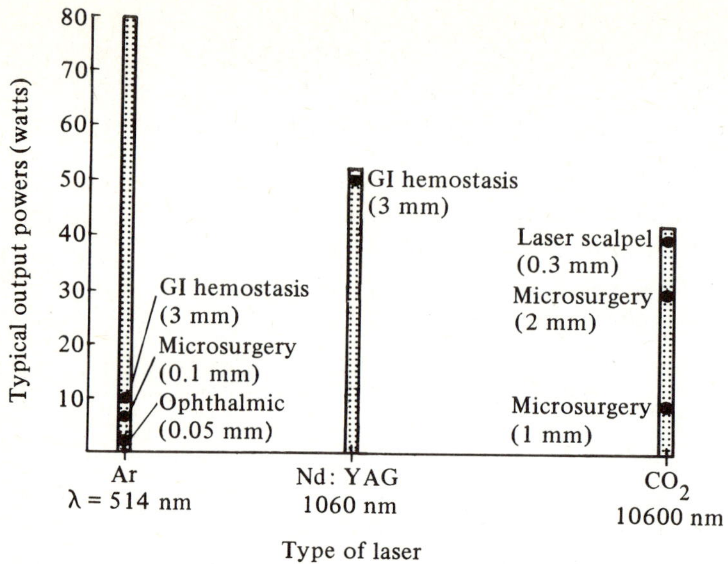

Figure 5.6 Typical laser types and output powers in watts. Ultimate tissue effects will be determined by power densities achieved by focusing to small spot sizes. Power density = Power (watts)/area cm^2

sector, two types of laser are presently available, which differ from one another in the wavelength of their respective beams (*Figure 5.6*). Goodall, Okuda and Gonzales[36] were the first to show that a CO_2 laser could be used through an open-ended rigid gastroscope to reduce bleeding from experimentally produced gastric lesions in the dog. For the use of the laser beam through *flexible* endoscopes, however, at present only the argon ion and the neodymium-YAG laser are suitable. Following comprehensive, preliminary experimental investigations in animals (detailed literature in Frühmorgen *et al.*[33]). Frühmorgen *et al.*[32] and Kieferhaber, Nath and Moritz[48] reported the first successful endoscopic management of bleeding in the human gastrointestinal tract using an argon and a neodymium-YAG laser respectively. The functional difference between these two types of laser beam is to be seen in their varying absorption behaviour. This is due to the fact that blood or highly vascular tissue absorbs the green-blue argon laser beam much more strongly than it does the infrared Nd-YAG laser[85].

The advantages of non-contact photocoagulation with the laser are:

(1) no contact with the tissue
(2) controllability under direct vision

(3) no flow of current through body tissue
(4) larger therapeutic range than electrocoagulation
(5) selective absorption (argon laser)
(6) self-limitation of the depth of penetration (argon laser).

Both laser systems have proved effective in clinical application. Comparative studies[23, 82] indicate that the Nd-YAG laser produces a greater haemostatic effect, but can involve deeper layers of the bowel wall and is thus associated with a potentially greater danger of perforation than is the argon laser.

Indications On the basis of the experience gained to date, the indications for laser coagulation are circumscribed bleeding and non-bleeding vascular anomalies (haemangioma, angiodysplasia, Osler's disease), bleeding ulcers, erosions and oesophageal varices, as also haemorrhage following therapeutic intervention (for example polypectomy).

Clinical results Owing to the considerable expense of the laser systems, reports on experience with appreciable numbers of patients are available from only a few centres. *Table 5.3* presents a selection.

Table 5.3 Results of laser-photocoagulations

Author	Laser	Coagulations	Unsuccessful	Rebleeds	Perforations
Brunetaud[9]	Argon	73	10	5	0
Frühmorgen[34]	Argon	294	3	3	0
Vallon[110]	Argon	68	5	15	0
Kiefhaber[49]	YAG	570	37	77	6
Rutgeerts[91]	YAG	14	1	4	0

With a success rate of better than 80 per cent in acute bleeding, laser coagulation appears to be the best endoscopic method of controlling gastrointestinal haemorrhage currently available. The value of endoscopic laser coagulation with respect to the rate of necessary surgical interventions and mortality of the patients has, however, not yet been established[90].

Controlled randomized studies are presently underway. In conjunction with a widespread clinical application of the laser, it must be borne in mind that the laser coagulators available at present are relatively immobile (fixed connections for water and three-phase current supply, large dimensions) and thus cannot be taken to the patient. It is also possible that the relatively high price will make the laser uneconomical for smaller hospitals with a low incidence of gastrointestinal bleeders.

Electrocoagulation

Conventional electrocoagulation using the high-frequency button electrode, such as is used, for example, to control bleeding after laparoscopic procedures, is considerably less expensive than the laser systems, and is not confined to a single location. Owing to a number of serious disadvantages, in the management of gastrointestinal bleeding, however, it has proved to be of value only for punctate bleeding from telangiectasia, angioma or dysplasia[72].

Only in individual cases has arterial bleeding been arrested[15]. During the coagulation process the electrode frequently adheres to the site of bleeding, and is made ineffectual by adhering coagulation material. The extravasating blood carbonizes and, if coagulation continues, this leads to an incalculable risk of perforation.

In recent years, various working groups have carried out animal experiments with the aim of finding a method of combining the advantages of electrocoagulation with those of laser-beam coagulation, while excluding their respective disadvantages.

In the interpretation of the experimental results, one problem is that the power outputs of the high-frequency surgical units of different makes cannot be directly compared with one another. Furthermore, the coagulative effect of the current applied is dependent upon the nature of the tissue (fluid and electrolyte content), which also changes during the coagulation process[7, 73].

Computer-controlled electrocoagulation A possible solution to this problem may be the computer-controlled electrocoagulation technique developed by Piersey *et al.*[79]. Here, the changes in the electrical properties of the tissue (resistance) during coagulation are measured with the aid of a computer and compensated for by adjustments to the current strength. This method and trials with electrofulguration[22] are still at the animal experimental stage.

Heater probe The heater probe[81], comprises a teflon-coated aluminium cylinder which can be heated to 160 °C by means of a heating filament contained within it. This device has been successfully employed to control bleeding from experimental ulcers induced in animals.

Electrohydrothermo probe Another possibility of making electro-coagulation safer and more effective is the electrohydrothermo probe developed by Frühmorgen's working group[57]. Prior to and during the coagulation process, water is pumped through the tip of the electrode. In this way, visualization of the bleeding point is considerably improved, and the adherence of coagulation material to the electrode completely avoided. Bleeding is arrested by pure coagulation, without carbonization of the extravasating blood, and the energy supplied is calculable. Initial successful attempts to produce haemostasis in bleeding patients make this method appear very promising, although here, too, a number of questions still remain to be answered before large-scale clinical application becomes possible[93].

Tissue adhesives

Spray-on tissue adhesives that can be applied through the endoscope[56, 83], such as the derivatives of acrylic acid which harden by polymerisation to form a fluid-proof plastic coating, are, to date, ineffective in controlling brisk bleeding[35]. In common with the endoscopic application of clotting factors[51], they are probably suitable only for the treatment of persistent, slight bleeding, but not for arterial haemorrhage, or bleeding oesophageal varices.

Therapeutic angiography

Catheter techniques may be used to slow or arrest unremitting haemorrhage particularly when the site of bleeding has been demonstrated by angiography[88]. Such techniques are particularly useful and often life-saving in patients who are poor surgical candidates such as the elderly, patients with multiple organ diseases, postoperative patients[4] and patients with decompensated cirrhosis bleeding from varices[100]. Operation may be completely avoided or at least delayed so that the patient can be adequately prepared for surgery[96]. Bleeding can be controlled by (1) infusion of vasoconstrictive drugs, (2) embolization of the bleeding vessel.

Vasoconstrictive therapy

The most effective vasoconstrictive drug is vasopressin, an octapeptide secreted by the posterior pituitary. Vasopressin has a short half-life action causing splanchnic arterial constriction with a consequent reduction in portal venous flow and pressure, and also bowel wall contraction which may help with clot formation at the site of bleeding. The vasoconstrictive effect of vasopressin lasts about 30 min after infusion has been discontinued and there is no rebound hyperaemia following cessation of therapy. Vasopressin is infused intra-arterially at a rate of 0.2–0.4 u/min for 20 min and then at a reduced dosage for up to 72 hours. The dosage may be increased intermittently to control any further acute episodes of bleeding. Vasopressin is most effective in controlling capillary-type bleeding and will control haemorrhage in up to 80 per cent of bleeds due to haemorrhagic gastritis. When bleeding occurs from segmental arteries as in a duodenal ulcer, the control rate is only 30 per cent and embolization is more effective. Haemorrhage from Mallory-Weiss tears has been successfully controlled by intra-arterial vasopressin in a small number of patients.

Temporary control of variceal haemorrhage is obtained in over 50 per cent of patients by superior mesenteric arterial infusion of vasopressin, but rebleeding is common and survival is not improved. In contrast to arterial bleeding which appears more readily controlled by selective intra-arterial infusion of vasopressin, intravenous vasopressin in equally good at controlling variceal haemorrhage as a mesenteric arterial infusion[13] and is simpler and safer. Failure to control arterial or variceal haemorrhage within 24 hours of starting intra-arterial vasopressin infusion suggests that other methods of controlling bleeding should be considered. Vasopressin is tachyphylactic, becoming progressively less effective. Prolonged use increases the risk of complications.

Complications of vasopressin therapy Vasopressin has a number of undesirable side effects. Its vasoconstrictive action is not restricted to the splanchnic arterial bed and coronary artery spasm leading to myocardial infarction may occur. Electrocardiography is mandatory in patients over 50 years of age prior to the use of vasopressin and the presence of cardiac ischaemia is a relative contraindication to vasopressin therapy. Arterial constriction may also lead to mesenteric infarction with gangrene and peripheral vascular insufficiency especially in the lower limbs. In cirrhotic patients where hepatic perfusion is already compromised, the reduction in portal venous blood flow may further depress hepatocellular function. Smooth muscle contraction causing abdominal cramps and defaecation is unpleasant for the patient, but demonstrates that the vasopressin has not become inactive during storage. Finally, the antidiuretic effect of vasopressin may cause serious hyponatraemia and fluid overload particularly if excessive intravenous dextrose is given.

The incidence of side effects is not reduced by the use of selective intra-arterial infusions of vasopressin as similar plasma concentrations of vasopressin are achieved by arterial or intravenous administration[97].

Transcatheter embolization

Embolization techniques are employed when (1) vasoconstrictive therapy fails to control haemorrhage, (2) the cause of bleeding is unlikely to respond to vasopressin therapy, (3) there is focal bleeding in the presence of a coagulation disorder.

Multiple agents are available for embolization including gelatine sponge, polyvinyl alcohol sponge, isobutyl-2-cyanoacrylate, balloons and wire coils[5]. Bleeding from duodenal or gastric ulcers and Mallory-Weiss tears may be arrested by embolizing the appropriate artery. Gastritis is best treated by vasopressin infusion as there is no localized blood supply.

Complications Provided the collateral blood supply is good and the bleeding artery is deeply catheterized complications should be few. The local vascular anatomy and collateral blood supply to the area of haemorrhage must always be assessed by diagnostic angiography prior to embolization, catheter position checked frequently for stability and embolic material introduced slowly to avoid reflux of emboli into other vessels[43]. The risk of ischaemia is increased by arteriosclerosis, previous surgery and possibly by concomitant vasoconstrictive therapy[109].

Transhepatic variceal obliteration

Following transhepatic portography the coronary and short gastric veins are catheterized and selectively embolized (*Figure 5.7a, b, c*). Control of haemorrhage is immediate but rebleeding frequently occurs

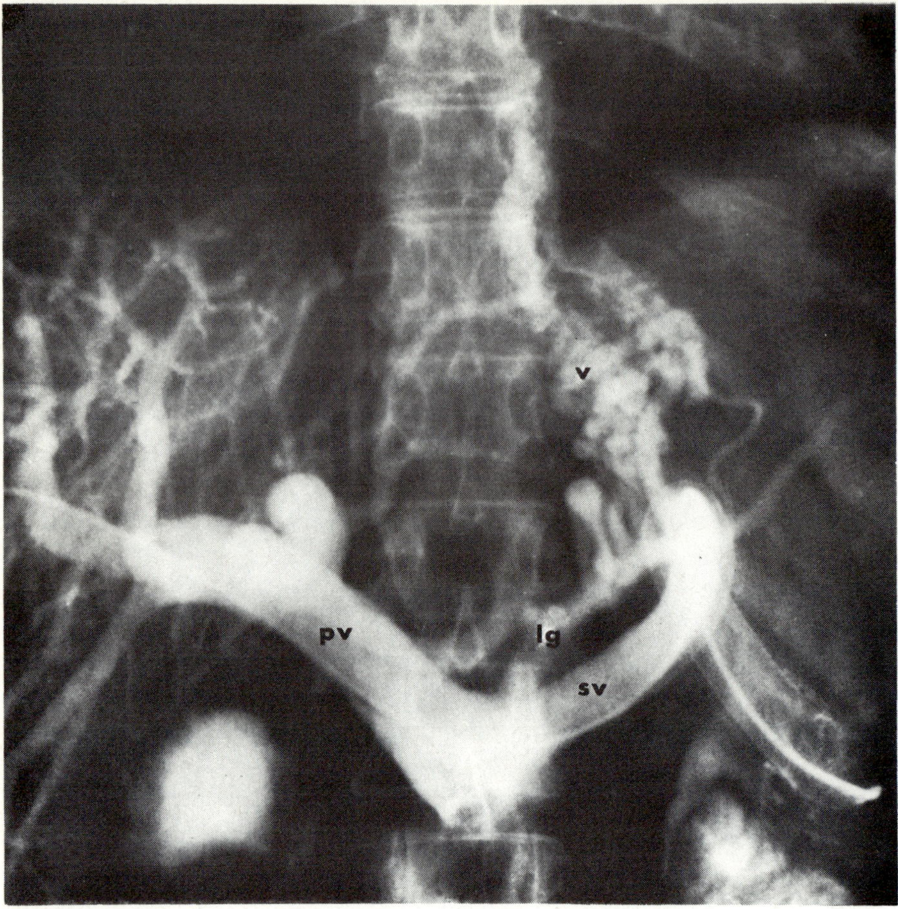

Figure 5.7a Transhepatic portogram demonstrates portal vein (pv), slenic vein (sv) and left gastric vein (lg) feeding oesophageal varices (v)

from the recanalized [53] or newly formed[100] varices. This renders the procedure unsuitable for prophylaxis and the principal indication is variceal haemorrhage which fails to respond to transfusion, vasopressin or the use of a Sengstaken-Blakemore tube.

Complications The most serious complication is intraperitoneal haemorrhage which is avoided by carefully sealing the needle track through the liver when withdrawing the catheter. Puncture of the biliary tree is common but does not lead to sequelae. A right-sided pleural effusion is usual if there is marked ascites but generally responds to conservative therapy. Splenic and portal vein thrombosis

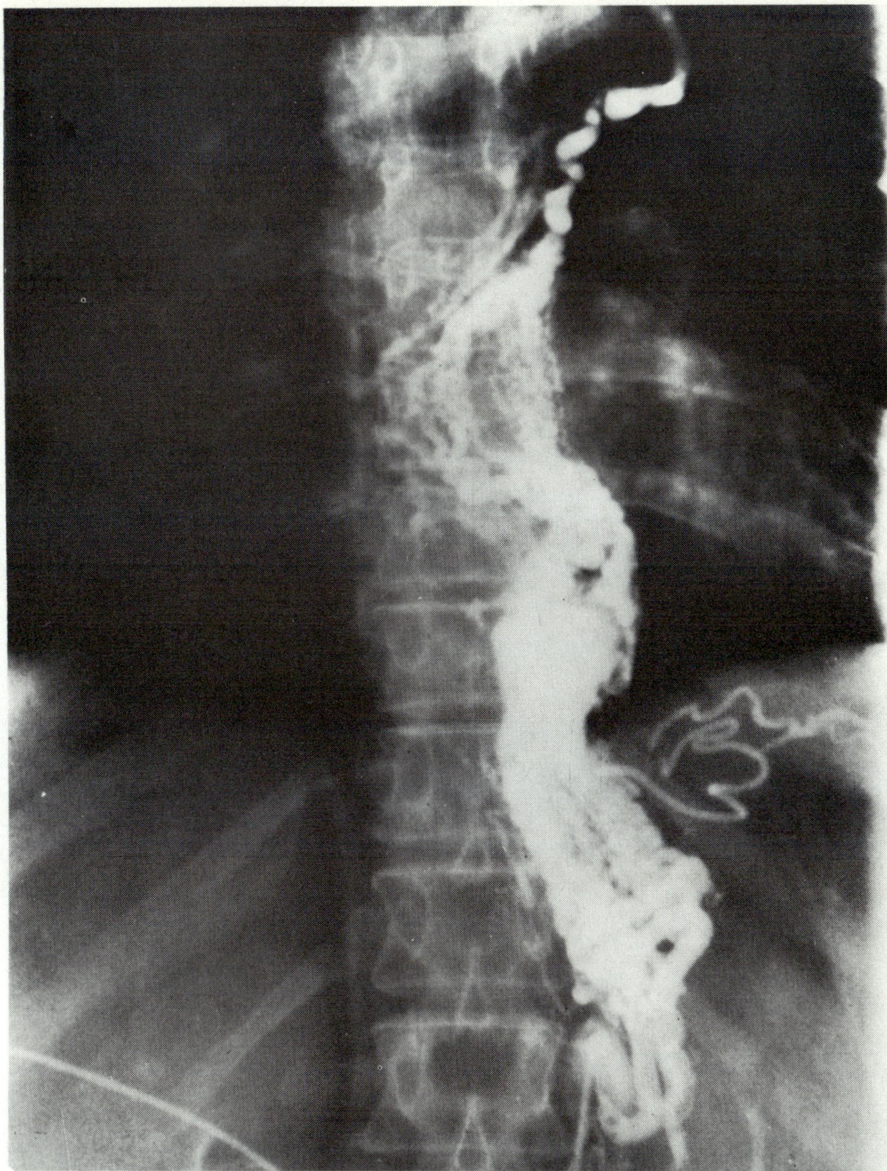

Figure 5.7b Selective left gastric injection demonstrates the extent of the oesophageal varices

occur in less than 5 per cent of patients. The theoretical complication of pulmonary embolization does not seem to occur despite the extensive communication between portal and systemic venous systems.

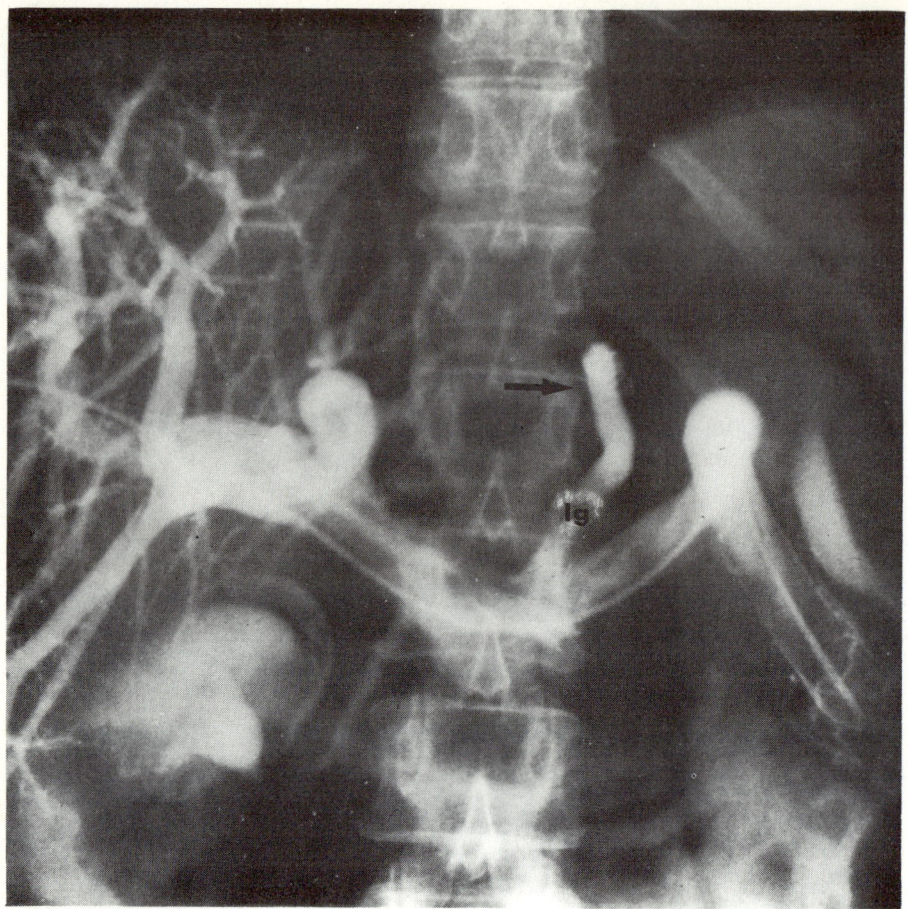

Figure 5.7c Following injection of gelatine foam and a wire coil (arrowed) the left gastric vessel fails to fill with contrast medium

Surgical therapy

An attempt should always be made to control gastrointestinal bleeding by conservative means if possible. If this is successful, surgical treatment of the source of bleeding can then be carried out under better conditions, thus resulting in an improved prognosis.

The decision to recommend surgical therapy is usually based on one or more of the following factors:

(1) the general state of health of the patient; that is, the effect of chronic or acute illness that may be aggravated by the acute blood loss;

(2) accurate diagnosis of the bleeding lesion, plus any other potential bleeding lesions known to be present;
(3) a history of past bleeding episodes, especially if documented to have arisen from the same or a similar lesion;
(4) severe, exsanguinating rate of bleeding;
(5) continued blood loss requiring five units replacement with instability of vital signs;
(6) recurrent bleeding after a brief interval especially from a gastric ulcer;
(7) availability of non-surgical methods of proven safety and effectiveness that may stop or slow bleeding and permit elective surgery.

The decision to operate or to continue medical therapy should be made by the entire responsible for patient management. Joint decisions by the physician and surgeon in attendance are unquestionably the most appropriate in this critical care situation[8].

For the various sources of bleeding, the following surgical procedures are available.

Bleeding from oesophageal varices

In common with the 'emergency shunt', the various operations aimed at 'shutting down' the veins are associated with a mortality rate of up to 60 per cent and should be considered only when every conservative treatment possibility has failed. It must, however, be pointed out that dissection of the oesophageal wall is extremely difficult after unsuccessful sclerotherapy. In such cases, a fundectomy or a subcardial gastric resection may be considered.

Prerequisites for shunt surgery in the bleeding-free interval (elective if possible) are[75]:

(1) compensated hepatic function;
(2) inactive liver disease;
(3) liver blood volume of between 1000 and 2500 ml;
(4) selective portal vein flow between 15 per cent and 40 per cent;
(5) exclusion of a haemodynamically effective stenosis of the coeliac axis.

All types of portosystemic shunts including the recently favoured mesocaval anastomosis[25, 27, 84] reduce portal blood flow. Liver arterialization[54, 55, 62] does not appear to be a convincing alternative procedure. Operations aimed at selective segmental decompression (selective distal splenorenal anastomosis after Warren[111, 112], spleno-caval anastomosis[38, 84]) reduce variceal pressure without affecting portal haemodynamics. The advantage of these techniques is the lower rate of encephalopathy, although the Warren shunt appears to be associated with a higher risk from thrombosis[6].

Prophylactic shunt is clearly of no value, as has been shown in three prospective studies[12, 42, 63].

Prognosis It is not easy to provide valid information as to the prognosis of shunt surgery, since frequently no differentiation is made between emergency and elective shunts, and the surgical techniques also vary considerably. In a group of 612 patients presenting with cirrhosis of the liver, in whom an elective portacaval shunt was performed, Orloff[68] reported a 5-year survival rate of 60 per cent and an encephalopathy incidence of 21 per cent.

The further problems still associated with shunt surgery are illustrated by Conn's remark made in 1974[17], which is still applicable today: 'To shunt or not to shunt; either to select better who should be shunted, or to shunt better those we select'.

Ulcers

Excision or ligature of the bleeding ulcer as the sole intervention, are associated with a high rate of recurrence, so that they should always be combined with a curative intervention. In the case of bleeding gastric ulcer, resection produces better results, while in duodenal ulcer and jejunal ulcer, selective proximal vagotomy (SPV) with local suturing of the bleeding point and possibly ligature of the supplying arterial vessels, appears to give good results[95]. The mortality rate of this emergency procedure is about 10 per cent[30, 67].

Recently, Griffith, Neumann and Welsh[37] have shown that ulcers presenting with an endoscopically recognizable 'visible vessel' in the floor of the ulcer, have a poorer prognosis and, almost without exception, lead to recurrent bleeding that cannot be controlled medically. The authors urge that such ulcers should be strongly considered for operation therapy at the first bleeding episode. Arterial bleeding from Dieulafoy ulcers and Mallory-Weiss tears, which are exceptionally resistant to conservative treatment, can be well managed solely with surgical suturing.

Erosions

So-called stress haemorrhage from acute erosions can be controlled by conservative treatment in almost 90 per cent of the cases. For the few cases that do not respond to medical treatment, subtotal gastric resection coupled with truncal vagotomy is, at the present time, the most successful treatment procedure[26, 30, 50].

References

1 ALLEN, H. M., BLOCK, M. A. and SCHUMANN, B. M. Gastroduodenal endoscopy —management of acute upper gastrointestinal hemorrhage. *Archives of Surgery*, **106**, 450–455 (1973)

2 ALLAN, R. and DYKES, P. A comparison of routine and selective endoscopy in the management of acute gastrointestinal haemorrhage. *Gastrointestinal Endoscopy*, **20**, 154–156 (1974)

3 AMSARI, S. and BALDWIN, D. S. Acute renal failure due to radiocontrast agents. *Nephron*, **17**, 28–40 (1976)

4 ATHANASOULIS, C. A., WALTMAN, A. C., RING, R. J., CARLISLE SMITH, J., JR. and BAUM, S. Angiographic management of post operative bleeding. *Radiology*, **113**, 37–42 (1974)

5 ATHANASOULIS, C. A. Therapeutic applications of angiography. *New England Journal of Medicine*, , 1117–1125 (1980)

6 BERCHTOLD, R. Der Warren Shunt. *Langenbecks Archiv für Klinische Chirurgie*, **342**, 153–157 (1976)

7 BLACKWOOD, W. D. and SILVIS, S. E. Standardization of electrosurgical lesions. *Gastrointestinal Endoscopy*, **21**, 22–24 (1974)

8 BOYCE, H. W. Upper gastrointestinal bleeding. Evaluation and treatment. *Practical Gastroenterology*, **IV**, 38–43 (1980)

9 BRUNETAUD, J.-M., MAFFIOLI, C., ENGER, A. and MOSCHETTO, Y. La photocoagulation par rayon laser à argon ionisé en endoscopie digestive. *IV World Congress of Digestive Endoscopy, Madrid 1978, Book of Abstracts*, 94. London/Madrid, Editorial Garsi (1978)

10 BRUNNER, H. and PANSER, G. Somatostatin in der Behandlung der akuten Ulkusblutung. *Wiener Klinische Wochenschrift*, **13**, 468–471 (1978)

11 BURCHARTH, F. and MALMSTRÖM, J. Experiences with the Linton-Nachlas and the Sengstaken-Blakemore tubes for bleeding esophageal varices. *Surgery, Gynecology and Obstetrics*, **142**, 529–531 (1976)

12 CALLOW, A. D., RESNIK, R. H., CHALMERO, T. C., ISHIHORA, A. M., GARCEAU, A. J. and O'HARA, E. T. Conclusions from a controlled trial of prophylactic portacaval shunt. *Surgery*, **67**, 97–103 (1970)

13 CHOJKIER, M., GROSZMANN, R. J., ATTERBURY, C. E., BAR-MEIR, S., BLEI, A. T., FRANKEL, J., GLICKMAN, M. G., KNIAZ, J. L., SCHADE, R., TAGGART, G. J. and CONN, H. O. A controlled comparison of continuous intra-arterial and intravenous infusion of vasopressin in haemorrhage from oesophageal varices. *Gastroenterology*, **77**, 540–546 (1979)

14 CLASSEN, M., HAGENMÜLLER, F., HOFFMANN, L., WURBS, D. and RASCHKE, E. Endoscopy in severe upper gastrointestinal bleeding. In *Gastrointestinal Emergencies*, edited by F. R. Baraney and A. Torsoli, 121–127. Oxford, Pergamon (1977)

15 CLASSEN, M. and WURBS, D. Therapeutische Endoskopie im Verdauungstrakt. *Berichte der Gesellschaft Innere Medizin*, **11**, 211–215 (1978)

16 CLASSEN, M., DANCYGIER, H. and FUCHS, H. F. Endoscopy in diagnosis of duodenal ulcer. *International Congress Series No.537, Advances in Ulcer Disease*, 282–285. Amsterdam, Excerpta Medica (1981)

17 CONN, H. O. Therapeutic portacaval anastomosis: to shunt or not to shunt. *Gastroenterology*, **67**, 1065–1071 (1974)

18 COTTON, P. D., ROSENBERG, M. T., WALDRAM, R. P. L. and AXON, A. T. R. Early endoscopy of oesophagus, stomach and duodenal bulb in patients with haematemesis and melanea. *British Journal of Medicine*, **2**, 505–509 (1973)

19 CRAFOORD, C. and FRENCKNER, P. New Surgical treatment of varicous veins of the oesophagus. *Acta Oto-larynology*, **27**, 422–429 (1939)

20 DENCK, H. Versorgung der akuten Blutung bei Leberzirrhose. *Wiener Zeitschrift für Innere Medizin*, **51**, 118–120 (1970)

21 DENCK, H. and OLBERT, F. Wandsklerosierung bei Ösophagusvarizen–prophylaktisch– bei akuter Blutung–im Intervall? In *Operative Endoskopie*, edited by L. Demling and W. Rösch, 27–32. Berlin, Acron Verlag, (1979)

22 DENNIS, M., PEOPLES, J., HULETT, R., AUTH, D. and PROTELLI, R. Control of experimental gastric bleeding with electrofulguration: Is it effective? Is it safe? *Gastrointestinal Endoscopy*, **24**, 194 (1978) (Abstract)

23 DIXON, J. A., BERENSON, M. M. and MCCLOSKEY, D. W. Neodymium–Yag laser treatment of experimental canine gastric bleeding. *Gastroenterology*, **77**, 647–651 (1979)

24 DORIN, M. Technical note on lasers in medicine and surgery. *Spectra-Physics Laser Technical Bulletin*, **9**, 1–7 (1979)

25 DRAPANAS, T. H. Interposition mesocaval shunt for treatment of portal hypertension. *Annals of Surgery*, **176**, 435–446 (1972)

26 DRAPANAS, T. H., WOOLVERTON, W. C., REEDER, J. W., REED, R. L. and WEICHERT, R. F. Experiences with surgical management of acute gastric mucosal hemorrhage. *Annals of Surgery*, **173**, 628–640 (1971)

27 DRAPANAS, TH., LOCICERO, J. and DOWLING, J. B. Hemodynamics of the interposition mesocaval shunt. *Annals of Surgery*, **181**, 523–525 (1975)

28 DRONFIELD, M., MCILLMURRAY, M. B., FERGUSON, R., ATKINSON, M. and LANGMAN, M. J. S. A prospective randomised trial of endoscopy and radiology in upper gastrointestinal tract bleeding. *Lancet*, **1**, 1167–1169 (1977)

29 EDER, M. and CASTRUP, H. J. Die gastrointestinale Blutung aus der Sicht des Chirurgen. *Chirurg*, **40**, 97–105 (1969)

30 FEIFEL, G. and HEBERER, G. Die Problematik der oberen akuten gastrointestinalen Blutung. *Chirurg*, **48**, 204–211 (1977)

31 FRAZER, G. M. The double contrast barium meal in patients with acute gastrointestinal bleeding. *Clinical Radiology*, **29**, 625–634 (1978)

32 FRÜHMORGEN, P., BODEM. F., REIDENBACH, H. D., KADUK, B. and L. DEMLING. The first endoscopic laser coagulation in the human gastrointestinal tract. *Endoscopy*, **7**, 156–157 (1975)

33 FRÜHMORGEN, P., BODEM, F., REIDENBACH, H.-D. and DEMLING, L. Was ist gesichert in der Laserkoagulation zur Stillung gastrointestinaler Blutungen? *Internist*, **19**, 707–712 (1978)

34 FRÜHMORGEN, P., REIDENBACH, H. D. and BODEM, F. Blutstillung durch Photokoagulation. In *Therapeutische Endoskopie*, edited by B. C. Manegold, 69–83. Baden-Baden, Witzstrockverlag (1979)

35 GILBERT, D. A., SAUNDERS, D. R., PEOPLES, J., SILLERY, J. and GULASCIK, C. Failure of iced saline lavage to suppress haemorrhage from experimental bleeding ulcers. *Gastroenterology*, **76**, 1138 (1979)

36 GOODALE, R. L., OKUDA, A. and GONZALES, B. Rapid endoscopic control of bleeding gastric erosions by laser radiation. *Archives of Surgery*, **101**, 211–214 (1970)

37 GRIFFITHS, W. J., NEUMANN, D. A., WELSH, J. D. The visible vessel as an indicator of uncontrolled or recurrent gastrointestinal haemorrhage. *New England Journal of Medicine*, **300**, 1411–1413 (1979)

38 GUHARAY, B. N., SAIN, P., SENGUPTA, K. P., MALLIK, K. K., BISWAS, S. and BASU, A. K. Graft interposition splenocaval shunt for total or selective decompression of portal hypertension. *Surgery*, **83**, 164–172 (1978)

39 HASTING, P. R., SKILLMAN, J. J., BUSHNELL, L. S. and SILEN, W. Antacid titration in the prevention of acute gastrointestinal bleeding. A controlled, randomized trial in 100 critical ill patients. *New England Journal of Medicine*, **298**, 1041–1045 (1978)

40 HOARE, A. M., BRADBY, G. V. H., HAWKING, C. F., KANG, J. Y. and DYKES, P. W. Cimetidine in bleeding peptic ulcer. *Lancet*, **2**, 671–673 (1979)

41 IHSE, I., LUNDERQUIST, A. and AKERMAN, M. Chronic bleeding from primary non-specific small intestinal ulceration localised by angiography. *Acta Chirurgica Scandinavica*, **144**, 189–192 (1978)

42 JACKSON, F. C., PERRIN, E. B., SMITH, A. G., DAGRADI, A. E. and NADAL, H. M. A clinical investigation of the portacaval shunt. II. Survival analysis of the prophylactic operation. *American Journal of Surgery*, **115**, 22–42 (1968)

43 JACOB, E. T., SHAPIRA, Z., MORAG, B. and RUBINSTEIN, Z. Hepatic infarction and gall bladder necrosis complicating arterial embolization for bleeding duodenal ulcer. *Digestive Diseases and Sciences*, **24**, 482–484 (1979)

44 KATON, R. M. and SMITH, F. W. Panendoscopy in the early diagnosis of acute upper gastrointestinal bleeding. *Gastroenterology*, **65**, 728–734 (1973)

45 KAYASSEH, L., GYR, K., KELLER, UL and STALDER, G. A. Somatostatin and cimetidine in peptic ulcer haemorrhage. *Lancet*, **1**, 844–846 (1980)

46 KELLER, R. T. and LOGAN, G. M. Comparison of emergency endoscopy and upper gastrointestinal series radiography in acute upper gastrointestinal haemorrhage. *Gut*, **17**, 180–184 (1976)

47 KERN, F. Severe upper gastrointestinal bleeding: diagnosis. In *Gastrointestinal Emergencies*, edited by F. R. Barany and A. Torsoli, 113–115. Oxford, Pergamon (1977)

48 KIEFHABER, P., NATH, G. and MORITZ, K. Endoscopical control of massive gastrointestinal haemorrhage by irradiation with a high-power neodymium YAG laser. *Progress in Surgery*, **15**, 140–155 (1977)

49 KIEFHABER, P., MORITZ, K. and NATH, G. Endoscopic control of acute gastrointestinal hemorrhage by irradiation with a high power Neodymium Y.A.G. Laser. *International Medical Laser Symposium*, (Detroit, March 29–31) (1979)

50 LINDKAER-JENSEN, ST., NIELSEN, O. V., PAGEL, J. and CHRISTIONSEN, L. Acute hemorragic gastritis–diagnosis and treatment. *Acta Chirurgica Scandinavica*, **142**, 246–250 (1976)

51 LINSCHEER, W. G. and FAZIO, T. L. Control of upper gastrointestinal hemorrhage by endoscopic spraying of clotting factors. *Gastroenterology*, **77**, 642–646 (1979)

52 LUK, G. D., BYNUM, T. E. and HENDRIX, T. H. R. Gastric aspiration in localisation of gastrointestinal hemorrhage. *Journal of the American Medical Association*, **241**, 576–578 (1979)

53 LUNDERQUIST, A., SIMERT, G., TYLEN, U. L. and VANG, J. Follow up of patients with portal hypertension and oesophageal varices treated with percutaneous obliteration of gastric coronary vein. *Radiology*, **122**, 59–63 (1977)

54 MAILLARD, J. N., BENHAMON, J. P. and RUEFF, B. Arterialization of the liver with portacaval shunt in the treatment of portal hypertension due to intrahepatic block. *Surgery*, **67**, 883–890 (1970)

55 MAILLARD, J. N., RUEFF, B., PRANDI, D. and SICOT, C. H. Hepatic arterialization and protacaval shunt in hepatic cirrhosis. *Archives of Surgery*, **108**, 315–320 (1974)

56 MARTIN, R. R., ONSTAD, G. R. and SUVIS, S. W. Endoscopic control of upper gastrointestinal bleeding with a tissue adhesive (MBR 4197) *Gastrointestinal Endoscopy*, **24**, 73–76 (1977)

57 MATEK, W., FRÜHMORGEN, P., KADUK, B., REIDENBACH, H.-D., BODEM, F. and DEMLING, L. Modified electrocoagulation and its possibilities in the control of gastrointestinal bleeding. *Endoscopy*, **11**, 253–258 (1979)

58 MATTES, P., LAUTERBACH, H. H. and RAPTIS, S. Prevention of stress ulcer by somatostatin in rats. *Langenbecks Archiv für Klinische Chirurgie*, **341**, 297–301 (1976)

59 MCALHANY, J. C., CZAJA, A. J. and VILLAREAL, Y. The gastric mucosal barrier in terminal injured patients: correlation with gastroduodenal endoscopy. *Surgical Forum*, **25**, 414–418 (1974)

60 MACDONALD, A. S., STEELE, B. J. and BOTTOMLEY, M. G. Treatment of stress-induced upper gastrointestinal haemorrhage with Metiamide. *Lancet*, **1**, 68–70 (1976)

61 MACGINN, F. P., GUYLER, P. B., WILEN, B. J. and STEER, H. W. A prospective comparative trial between early endoscopy and radiology in acute upper gastrointestinal haemorrhage. *Gut*, **16**, 707–713 (1975)

62 MATZANDER, U. Probleme bei der Arterialisierung des intrahepatischen Pfortaderkreislaufs nach porto-cavalen Anastomosen. *Langenbecks Archiv für Klinische Chirurgie*, **322**, 1155–1159 (1968)

63 MERIGAN, T. C., PLOTHIN, G. R. and DAVIDSON, L. S. Effect of intravenously administered posterior pituitary extract on haemorrhage from bleeding esophageal varices. *New England Journal of Medicine*, **266**, 134–135 (1962)

64 MOORE, J. D., THOMPSON, N. W., APPLEMAN, H. D. and FOLEY, D. Arteriovenous malformations of the gastrointestinal tract. *Archives of Surgery*, **111**, 381–389 (1976)

65 MORRIS, D. W., LEVINE, G. M., SOLOWAY, R. D., MILLER, W. T. and MARIN, G. A. Prospective randomized study of diagnosis and outcome in acute upper gastrointestinal bleeding. Endoscopy versus conventional radiology. *American Journal of Digestive Diseases*, **20**, 1103–1109 (1975)

66 MORRISSEY, J. F. Early endoscopy for major gastrointestinal bleeding – it should be done. *American Journal of Digestive Diseases*, **22**, 534–535 (1977)

67 MÜHE, E., GALL, F. and SCHICK, A. Die SPU zur Behandlung von Ulkuskomplikationen. *Gastroenterologisches Symposion: Die selektiv proximale Vagotomie – 'aktuelle Probleme'* (Köln) (1978)

68 ORLOFF, M. J., BELL, R. H., HYDE, P. V. and SHIVOLOCKI, W. P. Long-term results of emergency portacaval shunt for esophageal varices in unselected patients with alcoholic cirrhosis. *Annals of Surgery*, **192**, 325–337 (1980)

69 PALMER, E. D. Observations on the vigorous diagnostic approach to severe upper gastrointestinal hemorrhage. *Annalen der Inneren Medizin*, **36**, 184–189 (1952)

70 PALMER, E. D. The vigorous diagnostic approach to upper gastrointestinal tract hemorrhage. *Journal of the American Medical Association*, **207**, 1477–1480 (1969)

71 PALMER, E. D. *Upper Gastrointestinal Hemorrhage*. Springfield, Ill., C.C. Thomas (1970)

72 PAPP, J. P. Endoscopic electrocoagulation in upper gastrointestinal hemorrhage. *Journal of the American Medical Association*, **230**, 1172–1173 (1974)

73 PAPP, J. P., FOX, J. M. and NALBANDIAN, R. M. Experimental electrocoagulation of dog esophageal and duodenal mucosa. *Gastrointestinal Endoscopy*, **23**, 27–28 (1976)

74 PAQUET, K. J. ALBRECHT, M. and KLIEMS, G. Wandsklerosierung bei Ösophagusvarizen – prophylaktisch – bei akuter Blutung – im Intervall. In *Operative Endoskopie*, edited by L. Demling, W. Rösch, 33–46. Berlin, Acron Verlag (1979)

75 PAQUET, K. J. Indikationen zur Shunt-Operation. *Deutsche Medizinische Wochenschrift*, **105**, 676–677 (1980)

76 PAUL, F., SEIFERT, E., LESCH, P., BÄR, UL and OTTO, P. Analyse von Komplikationen notfallmäßiger endoskopischer Untersuchungen des proximalen Magen-Darm-Trakts. In *Fortschritte der Endoskopie*, edited by R. Ottenjann, 99–103. Stuttgart, Schattauer (1974)

77 PHILLIP, J., CLASSEN, M. and GUNSELMANN, W. European Emergency Endoscopy Study. *Endoscopy*, Supplement: *IV European Congress of Gastrointestinal Endoscopy*, 102. Stuttgart, Georg Thieme Verlag (1980) (Abstract)

78 PICHARD, R. G., SONDERSON, I. and SOUTH, M. Controlled trial of Cimetidine in acute upper gastrointestinal bleeding. *British Medical Journal*, **1**, 661–662 (1979)

79 PIERCEY, J. R. A., AUTH, D. C., SILVERSTEIN, F. E., WILLARD, H. R., DENNIS, M. B., ELLEFSON, D. M., DAVIS, D. M., PROTELL, R. I. and RUBIN, C. E. Electrosurgical treatment of experimental bleeding canine gastric ulcers: Development and testing of a computer control and a better electrode. *Gastroenterology*, **74**, 527–534 (1978)

80 PRIEBE, H. J., SKILLMAN, J. J., BUSHNELL, L. S., LONG, P. C. and SILEN, W. Antacid versus Cimetidine in preventing acute gastrointestinal bleeding. *New England Journal of Medicine*, **302**, 426–430 (1980)

81 PROTELL, R. I., RUBIN, C. E., AUTZ, D. C., SILVERSTEIN, F. E., TEROU, F., DENNIS, M. and PIERCEY, J. R. A. The heaterprobe – a new endoscopic method for stopping massive gastrointestinal bleeding. *Gastroenterology*, **74,** 257–262 (1978)

82 PROTELL, R. L., SILVERSTEIN, F. E., AUTH, D. C., DENNIS, M. B., GILBERT, D. A. and RUBIN, C. E. The Nd-YAG-Laser is dangerous for photocoagulation of experimental bleeding gastric ulcers when compared with the Argon Laser. *Gastroenterology*, **74,** 1080 (1978)

83 PROTELL, R. L., SILVERSTEIN, F. E., GULACSIK, C., MARTIN, T. R., DENNIS, M. B., AUTH, D. C. and RUBIN, C. E. Failure of cyanoacrylate tissue glue (Flucrylate™, MBR 4197) to stop bleeding from experimental canine gastric ulcers. *American Journal of Digestive Diseases*, **23,** 903–908 (1978)

84 RAIA, S., MITTELSTAEDT, W., MIES, S., DE SILVA, A. D., MONTEIRO, C. and RAIA, A. Selektive Druckentlastung des Pfortadersystems bei blutenden Ösophagusvarizen. *Chirugische Praxis*, **23,** 51–60 (1977/78)

85 REIDENBACH, H. D., BODEM, F., FRÜHMORGEN, P., BRAND, H. and DEMLING, L. The plastic light guide in endoscopic laser photocoagulation. *Endoscopy*, **7,** 196–201 (1975)

86 RÖSCH, W., FRÜHMORGEN, P., ZEUS, J., RUPPIN, H., PHILLIP, J. and KOCH, H. 24-Stunden-Notfallendoskopieservice: Erste Erfahrungen. *Aktuelle Gastrologie*, **4,** 225–227 (1975)

87 RÖSCH, W. Notfallendoskopie – diagnostische und therapeutische Möglichkeiten. *Internist*, **21,** 25–29 (1980)

88 ROSCH, J., DOTTER, C. T. and BROWN, A. J. Selective arterial embolization. A new method for controlling acute gastrointestinal bleeding. *Radiology*, **102,** 303–306 (1972)

89 ROHDE, H., TROIDL, H., LORENZ, W., FISCHER, M. and VESTWEBER, K. H. Neue Ansätze zur Frage: Hat die Notfallendoskopie für den Chirurgen Bedeutung? *Medizinische Klinik*, **73,** 773–780 (1980)

90 ROHDE, H., THON, K., FISCHER, M., OHMANN, CH. and LORENZ, W. Early endoscopy combined with endoscopic neodymium-YAG-Laser therapy in patients with actively bleeding lesions. In *IV European Congress of Gastrointestinal Endoscopy*, 107, Stuttgart, G. Thieme Verlag (1980)

91 RUTGEERTS, P., VANTRAPPEN, G., BROECKAERT, L., JANNSENS, J. and COREMANS, G. The efficiency of Neodymium-YAG-Laser photocoagulation in the treatment of upper gastrointestinal hemorrhage. In *Endoscopy*, Supplement: *Gastrointestinal Endoscopy*, edited by M. Classen, H. Henning and E. Seifert, 107. Stuttgart, G. Thieme Verlag (1980)

92 SANDLOW, L. J., BECKER, G. H., SPELLBERG, M. A., ALLEN, H. A. BERG, M., BERRY, L. H. and NEWMAN, E. A. A prospective randomized study of the management of upper gastrointestinal hemorrhage. *American Journal of Gastroenterology*, **61,** 282–289 (1974)

93 SCHAPIRO, M. Watering down electrocoagulation for GI bleeding. (Selected summaries) *Gastroenterology*, **79,** 169 (1980)

94 SCHILLER, K. F. R., TRUELOVE, S. C., WILLIAMS, D. G. Haematemesis and melanea, with special reference to factors influencing the outcome. *British Medical Journal*, **2,** 7–14 (1970)

95 SEUFERT, R. M., ENCKE, A. Akute Diagnostik und Therapie bei großen Blutungen aus Ösophagus, Magen und oberem Dünndarm. *Medizinische Welt*, **31**, 700–705 (1980)

96 SHERMAN, I. M., SHENOY, S. S., CERRA, F. A. Selective intra-arterial vasopressin: clinical efficacy and complications. *Annals of Surgery*, **189**, 298–302 (1979)

97 SIMMONS, J. T., BAUM, S., SHEEHAN, B. A., RING, E. J., ATHANASOULIS, C. A., WALTMAN, A. C., COGGINS, P. C. The effect of vasopressin in hepatic arterial blood flow. *Radiology*, **124**, 637–640 (1977)

98 SIMONIAN, D. J., CURTIS, L. E. Treatment of hemorrhagic gastritis by antacid. *Annals of Surgery*, **184**, 429–434 (1976)

99 SMITH-LAING, G., CAMILO, M. E., DICK, R., SHERLOCK, S. Percutaneous transhepatic portography in the assessment of portal hypertension. Clinical correlations and comparison of radiographic techniques. *Gastroenterology*, **78**, 197–205 (1980)

100 SMITH-LAING, G., SCOTT, J., LONG, R. G., DICK, R. and SHERLOCK, S. The role of percutaneous transhepatic variceal obliteration in the management of haemorrhage from gastro-oesophageal varices. *Gastroenterology*, **80**, (In press)

101 SOEHENDRA. N. Fiberscopy sclerosing of esophageal varices. In *Operative Endoskopie*, edited by L. Demling and W. Rösch, 47–52. Berlin, Acron Verlag (1979)

102 SOS, T. A., LEE, J. G., WIXON, D. and SNIDERMAN, K. W. Intermittent bleeding from minute to minute in acute massive gastrointestinal haemorrhage: arteriographic demonstration. *American Journal of Roentgenology*, **131**, 1015 –1017 (1978)

103 STADELMANN, O., KAIP, E. and MIEDERER, S. E. Endoskopie des oberen Verdauungstrakts. Fortschritte, Grenzen, Risiken. *Fortschritte der Endoskopie*, edited by R. Ottenjann, 1–5. Stuttgart, Schattauer (1974)

104 STELZNER, F. and LIERSE, W. Der angiomuskuläre Dehnverschluss der terminalen Speiseröhre. *Langenbecks Archiv für Klinische Chirurgie*, **321**, 35–64 (1968)

105 STROHMEYER, G. and KIENE, K. Konservative Therapie der Ösophagusvarizenblutung. *Intensivmedizin bei gastroenterologischen Erkrankungen*, edited by H. Schönborn, M. Neher, H. P. Schuster and G. Manegold, 81–86, Stuttgart, G. Thieme Verlag (1980)

106 SWARTZ, R. D., RUBIN, J. E., LEEMING, B. W. and SILVA, P. Renal failure following major angiography. *American Journal of Medicine*, **65**, 31–37 (1978)

107 TERBLANCHE, J., NORTHOVER, J. M. A., BORMAN, P., KOHN, D., BARBLZAT, G. O., SELLARS, S. L. and SAUNDERS, S. J. A prospective evaluation of injection sclerotherapy in the treatment of acute bleeding from esophageal varices. *Surgery*, **85**, 239–245 (1979)

108 TEVES, J., CECILIA, A., BORDAS, J., RIMOLA, A., BRU, C. and RODES, J. Esophageal tamponade for bleeding varices. Controlled trial between the Sengstaken-Blakemore tube and the Linton-Nachlas tube. *Gastroenterology*, **75**, 566–569 (1978)

109 TWIFORD, T. W. JR., GOLDSTEIN, H. M. and ZORNOZ, A. J. Transcatheter therapy of gastrointestinal arterial bleeding. *American Journal of Digestive Diseases*, **23**, 1046–1056 (1978)

110 VALLON, A. G., COTTON, P. B., ARMEGOL MIRO, J. R., LAURENCE, B. H. and SALORD ORES, J. C. Randomized study of endoscopic Argon Laser photocoagulation in bleeding peptic ulcers. In *Endoscopy*, Supplement: *Gastrointestinal Endoscopy*, edited by M. Classen, H. Henning and E. Seifert, 106. Stuttgart, G. Thieme Verlag (1980)

111 WARREN, W. D., ZEPPA, R., FOMON, J. J. Selective trans-splenic decompression of gastroesophageal varices by distal splenorenal shunt. *Annals of Surgery*, **166,** 437–455 (1967)

112 WARREN, W. D. Preoperative assessment and choice of operative procedure for portal hypertension. In *Surgery of the Liver, Pancreas and Biliary Tract*, edited by J. S. Najarion and J. P. Delonay, 629. New York, Stratton Intercontinental Medical Book (1975)

113 WILLIAMS, K. G. D. and DAWSON, L. Fibreoptic injection of oesophageal varices. *British Medical Journal*, **2,** 766–767 (1979)

114 WODAK, E. Die konservative Behandlung von Ösophagusvarizen. *HNO*, **13,** 131–133 (1965)

115 WURBS, D., HEUECK, A., DAMMERMANN, R. and CLASSEN, M. Ösophaguswand-sklerosierung mit flexiblen Endoskopen. *Notfallmedizin*, **6,** 135–143 (1980)

6
Menetrier's disease

B. T. Cooper and V. S. Chadwick

Introduction

Menetrier's disease[98] is a bizarre but fascinating disorder which has intrigued physicians and surgeons for almost 100 years. Many clinicians will never see a case and yet most will be familiar with the gross morphological features and would include it in a list of causes of protein-losing enteropathy. The aetiology of Menetrier's disease is unknown and the management controversial, even though more than 300 cases have been reported in the literature.

An exact definition of Menetrier's disease is difficult, since in published case reports detailed histological descriptions were not always presented and, indeed, strict histological criteria have never been established. Giant rugal folds in the stomach can be produced by a variety of disorders and it is possible that Menetrier's disease itself (with 'typical' histological features) may be a response of the gastric mucosa to a variety of endogenous or exogenous stimuli, so that a single aetiological agent or factor will never be implicated. Similar disorders occur in a variety of animals and in some an infective agent has been isolated. A transient form of the disease is seen in children and may have an allergic pathogenesis. The disease may progress to chronic atrophic gastritis and there may be a risk of malignant transformation to adenocarcinoma. The excess gastric protein loss and the finding of circulatory antibodies to dietary antigens probably reflect increased gastric mucosal permeability, though the morphological basis for this is not very clear.

Considerable confusion exists in relation to the nomenclature of this disorder. Menetrier[98] described a group of patients with discrete gastric polyps (*polyadenomes polypeux*), and another with enlarged gastric rugae resembling cerebral convolutions (*polyadenomes en nappe*). The latter condition later became known as Menetrier's disease. The term giant hypertrophic gastritis[127, 128] based on the endoscopic appearances has little pathological basis. Mucus cell hyperplasia and not hypertrophy is the characteristic histological feature[154] and there are few features of gastritis, any inflammatory infiltrate being patchy, absent or of variable cell type[154]. The term hyperplastic

Table 6.1 Synonyms for Menetrier's disease

Giant hypertrophic gastritis (gastropathy)

Hypertrophied gastric mucosa

Giant rugal hypertrophy

Giant fold gastritis

Giant hypertrophy of the gastric mucosa

Exudative gastropathy

Protein-losing gastropathy

Tumour-simulating gastritis

Gastritis polyposa

Adenopapillomatosis gastrica

gastropathy is more appropriate, but the eponym Menetrier's disease has stood the test of time and is preferable to some of the other terms in occasional usage (*Table 6.1*). The purpose of this review is to assess the current position with regard to the clinical and pathological features, pathophysiology and management of Menetrier's disease.

Radiology

The stomach in Menetrier's disease has usually been studied by barium meal, although there is one report of thick gastric folds being demonstrated by CAT scanning[80]. The radiological appearance of the stomach frequently gives the first indication of the disease and is characterized in every case by giant thickened gastric rugae[114].

Reese, Hodgson and Dockerty[114] have reviewed the barium meals of 18 patients with Menetrier's disease, thus forming the largest series. They concluded that while no feature was pathognomonic, four abnormalities are highly suggestive of Menetrier's disease – first: thick gastric folds; second: the configuration of the stomach in involved areas; third: thickening of the stomach wall in involved areas; and fourth: the pattern caused by the mixture of barium and mucus. The radiological differential diagnosis is that of thick folds which may be caused or mimicked by a wide variety of other disorders (*Table 6.2*). The thick folds are usually large, tortuous and 1–2 cm in height and often better delineated with air contrast[114]. They cannot be effaced by the palpating hand during fluoroscopy, or by over-distension of the stomach with gas or barium[55, 114]. This may enable giant folds to be distinguished from prominent normal folds[46, 116]. However, one author

Table 6.2 Radiological differential diagnosis of large gastric folds

Zollinger-Ellison syndrome[130, 134]

Hypertrophic hypersecretory gastritis[18, 107, 130, 134, 138]

Carcinoma[43, 88, 114, 134]

Lymphoma[43, 88, 114, 134]

Polyps[43, 49, 55, 153]

Leiomyoma/leiomyosarcoma[43, 55, 88]

Neurofibroma[43, 88]

Lipoma[43, 88]

Acute or chronic gastritis[43, 114]

Eosinophilic gastritis[43, 55]

Tuberculosis[43, 88]

Syphilis[43, 88]

Histoplasmasis and other fungal disorders[43, 45, 88]

Aberrant pancreatic tissue[43]

Bezoars[35, 43]

Blood clot[35]

has described the folds as effaceable with intragastric gas[43]. Frequently the folds have a polypoid appearance[23, 77, 123] or appear as mucosal masses[2, 103]. Antral involvement may take the form of polypoid lesions or thick folds[25, 125].

Between the large folds are sulci 1–2 cm deep into which barium may run, forming coarse septal lines, giving a spiculated appearance. These are typically seen on the greater curve and are characteristic of the disease[114]. Occasionally the appearance of barium in the sulci can mimic gastric ulcer[43, 55]. The gastric wall is frequently thickened at more than 1 cm[114]. The mucosal pattern is often normal although mucosal nodules may form circumscribed elevations which are visible radiologically[43]. Barium mixes with the copious mucus in the lumen of the stomach to give a characteristic reticulated appearance[55, 114]. The body is the usual site of involvement especially the proximal half[55]. The greater curve is nearly always markedly abnormal[31, 38 55, 106, 114, 123]. Earlier workers thought that the antrum was spared[114] but it is now realised that antral involvement is quite common[25, 86, 88, 125]. Olmstead Cooper and Madewell[106] found antral involvement in six of 13 cases. A few patients have been described with prominent duodenal folds[8, 31], and patients have been described with a malabsorption pattern on follow-through, i.e. dilation of the small intestine and flocculation of barium[100, 115].

Gastroscopy and biopsy

The earlier literature contained many descriptions of the appearance of hypertrophic gastritis as seen with the rigid gastroscope[7, 126], but few, if any, of these patients had Menetrier's disease. There are many more recent descriptions of the stomach in Menetrier's disease as viewed with fibreoptic gastroscopes.

The characteristic features described by all workers is the extremely prominent, thick, tortuous gastric folds which are usually seen in the body, but especially along the greater curve. These folds cannot be flattened by air insufflation[2, 117]. The fundus may also be involved with thick folds[25]. Thick folds[43, 90] or polyps[8, 25] may be seen when the antrum is involved. Prominent hyperaemic duodenal folds have been described[8].

The rugal configuration has been likened to the contours of the brain[43, 93]. The mucosa is dull or reddened, oedematous, and may be cobblestoned, frequently giving a nodular appearance[2, 30, 92, 117, 125], and in some areas there may be obvious polypoid lesions[17, 66, 123]. There may be patchy hyperaemic[8, 47] or haemorrhagic areas[43, 92, 157]. Superficial erosions are often seen[8, 10, 38, 43, 79, 125]. Copious viscous mucus, coating the folds or free in the gastric lumen, is a usual finding[10, 30, 125, 134, 157]. Associated features that may be seen are gastric ulcers[72], evidence of haemorrhage with adherent clot[38] and carcinoma[119].

There are no pathognomonic gastroscopic features of Menetrier's disease, so other causes of giant folds (*see Table 6.2*) cannot be excluded. Multiple endoscopic biopsies of affected areas may allow definitive diagnosis of Menetrier's disease, providing muscularis mucosa is included in the specimen. However, this can be difficult because of the thickness of the mucosa[125, 127, 130]. Endoscopic biopsies have been reported as normal[35, 117] or showing nonspecific changes[130, 134, 157]. Moreover infiltrative carcinoma could be missed. To increase the change of getting a thick enough biopsy for diagnosis and to exclude malignancy, some workers have used a suction biopsy capsule[10, 47, 69], but even this may not give a deep enough specimen in every case[10, 69, 97]. Exfoliative and brush cytology plays no part in the diagnosis of Menetrier's disease and can miss infiltrative carcinoma[2, 125].

Pathology – macroscopic

The macroscopic pathology of Menetrier's disease is well described in the reviews by Kenney, Dockerty and Waugh[75] (20 cases), Butz[23] (14 cases), Reese, Hodgson and Dockerty[114] (18 cases), and Olmstead, Cooper and Madewell[106] (13 cases). However, the description of gross appearances of the stomach in the disease by Feiber[43] has not been bettered:

> 'Hypertrophic gastritis can be recognised grossly by the large, thickened, tortuous, nodular folds of the mucosal rugae. These folds may take on a polypoid, lobular, globular or papillomatous appearance, arranged in rows in the transverse or longitudinal axis of the stomach. Not infrequently they bear a likeness to cerebral convolutions. The sulci between the folds are deep. Accurate measurements of hypertrophied rugae are technically difficult. Best estimates of the average height and width are between 0.5 and 3.5 cm. The surface may appear any shade from pink to red to violet . . . Closer inspection of the surface of a rugal fold may reveal finely or coarsely granular tissue. The coarsely granular tissue resembles warts, cobblestones or mammillations. The consistency of these rugal folds, when palpated from outside of the stomach, is soft and freely movable and gives the sensation of a bag of worms. The stomach is "boggy and heavy"'.

Polypoid lesions projecting from the folds may be seen[31, 130] which Butz[23] described as tapering, finger-like projections which are soft to touch. The mucous membrane may be up to 5 mm in thickness[114] and the gastric wall may be 40 mm thick[15]. The mucosa is congested and dusky[23] or inflamed[69] and the mucosal surface is covered with tenacious mucus[23,31]. Intramural cysts may be visible[106]. The mucosa is freely movable on the submucosa[23]. The submucosa is grossly normal[106] or oedematous and congested[23], whereas the muscularis propria and serosa appear to be normal[23, 35, 106].

In the majority of cases, the stomach is diffusely involved with the greater curve being most severely involved[23, 75, 106, 114]. However, localised 'plaques' of the disease have been reported in any part of the body or fundus[23, 35, 75, 106, 142] and the demarcation between normal and abnormal stomach is very sharp[23, 75]. However, apparently uninvolved mucosa may be thickened and have a lobulated surface[106]. Lesser curve involvement was not described in some series[75,114], but was described in others[106]. Although antral involvement was noted in two patients by Maimon, Bartlett and Humphreys[93], antral sparing was thought to be characteristic of the disorder[114]. It is now realised that the antrum is frequently involved with either large folds or polyps[15, 31, 69, 80, 106, 113, 135]. Small intestinal involvement has not been described pathologically. Gastric ulcers[69, 75, 85, 113, 114, 130, 147] and gastric carcinomas (*see* p. 164) have been seen in association with Menetrier's disease.

Pathology – microscopic

The most detailed histological descriptions are by Kenney, Dockerty and Waugh[75] (20 cases), and Butz[23] (14 cases). The most distinctive feature seen in every case is thickening of the mucosa as a result of elongation of the gastric pits and glands.

It is generally accepted that there are increased numbers of mucus-producing cells in the glands and that the glands become cystic in the middle or deep third of the mucosa. These mucous cells and cysts may contain PAS positive material[64, 130]. These cysts are thought to be the cardinal diagnostic histological feature of Menetrier's disease[23]. The glands may be straight with some terminal tortuosity[23] or branched and very tortuous[28]. Although Butz[23] reports hyperplasia and hypertrophy of the mucus elements in the glands, most authors conclude that the glandular elongation is due to hyperplasia of mucus-producing cells[23, 28, 31, 35, 64, 106, 108, 113, 130, 154]. Butz[23] felt that mucous cell hyperplasia was most marked in areas of the stomach which did not produce acid. Most workers describe relative or absolute paucity of parietal and peptic cells with replacement by mucous cells[35, 93, 113, 117, 130], but a few have reported normal parietal and peptic cells in the glands[75, 114] which are in normal proportion to each other and to mucous cells[114, 142]. It is possible that parietal and peptic cells may undergo metaplasia to mucus-producing cells[113]. The mucosal cells may be normal or may show intestinal metaplasia[23, 31, 35, 93, 113, 117]. Frank intestinal metaplasia seems to occur more in areas where there is inflammatory infiltration[154]. Mild inflammatory cell infiltration of the mucosa is often seen in the epithelium and lamina propria. It may consist of lymphocytes[28, 35, 113], neutrophils[23, 35, 75, 113], plasma cells[23, 28, 31, 75, 113] or eosinophils[28, 31, 135]. Cell infiltration may be very patchy[106] and neutrophils may be seen in the crypts[23]. Mucosal erosions are quite often seen[23, 93, 113]. Noncaseating granulomas have been described in the mucous membrane in two cases[47, 113].

The lamina propria, apart from the cellular infiltrate, may be oedematous[23, 117]. A characteristic and important feature is the penetration of the muscularis mucosa by elongated glands which may balloon out into the submucosa[23, 35, 39, 53, 75, 93]. It is not a reliable diagnostic sign as it may be absent; for example it was not reported in any of 18 cases in one series[114]. The penetration by the glands can lead to fragmentation of muscularis mucosa and can be misdiagnosed as malignancy[29, 35, 68]. The muscularis may also be thickened, oedematous, and infiltrated with chronic inflammatory cells[23, 75]. A further characteristic feature, which is not always seen, is smooth muscle fibres extending from the muscularis into the lamina propria and to the apices of the gastric glands[15, 23, 35, 68, 75]. The core of the thick folds seen macroscopically consists of oedematous or minimally fibrotic submucosa carrying blood vessels covered with thickened muscularis mucosa[23, 106]. The submucosa is usually oedematous with dilated blood vessels or lymphatics[23, 28, 75, 113]. The muscularis propria and the serosa are normal[23]. Adjacent lymph nodes may show reactive hyperplasia[43]. Antral mucosa may be normal or show typical histological changes of Menetrier's disease[106]. If polyps are present in the antrum, they consist of mucus-producing epithelium on small smooth muscle stalks[31]. One case has been reported with atrophic gastritis of the antrum in association with Menetrier's disease of the gastric body[93]. Atrophic gastritis has also been described as an end stage of Menetrier's disease[8, 47, 79], in the fundus in association with Menetrier's disease and an adenocarcinoma[30], and overlying thick folds in the gastric body itself[69].

Small intestinal histology obtained by peroral jejunal biopsy from patients with the disease is usually normal[6, 10, 54, 130, 157] although there is one report of oedema of the jejunal lamina propria, with dilated submucosal lymphatics; similar changes were seen in this patient's rectal biopsy[27].

In conclusion, the diagnosis of Menetrier's disease should be made only when the typical histology has been demonstrated on an adequate gastric biopsy, i.e. one that includes muscularis mucosa. The diagnostic features of the disorder which should always be seen are elongated gastric pits and glands due to mucous cell hyperplasia which leads to an increase in mucosal thickness. The glands may become cystic in the middle or lower thirds. Other important diagnostic features which are not seen in every case are penetration of the musclaris mucosa by the gastric glands, and smooth muscle fibres passing from the muscularis mucosa to the apices of the gastric glands.

Electron microscopy

Only two papers have reported the ultrastructure of the gastric mucosa in Menetrier's disease[17, 26]. A few abnormalities were reported. Great numbers of secretory vacuoles were present in the mucus-producing cells, ranging from 0.8 to 1.5 µm in diameter[26]. In these cells the mitochondria were numerous and the Golgi apparatus was abundant. The intercellular spaces were dilated[17] and a striking feature was intense micropinocytosis of the endothelial cells of the capillaries underneath the mucus-producing cells which Chambourlier *et al.*[26] postulated might be one mechanism involved in protein loss. Parietal cells were noted to be not very numerous in the glands, but were ultrastructurally normal[17].

Histochemistry

There is only one detailed histochemical study of the gastric mucosa in Menetrier's disease[17]. However, many groups have noticed that the simple mucous cells of the surface and glands as well as the gland cysts themselves, contain a large amount of PAS positive material which is neutral mucin[17, 26, 64, 89, 130]. The superficial epithelial cells contain no sialated or sulphated mucin but the isthmus cells can produce sialated mucin[17], whereas the gland cells produce a little sulphated mucin[17, 26]. Droplets have been described in the superficial epithelial cells in the fundus and antrum in one case[89]. These droplets were either empty or contained protein, mainly plasma protein but possibly some haemoglobin as well.

Brocheriou *et al.*[17] have studied histochemically the distribution and activities of various enzymes in the gastric mucosa of one patient. Those studied were alkaline and acid phosphatase; adenosinetriphosphatase; malate, isocitrate, lactate, succinate, UDPG, β-hydroxybutyrate, glucose 6-phosphate, and 6-phosphogluconate dehydrogenases; nonspecific esterase; NAD and NADPH. All enzymes, with the exception of adenosinetriphosphatase and alkaline phosphatase, were present in the surface and glandular mucosal cells and in the parietal cells. However, the activities of enzymes in the surface mucosal cells were less marked then in the glandular mucosal cells, with the exception of the Krebs cycle enzymes, malate and isocitrate dehydrogenases, whose activities were more marked. The parietal cells stained very strongly for the phosphogluconate pathway enzymes, glucose 6-phosphate and 6-phosphogluconate dehydrogenases. Alkaline phosphatase and adenosinetriphosphatase activities were seen only in the base of the mucosal cells and in the capillary endothelial cells in the lamina propria. The significance of these histochemical findings in terms of pathogenesis of the disorder is unclear and more study of the intracellular enzymes of the gastric mucosa is required.

Immunofluorescent microscopy

There is only one study on the immunoglobulin-containing cells in the gastric mucosa[59]. Using monospecific fluorescent antisera, the areas of IgG and IgA-containing cells in gastric fundus biopsies from six patients were within normal limits but the areas of IgM-containing cells were significantly increased. There was no correlation between serum levels and tissue amounts of IgM. Antral biopsies from three patients were studied showing normal amounts of IgG and IgA-containing cells. In one biopsy, the area of IgM-containing cells was increased, whereas the areas of IgM cells were normal in the other two biopsies. On the basis of these finding a role for IgM in the pathogenesis of the disorder has been suggested.

Cell turnover

Only two studies on the cell turnover in the gastric mucosa of Menetrier's disease have been published. Hansen *et al.*[59] studied four patients measuring DNA synthesis by labelling antral and fundal mucosa *in vitro* with tritiated thymidine and preparing autoradiographs. Labelled cells were found mainly in the lower part of the gastric foveoli and in the isthmus of the gastric glands. They found that the percentage of labelled cells in the fundal and antral mucosa was higher in the cases of Menetrier's disease than in normal controls. The percentage of labelled cells was considered to be approximately proportional to the growth rate of the cell population assuming a similar duration of DNA-synthetic phase in the patients studied. However, the differences were not statistically significant. This aspect of the paper is confusing because in the discussion it was concluded that in two of the patients the epithelial proliferation rate was normal, which was at variance with statements in the results section. Unfortunately, their control data were not published to allow the reader to make his own conclusion. There is one other piece of evidence suggesting an increased epithelial cell proliferation rate in the gastric foveoli in Menetrier's disease. Castrup[24] found the tritiated thymidine uptake of epithelial cells in the fundal mucosa from one patient with Menetrier's disease was 2.5 times normal compared to 1.6 and 1.75 times normal in Zollinger-Ellison syndrome and atrophic gastritis respectively. The time between epithelial cell mitoses in Menetrier's disease was one third the length of time in normals. He concluded that the epithelial cell hyperproliferation which occurred might lead to an increased risk of gastric carcinoma (*see* p. 164).

Clearly further work on the kinetics of the epithelial cells in Menetrier's disease is needed. However, the direct evidence, such as it is, taken with the histological appearance of the mucosa suggests that the rate of epithelial cell proliferation is increased in the disorder.

Gastric function

It might be predicted that the gross derangement of mucosal structure seen in Menetrier's disease would be accompanied by altered gastric function. The decrease in specialised parietal cells and increase in mucus-secreting cells may account for the gastric hyposecretion[27] and increase mucus secretion[17,38] most often described. The situation is complicated by a dramatic change in gastric permeability so that back diffusion of H^+ ions occurs and secreted H^+ ions are neutralised by mucus and exudative protein accentuating apparent hypochlorhydria[8]. Altered mucosal permeability to protein probably explains the excess gastric protein loss and may explain the finding of circulating antibodies to dietary antigens[8] which presumably have crossed the gastric mucosal barrier, normally the 'tightest' epithelium in the gastrointestinal tract[33]. It is clear that the mucosal hypertrophy and hyperplasia, acid hyposecretion and excess protein loss characteristic of Menetrier's distinguish it from the mucosal hypertrophy, hyperplasia, acid hypersecretion and absence of gastric protein loss of hypertrophic, hypersecretory gastropathy (HHG)[138] itself distinct from the Zollinger-Ellison syndrome. However, several cases[43, 93, 107] appear to have features of both disorders and have been labelled hypertrophic, hypersecretory, protein-losing gastropathy (HHPG)[18, 107] and predictably hyperplasia of all gastric epithelial cell types was present at autopsy. Thus, while the Zollinger-Ellison syndrome is characterized by hyperplasia in response to gastrin from a G cell tumour or antral G cell hyperplasia, HHPG, HHG and Menetrier's disease probably represent a spectrum of disorders resulting from hyperplasia or mixed hyperplasia and hypoplasia of gastric epithelial cells in response to unknown stimuli. The functional expression of the altered cell populations probably account for the clinical and pathophysiological differences between these disorders. Since the morphological picture may change with time (viz. progression of Menetrier's disease to chronic atrophic gastritis), so complete achlorhydria and a reduction of protein loss may develop in some patients.

Gastric acid secretion

Among 120 cases (approximately 100 pre-1970) reviewed by Scharschmidt[125] approximately one-half had acid-secretion studies and in three-quarters of these, acid production was diminished or absent. In approximately 100 cases reviewed by the authors (all since 1970) seventy had acid-secretory studies usually consisting of basal acid output (BAO) and maximal acid output (MAO) (histamine, histalog, pentagastrin etc.) determinations. Achlorhydria was present in 22, hypochlorhydria in 33, normochlorhydria in 13 and there were two cases of HHPG[18, 107]. Those patients with hypochlorhydria often had negligible BAO but some response to stimulation. Total volumes of gastric fluid were normal[69] or increased[130, 157] but were most often not reported. Corrections for acid back-diffusion as recommended by Sanner, Saltzman and Mueller[123] on the basis of methodology devised by Ivey and Clifton[65] were rarely performed. In a single case[157] prednisolone therapy (60 mg for 3 weeks, 20 mg for 6 months) increased BAO from 0 to 4.5 mmol/h; MAO from 1 to 16.08 mmol/h and reduced basal volume from 195 to 60 ml/h. In the six paediatric cases reported by Burns and Gay[22], there is no mention of gastric acid nor was it measured in the 'reversible' cases of Menetrier's disease reported by Lesser *et al.*[88] and Jarnum and Jensen[66] or in those with clinical remission, or eventual development of atrophic gastritis[8, 47]. There is in fact one child on record with achlorhydria[36]. Thus, normal low or absent acid secretion may be found in Menetrier's disease, but the hypoacidity may be more apparent than real.

The natural history of acid secretory function has not been adequately studied but high-dose steroid therapy may increase acid production (or decrease back-diffusion) and the ultimate development of chronic atrophic gastritis finally establish achlorhydria. The mechanism of acid hyposecretion after correction for buffering by protein and back-diffusion is probably related to the decreased parietal cell numbers though this has not been established experimentally. However, among 20 reports where serum gastrin levels have been measured (since 1970), normal levels were reported in half and elevated levels in half, suggesting no failure of endocrine drive for acid secretion, or for that matter for trophic effects on parietal cells. In one case[8] previously elevated serum gastrin became normal with progression of the disease to involve the antrum, suggesting that the conditions necessary for elevated serum gastrin are reduced acid secretion and antral-sparing by the disease (compare pernicious anaemia).

Though references to acid secretion are numerous, scant attention has paid to pepsin, though uropepsin excretion was reported to be increased in association with histamine-fast achlorhydria in two patients[27].

Gastric protein loss

It is of considerable historical interest and importance that the elucidation of the mechanism of hypoproteinaemia in Menetrier's disease by Citrin, Sterling and Halsted[31] was the first demonstration of gastrointestinal protein loss as the cause of hypercatabolism of serum proteins without urinary protein loss (idiopathic hypercatabolic hypoproteinaemia). They used[131]I-albumin administered intravenously and found an increased rate of albumin turnover with considerable protein-bound radioactivity in aspirated gastric juice implicating the stomach as the site of excessive protein loss. This important observation led to similar studies of gastrointestinal protein loss in a variety of intestinal disorders now collectively termed protein-losing enteropathies[150, 152]. Among 120 cases (1919–73) reviewed by Scharschmidt[125] serum albumin was measured in 60 cases and was below 3.5 g/100 ml in 80 per cent (average 2.8; range 1.3–5.8). Similar levels and ranges have been reported in the 100 or so cases in the 1970–80 literature. There is general agreement that the half-life of serum albumin is reduced, that protein content of gastric juice is increased and that serum albumin returns to normal following gastrectomy. Electrophoresis of gastric juice in Menetrier's disease[51, 73] showed not only an increased albumin but also large globulin peaks suggesting a nonselective protein loss.

More than 20 studies of radioactively labelled protein turnover or loss in some 55 patients have been reported using a variety of different isotopic forms (iodine-125, iodine-131, chromium-51) of albumin, other proteins like ^{125}I-labelled fibrinogen, transferrin and immunoglobulins (IgG or IgM) or inert polymers such as ^{131}I-polyvinylpyrrolidone (PVP) and ^{59}Fe-dextran. Several of these studies are worthy of mention. Riegel, Del Vecchio and Gillson[117] (one case) demonstrated an albumin half-life of 4 days (normal: 15–30), gastric protein loss of 0.57 g/12 hours, but maintenance of normal serum proteins except for low caeruloplasmin. Jarnum and Jensen[66] (10 cases) measured the plasma turnover of albumin, transferrin, IgG and IgM and found normal or slightly increased synthetic rates and increased fractional catabolic rates (FCR) (per cent intravascular pool catabolised per day) which were equivalent for albumin, transferrin and IgG, confirming nonselective losses but a disproportionally higher FCR for IgM. This last was only partly explained by gastric IgM loss and suggested possible involvement of IgM antibodies in the pathogenesis of the disorder. Jones et al.[69] studied albumin metabolism in five patients with mild disease and normal serum albumins. FCR was increased in four out of five and was reduced by subtotal gastrectomy in two. Scott et al.[130], using ^{131}I-labelled albumin, showed increased albumin turnover, decreased half-life of 4.2 days (N: 14–23); using ^{51}Cr-labelled albumin, the total ^{51}Cr recovery in stool was 53 per cent in 96 hours

(N: 1–2 per cent) and there was a four-fold increase increase in gastric protein concentrations, to 8 mg/ml (N < 2 mg/ml). Hansen *et al.*[59] using ^{59}Fe-labelled iron dextran, ^{131}I-labelled albumin and IgG showed in six patients, ^{59}Fe clearances of 2.4 to 8.9 per cent of intravascular pool per day (N: 0.8 per cent) and increased FCRs for albumin, range 13–22 (N: 7–10 per cent per day) and IgG, range 12–20 (N: 4–10 per cent per day). These studies illustrate the essential abnormalities in protein metabolism characteristic of Menetrier's disease viz: normal or reduced serum albumin, increased FCR of plasma albumin and other plasma proteins, normal or increased synthesis of plasma proteins, increased protein concentration in gastric juice (nonselective) and increased recovery of ^{51}Cr in faeces after intravenous administration of ^{51}Cr-labelled albumin. The different tests described above, though all concerned with demonstrating protein loss into the gut do not all give the same information. The simplest test for protein-losing enteropathy is the i.v. [51]Cr albumin test with faecal counting of excreted ^{51}Cr over 96 hours. This test is abnormal in all reported cases of Menetrier's (where measured) with values usually in the range of 6–50 per cent (N: 1–2 per cent), but of course does not confirm that the stomach is the site of gastrointestinal protein loss, unless gastric aspiration with ^{51}Cr counting is performed. In clinical practice, however, the clinical and morphological features of Menetrier's disease in the stomach, a total protein determination on gastric juice with or without electrophoresis and an i.v. [51]Cr test will suffice. The ^{51}Cr test can be repeated at intervals to assess response to therapy or spontaneous fluctuations in the disease. ^{131}I-labelled protein turnover studies are clinically less easy to perform, depend on plasma disappearance of the isotope, and once lost into the gut the ^{131}I is released by digestion, largely reabsorbed, and does not appear in stool.

Gastric perfusion to measure protein loss is a research investigation but is particularly useful when comparing the effects of therapeutic agents on gastric protein loss. Thus, Brassinne[14] measured gastric albumin clearance in normal subjects (11 per cent daily degradation/ day), and in patients with gastric or duodenal ulcers (11 per cent) pernicious anaemia (21 per cent) and Menetrier's disease (27 per cent), using careful corrections for losses due to digestion, haemorrhage and pyloric emptying. He found protein loss to be independent of the rate of gastric acid secretion, an observation confirmed by Berenson, Sannella and Freston[8]. Russell *et al.*[121] showed that gastric clearance (ml plasma/24h) of ^{51}Cr-albumin was reduced from 144 to 25 by trimethaphan, to 48 by atropine, and to 41 by vagotomy. Krag *et al.*[81] demonstrated a five-fold reduction in albumin and IgA secretion in response to cimetidine using a gastric perfusion technique. While direct perfusion techniques are particularly valuable in assessing the value of drugs, they are not essential; for instance high-dose prednisolone therapy, in one patient[157] reduced ^{59}Fe-dextran faecal plasma clearance from 7.6 to 1.8 (N: 1.0 per cent plasma volume per day) and ^{125}I-labelled albumin degradation from 0.31 to 0.14 (N: 0.1 g/kg per day), while serum albumin rose from 1.7 to 3.8 (N: >3.6 g per cent).

All these studies indicate the site, magnitude and degree of selectivity of the protein loss in Menetrier's disease but provide no information as to the mechanism of protein loss.

Mechanisms of increased gastric protein loss

Inflammatory conditions of the GI tract are associated with the production of a protein-rich exudate, containing plasma albumin and globulins which gain access to the inflammatory site because of increased capillary permeability, and enter the gut lumen through areas of mucosal ulceration. This mechanism probably accounts for the protein loss in simple gastric ulcer or carcinoma[151]. In Menetrier's disease the degree of inflammation as assessed by the number of inflammatory cells in the lamina propria is variable but may be minimal and ulceration is not usually present[35, 106]. Loss of protein into the gut also occurs when there are abnormalities of lymphatics[150] (hypoplasia, ectasia or passive congestion) *but* such abnormalities are not features of Menetrier's disease though lymph node enlargement and lymphatic hyperplasia have been reported[93]. Mucus contains various glycoproteins and such mucus secretion accounts for some of the protein loss in the disorder[64]; but this does not explain the nonselective loss of plasma proteins into the gastric lumen.

The normal gastric mucosal barrier shows restrictive permeability to luminal acid and dietary substances and prevents the loss of plasma constituents into the lumen[33]. The passive permeability properties of the gastric epithelium are altered in Menetrier's disease. Gastric perfusion studies, using tubes with electrodes to measure mucosal potential differences (PD) have shown a reduced PD and increased lumen to plasma flux of ^{58}Co-labelled vitamin B_{12}[81] suggesting more permeable (or 'leaky') tight junctions between gastric epithelial cells. This increased permeability was reflected in high albumin and IgA accumulation rates in perfusion fluid. All these changes were restored towards normal by cimetidine, suggesting that H_2-receptor blockade has either a direct effect on mucosal permeability or an indirect effect via reduction in H^+ ion production. Unfortunately, there have been no studies using radiolabelled molecular probes and autoradiography to visualize the route taken by macromolecules across the mucosa so the tight junction theory has not been confirmed. Other drugs, such as trimethaphan, atropine[121] and tranexamic acid[77], which reduce protein loss, and procedures such as vagotomy may or may not influence mucosal permeability, but could reduce protein loss simply by an effect on mucosal blood flow or capillary permeability. The increased plasminogen activation demonstrated in gastric mucosal biopsies in Menetrier's disease by Kondo et al.[77,78] might be the basis of a pathogenetic mechanism implicating increased vascular permeability, but the effect of plasmin on epithelial cell permeability has not been studied.

The increased gastric mucosal permeability probably allows absorption of dietary antigens[8] and explains the finding of circulating antibodies to milk, gliadin and bovine serum albumin. Similar mechanisms have been postulated in aphthous stomatitis, coeliac disease and colitis[76]. The fact that in Menetrier's disease, progression to atrophic gastritis with infiltration of lymphocytes and plasma cells results in a reduction in protein loss and disappearance of food antibodies, emphasizes that the altered permeability of the gastric mucosa in Menetrier's disease is related to the morphology of this condition. In this respect, dilated intracellular spaces (between mucin-producing cells) with intense micropinocytosis by capillary endothelial cells underneath the epithelium reported by Brocheriou[17] might explain the altered permeability.

Endocrine function

Plasma gastrin levels may be elevated[8, 38, 44, 115, 123, 130] or normal[26, 44, 59, 90, 121, 134] in Menetrier's disease. By and large, hypochlorhydria with the disease sparing the antrum[38] is associated with hypergastrinaemia, and when the antrum is involved gastrin levels are normal. It has been suggested that the reduction in parietal and chief cell numbers may be due to resistance to the trophic effects of gastrin but this is purely conjectural. On the other hand, the hyperplasia of epithelial cells other than parietal and chief cells could reflect a mucosal response to a trophic hormone other than gastrin. In spite of this attractive theory, plasma levels of thyroid hormones, aldosterone, cortisol, insulin, ACTH, growth hormone, calcitonin and parathormone[26] and of VIP, GIP, motilin, PP (Chadwick and coworkers unpublished observation) were all within the normal range, and associated endocrine disorders or similar gastric mucosal changes in endocrine disorders have not been reported. The very rare reports of endocrine adenomas in association with Menetrier's disease[73, 158] must be viewed with suspicion since few clinical details are available.

Intrinsic factor secretion and vitamin B_{12} absorption

It is surprising that so little attention has been paid to the problem of intrinsic factor secretion and vitamin B_{12} absorption in Menetrier's disease. Frank[47] performed serial standard Schilling tests in a single patient studied from 1959 (absorption 24 per cent) through 1962 (10 per cent) and 1963 (13 per cent) until the spontaneous development of atrophic gastritis in 1966 (1.3 per cent increasing to 13.1 per cent with intrinsic factor). This single study suggested that intrinsic factor secretion was adequately maintained even though acid secretion was markedly reduced (BAO 0.36 mmol/h; MAO 0.95 mmol/h) early in the course of this patient's illness. An alternative explanation, based on the observation by Krag *et al.*[81] that the gastric mucosa in Menetrier's disease is four to five times more permeable to B_{12} than normal, would be that gastric absorption of B_{12} (non-IF dependent) might be increased in this condition, thus masking a true intrinsic factor deficiency. In any event, a normal Schilling test in one patient was reported by Chambourlier *et al.*[26] who detected intrinsic factor in stimulated but not basal gastric juice, and normal serum B_{12} levels in patients were reported by Winney, Gilmour and Matthews[157], Berenson, Sannella and Freston[8] and Cooper and Chadwick (unpublished observations). Intrinsic factor antibodies were measured only by Frank and Kern[47] and were negative. There are no reports of vitamin B_{12} deficiency states in association with Menetrier's disease[100].

Gastrointestinal blood loss and iron deficiency

In Menetrier's disease significant anaemia is unusual, but biochemical evidence of iron deficiency is more frequent[125]. Faecal occult bloods were positive in 27 out of 48 cases reported since 1970, and frank gastrointestinal bleeding was reported in nine patients. Dickinson and Axon[38] reported a single patient who presented with melaena, and Mahmood, Ali and Nash[92] described a patient who died from a massive gastric haemorrhage. Dramatic haemorrhage may thus occur but is very unusual. A friable haemorrhagic gastric mucosa[157] or a diffuse superficial erosive gastritis[38] may be seen at gastroscopy; on the other hand the finding of hyperaemic folds only[47] is more characteristic. It is not surprising that blood may be found in aspirated gastric juice[26]. Iron deficiency with a low serum iron may represent non-haem iron loss and may be resistant to iron replacement therapy[132].

Absorption and nutrition

Weight loss is seen in 60 per cent of cases at presentation and may be as great as 20 kg. Therefore, some patients are severely nutritionally compromised by the disease.

Serum proteins

Total protein was first noticed to be depressed by Harris[61] and this observation was soon confirmed by Maimon, Bartlett and Humphreys[93] and Balfour *et al.*[3]. It is now realized that most of this depression is due to a low level of serum albumin although globulin may be depressed as well. The incidence of depressed serum albumin in the disorder is 70 per cent[66] or 80 per cent[125]. Protein loss from the stomach and protein turnover have been discussed earlier.

Faecal fat excretion

The faecal fat excretion has been normal in most of the cases studied[3, 6, 47, 54, 73, 117, 121, 157]. However, one alcoholic with Menetrier's disease has been shown to have a modest elevation of faecal fat excretion at 10 g/day[6]. Another patient with Menetrier's disease was found to have steatorrhoea secondary to chronic pancreatitis which was corrected by replacement therapy[115].

Xylose absorption

All but one of the few cases studied have had normal xylose absorption[6, 10, 26, 27, 130, 157]. There is one case on record with reduced xylose absorption[117].

Glucose absorption

Apart from those patients with diabetes mellitus (*see* p. 167), patients with Menetrier's disease have a normal glucose tolerance test[10, 157].

Serum folate

Serum folate levels have been measured only in seven cases. In two the levels were normal[157] (Cooper and Chadwick, unpublished observation), and in five the level was low[6, 147]. It is not immediately apparent why this should be so. Belaiche *et al.*[6] provided evidence of folate loss from the stomach in their own four cases, but it would be expected that the folate is reabsorbed from the small intestine. However, all four patients were chronic alcoholics and folate malabsorption has been described in this group of patients[57].

Calcium metabolism

One patient had a low serum calcium which recovered after total gastrectomy[26], and one alcoholic patient had evidence of calcium malabsorption whereas three other alcoholic patients had normal calcium absorption[6]. No biochemical, histological or radiological osteomalacia has ever been described.

Other haemological and biochemical tests

Haemoglobin is frequently depressed due to blood loss and iron deficiency (*see* p. 161) and the red cell indices and the blood film may reflect this. The white cell count is usually normal but may be elevated with a polymorphonuclear leucocytosis[17, 43]. An eosinophilic leucocytosis up to 12 per cent is not uncommon[15, 26, 28, 31, 47, 79]. The platelet count and ESR when measured have been normal.

Liver function tests, apart from serum proteins, have been normal except for two cases with an elevated aspartate aminotransferase at presentation[17] (Cooper and Chadwick, unpublished observation). The authors' own case also had an elevated alkaline phosphatase at presentation but these liver enzyme abnormalities settled over the course of the illness. There is no information available on levels of other vitamins or trace elements in the blood.

Clinical features and natural history

Age of onset

Menetrier's disease can present in childhood (*see* p. 163) or, more commonly, in adult life. In adults the sex incidence is approximately three males to one female[43, 125]. In adults the age of presentation ranges from 20 to 77 years[43]. Reviews of 50 cases[43] and 120 cases[125] respectively from the literature concluded that the peak incidence was in the fourth, fifth and sixth decades. However, in females the peak incidence is in the fourth decade whereas in males it is in the sixth decade[125].

Genetic aspects

Nothing is known about any hereditary basis for the disease. There is no evidence for an increased incidence of the disorder among relatives of affected individuals although there is one report of possible Menetrier's disease in a set of twins[25]. The nature of the disorder makes any form of inherited abnormality unlikely. In the one patient reported, the chromosome count was normal and the HLA groups were A2, A24, B12 and B13[26].

Racial aspects

The disease has been described in white Caucasians from all parts of Europe and North America, in American negroes and in Japanese.

Indeed, it has been claimed that Menetrier's disease is very common among Japanese[141]. This racial mix probably represents areas of developed medical services rather than any inherent racial predisposition.

Onset and clinical features

The onset of the disorder is usually insidious and gradual although occasionally it is more acute. There is usually no precipitating factor although a number of cases have been reported whose symptoms have closely followed an episode of apparent hypersensitivity to foods or drugs[47, 86, 88, 130].

The clinical picture is summarised by Feiber in his review of 50 published cases[43]. Later cases have not radically altered this picture. He found that the most important symptoms were epigastric pain, 74 per cent; weight loss, 60 per cent; and vomiting, 40 per cent. The average duration of symptoms to diagnosis was two years[43] with a range of one week[92] to more than 20 years[23, 135].

The epigastric pain is variable in intensity and duration and may be described as burning, pressing, cramping or stabbing. It is frequently dyspeptic, following 1–2 hours after food, and may be relieved by food or alkalies. Anorexia is very common and weight loss averages about 6 kg[43] although weight loss may on occasions be excessive, exceeding 20 kg[47, 61]. A more recent review found weight loss in only 30 per cent of a series of 120 published cases[125]. Vomiting is usually associated with nausea and may produce blood. Some evidence of gastric blood loss may be seen in 20 per cent[43], but severe gastrointestinal haemorrhage is unusual although it may be a presenting complaint[19, 38, 92, 155]. One important symptom not stressed by Feiber was oedema. It is reported as a symptom on presentation in up to 40 per cent of cases reported since 1965 and may even be the sole complaint[26, 103, 130, 135, 157]. Diarrhoea is not uncommon and was a complaint at presentation in almost 20 per cent of cases reported since 1965. The stools are usually unremarkable but may show melaena[43]. However, in one case, large amounts of mucus were passed per rectum[117]. More unusual complaints at presentation were postcoital pain[69] and heartburn with chest pain[72]. Refractory iron deficiency anaemia has been the sole presenting complaint in one case[132]. The commonest sign is localized epigastric tenderness[43]. Peripheral oedema may be demonstrable in up to 25 per cent of cases[125]. A few patients may have ascites[30, 54, 77] or a pleural effusion[30]. More unusual signs are cervical lymphadenopathy[54] koilonychia[41], epigastric mass[53, 56] and finger clubbing[21, 32].

Natural history

Scharschmidt[125] in his review of 120 published cases found that about two-thirds of patients underwent some form of gastric resection for symptoms and/or cancer risk. The great majority of patients who did not undergo resection continued to have symptoms. The longest follow-up of any patient so far reported, was 16 years and this man had symptoms over this time until his death from hepatic cell carcinoma[125]. However, some cases do appear to have remissions and relapses over short periods of time with no change in the appearance of the stomach radiologically[72, 141]. Progression of the disorder to previously uninvolved areas of the stomach while the patient is under observation has been reported[30, 43, 52]. The very long history of some patients before diagnosis[23, 135] illustrates the potential chronicity of the disorder.

Well-documented cases of spontaneous remission have been reported. Frank and Kern[47] reported a case which was followed up for 5 years with no relief in symptoms, after which the barium meal appearance started to improve. Over the next 3 years the gastric mucosa changed to atrophic gastritis with relief of symptoms, the appearance of intrinsic factor deficiency and the disappearance of gastric protein loss. Berenson, Sannella and Freston[8] reported a case who was followed up for 4 years after the diagnosis. However, from 12 to 18 months after diagnosis, she developed atrophic gastritis with symptomatic improvement, disappearance of gastric protein loss, decreased serum gastrin, and slightly increased gastric acid output. Berman and Spiegel[10] reported a case whose symptoms and gastric protein loss disappeared over the 5 months after diagnosis but the barium meal still showed prominent gastric folds. Others have reported cases of transient Menetrier's disease; Jarnum and Jenson[66] reported three cases but provided no clinical details. Lesser *et al.*[88] reported a case of rapid onset but well-documented Menetrier's disease with gastrointestinal protein loss, who was well 2 months after the onset of the illness with a normal serum albumin and a marked improvement in the size of her gastric folds. At 4 months, she had virtually normal gastrointestinal protein loss. However, none of these transient cases had gastric biopsies after recovery. As will be discussed later, some of the therapeutic responses claimed for certain drugs may well be explicable by spontaneous remission of the disorder.

Menetrier's disease in children

Degnan[36] reported the first case of Menetrier's disease in childhood although he did not recognise it as such. The patient, a 3-year-old negro boy, was admitted with a week's history of abdominal swelling and anorexia. He had peripheral oedema, peripheral blood eosinophilia, hypoalbuminaemia and large gastric folds on barium meal. He was asymptomatic with normal serum proteins 19 days later.

Since then 12 more cases have been recorded[11, 22, 62, 71, 84, 87, 104, 111, 122, 129]. The original case illustrated the important features seen in most of the cases, namely the male preponderance, the short history, the oedema at presentation, the peripheral blood eosinophilia, and the self-limiting nature of the disorder. As in adult Menetrier's disease, most of the cases, 10, were male. The age of onset ranged from 3 to 14 years (mean 5½ years) and the length of the histories varied from 1–12 weeks (mean 3¾ weeks). The onset was acute and the common symptoms were nausea and vomiting in 10 cases, peripheral oedema in 10, and abdominal pain in seven. Other symptoms were anorexia, diarrhoea and listlessness, and evidence of gastrointestinal bleeding was seen in three cases[11, 84, 104]. Oedema was the commonest sign and both pleural effusions[87, 111] and ascites[84, 122] were seen. In 12 cases laboratory data were available, showing anaemia in six, peripheral blood eosinophilia in 11, and hypoalbuminaemia in 10. Excessive gastrointestinal protein loss[11, 104, 111] and achlorhydria[36] have been demonstrated. The barium meal appearances were the same as those in adult Menetrier's disease[71] and although the antrum was usually spared, antral involvement does occur[129]. The histology of the stomach was similar to that seen in adult Menetrier's disease[11, 62, 71, 84, 87, 104, 111].

As in adults the duodenal folds can be prominent radiologically[111]. Small intestinal structure and function were normal as shown by a normal jejunal biopsy[87], xylose tolerance test[87] and faecal fat excretion[129].

In nine of the reported cases the disease underwent spontaneous resolution with rapid loss of symptoms, normal serum proteins and a normal barium meal appearance in 16 days to 6 months after presentation (mean 2½ months). The permanent nature of the recovery was shown by Pittman who reported that his patient was perfectly well with normal serum proteins 12 years after presentation[111a]. One child failed to improve over one year's follow-up[104] and another, while improving symptomatically at 10 days after admission, was not followed up long enough to show complete recovery (case 1 of Kadlec *et al.*[71]). The remaining two patients had gastric resections because of suspected lymphoma (case 1 of Lachmann *et al.*[84]) and because of symptoms[11]. Three of the nonresected cases had diagnostic laparotomies[84, 87, 104].

The aetiology of the childhood form of the disease is unknown. However, the sudden onset, peripheral blood eosinophilia and the usually transient nature of the illness has led to the view that it is a hypersensitivity reaction[71, 129]. Indeed, it has been suggested that it is a variety of eosinophilic gastroenteritis[131]. Cytomegalovirus has been found in the gastric mucosa of two cases leading to the proposal that the disorder has a viral aetiology[84, 87] but it seems more likely that the presence of the virus was incidental and unconnected with the Menetrier's disease.

Menetrier's disease and carcinoma of the stomach

One of Menetrier's original cases was described in association with a gastric adenocarcinoma[98]. Since that time, many reports of the association have appeared[13, 30, 40, 42, 48, 50, 93, 94, 95, 96, 99, 105, 109, 110, 119, 120, 123, 135, 136, 137, 139, 141, 143, 144, 145, 146, 149, 156]. However, there has been considerable dispute as to whether there is an increased risk of carcinoma in Menetrier's disease. Some authors claim it is a premalignant condition[4, 43, 94, 109, 135, 141] whereas others claim it is not[9, 23, 53, 114].

The dispute has arisen because many of the cases have not been shown to have the typical histology or other features of Menetrier's disease and because some workers have been sceptical about the nature of the thick folds found when Menetrier's disease and carcinoma coexist. It is well known that thick gastric folds can be caused by gastric carcinoma[9, 116] so it has been proposed that the whole clinical picture can be caused by the carcinoma alone. Indeed, it has been suggested that if Menetrier's disease is diagnosed in the presence of a gastric carcinoma then the diagnosis of Menetrier's disease is incorrect[39]. Chusid, Hirsch and Colcher[30] were the first to review the literature in an attempt to clarify the situation. They found 12 cases of carcinoma and Menetrier's disease to that date and concluded that the carcinoma risk was 8 per cent. Unfortunately, although this paper has been widely quoted, the conclusion may be misleading because the authors were rather uncritical and included some very suspect cases of Menetrier's disease[125]. Sanner, Saltzman and Mueller[123] concluded that the carcinoma risk was 21 per cent, but their paper is open to the same criticism as that of Chusid, Hirsch and Colcher[30].

The true incidence of gastric adenocarcinoma in Menetrier's disease is unknown, and likely to remain so for some time because a majority of cases of Menetrier's disease in the literature have had a gastric resection soon after diagnosis[125]. Few of the nonoperated cases have been followed up for any length of time. Because of the lingering doubts about the nature of many of the cases of coexistent Menetrier's disease and gastric carcinoma, the only cases which might shed some light on the subject are those developing carcinoma while under follow-up for well-documented Menetrier's disease. Unfortunately in many of these cases, the diagnosis of Menetrier's disease was only made on the radiological or visual appearances of the stomach[30, 93, 96, 135, 145, 156]. There are only two reports of patients developing gastric carcinoma more than a year after the diagnosis of histologically proven Menetrier's disease, the cases of van Loewenthal, Steinitz and Friedlander[149] (5½-year follow-up), and of Chusid, Hirsch and Colcher[30] (5-year follow-up). Other cases have been described, but the carcinoma was discovered within 12 months of the diagnosis of Menetrier's disease[119, 123] so the possibility of there being a carcinoma present all the time cannot entirely be excluded. If all cases of gastric carcinoma developing in known cases of Menetrier's disease, however diagnosed, are included, it has been estimated that the carcinoma risk is 10 per cent[125]. Circumstantial evidence to support this increased risk is, firstly, the observation that Menetrier's disease can end in atrophic gastritis[8, 47], which itself has a carcinoma risk of approximately 10 per cent after 10 years[133, 140]. Secondly, the gastric epithelial cell proliferation rate is increased in Menetrier's disease[24, 59] as it is in atrophic gastritis[24] and this could predispose the development of gastric carcinoma.

The possibility that some patients might have an inherited susceptibility to gastric carcinoma is raised by the report of a patient with coexistent gastric carcinoma and Menetrier's disease whose father and brother also developed carcinomas of the stomach[120]. There was no evidence that either had Menetrier's disease.

All the gastric malignancies have been adenocarcinomas with no unusual histological features. Most cases showed carcinoma in an area of Menetrier's disease but there are two reports of carcinoma in an area of the stomach away from that part of the stomach involved in the Menetrier's disease[114, 120]. Only one of the patients has been female[136]. Patients presented with carcinoma in the sixth or seventh decade, with the exception of one man presenting at the age of 46[123] and another at the age of 76[42]. Many cases were discovered as an incidental finding, but where the carcinoma followed previously diagnosed Menetrier's disease, the clinical features of the carcinoma were in no way unusual. The response to therapy and the survival of the patients appear no different from others with gastric carcinoma.

Diseases associated with Menetrier's disease

A number of other tumours as well as other diseases have been described in patients with Menetrier's disease. These associations seem likely to be fortuitous and shed no light on the nature or pathogenesis of Menetrier's disease; however, it is important to document these associations for information purposes.

Other tumours

Malignant
Individual cases of carcinoma of breast[52], cervix[121], bronchus[66], pancreatic acini[90], pancreatic islet cells[114] and hepatic cells[125] have been documented. Interestingly, the hepatoma presented with a gastric metastasis mimicking a malignant gastric ulcer. Histiocytic lymphoma of the stomach[37] and carcinoid tumour of the stomach[124] have been recorded.

Benign
Menetrier's disease has been described in patients with adenomas of large bowel[5, 23, 25, 35, 39, 52]; small intestine[54]; pancreatic islet cells[23, 75]; adrenals[23]; kidney[23]; parathyroid[75]; thyroid[26] and pituitary[75]. Kenney, Dockerty and Waugh[75] described multiple endocrine adenomas in three patients, but unfortunately no details of patients or adenomas were described.

Other diseases

Other gastrointestinal disorders apart from tumours described in patients with Menetrier's disease are hiatal hernia[35], gastric ulcer[72, 85,

[130, 147], duodenal diverticulosis[121], jejunal diverticulosis[47], ulcerative colitis[157] and chronic calcific pancreatitis[115]. Gastric obstruction has been described as a result of the prolapse of hypertrophied gastric mucosa through the pylorus[41, 85], and through the stoma after a Billroth II partial gastrectomy[25, 52]. Intussusception due to a coexistent caecal adenoma has been reported[52]. Two cases of cirrhosis without histological details have been described[11, 117].

Diabetes mellitus is an occasional finding in Menetrier's patients[11, 54, 66, 73]. One of the diabetic cases had a type II hyperlipidaemia[54]. Scharschmidt[125] has pointed out that patients with Menetrier's disease seem to have an unusually high incidence of premature cardiovascular and/or thrombotic disease.

Alcoholism is sometimes a feature of patients[6, 15, 30, 43, 92] and a few patients give a history of atopy[31, 54, 79, 80, 86].

Pathogenesis of Menetrier's disease

Though the cause of Menetrier's disease is unknown, there are many aetiological theories (*Table 6.3*). At the outset it seems prudent to consider the possibililty that the hyperplastic mucosal changes in Menetrier's disease represent a form of tissue response to a variety of different stimuli rather like the situation in atrophic gastritis, and there is no single aetiological agent or factor. Since the transition from florid

Table 6.3 Older aetiological theories (After Feiber[43])

Gastric irritants, e.g. alcohol, nicotine

Dietary indiscretions or irregular eating habits

Vitamin deficiency

Allergy

Bacteria, viruses, toxins

Neurogenic factors

Congenital abnormality

Inherited disorder

Endocrine or metabolic abnormalities

Mechanical factors

Menetrier's to atrophic gastritis is well documented, this adds credence to this hypothesis. Various models of protein-losing gastropathy may be found in the veterinary literature, some having clinical, radiological, morphological and functional similarities to Menetrier's disease. In some of these the aetiology has been established so that a brief review of these seems appropriate, before considering pathogenesis in man.

Veterinary models

An inherited form of gastric rugal hypertrophy has been reported in inbred mice[1]. Acute protein-losing gastropathy in dogs may be produced by feeding the chemical dithiothreitol[34, 101] and a similar condition in monkeys is reported following shale oil ingestion[91]. Brownstein *et al.*[20] described severe chronic hypertrophic gastritis in 14 snakes infested with *Cryptosporidium*, the disease running a protracted course with fatal outcome. Histological examination of the stomach revealed cystic hyperplasia of mucus cells with atrophy of specialized cells and developmental forms of this organism could be identified in the gastric mucosa. Infestations with Nochtia nochti in monkeys[12] and Trichostronglyus axei[70] and Haboronema megastoma[102] in horses also caused protein-losing gastropathy. Van der Gaag[148] described a 7-year-old boxer dog with protein-losing gastropathy, with clinical, radiological and histological features resembling Menetrier's disease, and van Kruiningen[83] reported four Basenji dogs with gross gastric morphology resembling Menetrier's disease but with preservation of parietal and chief cells microscopically. No aetiological agents were identified in these dogs. While it is not likely that any of these animal models really provide a clue to the aetiology of Menetrier's disease in man, they do suggest that genetic, chemical, infective and other factors can produce a gastric lesion in animals with some features resembling Menetrier's disease.

Genetic and environmental factors

Apart from concordance in a single set of twins[25] no definite genetic factors can be implicated. The unequal sex distribution (males 3 × females) in reported series may reflect other factors such as environmental exposure. Epidemiology of the condition does not help; it has been found in widely separated geographical regions, but especially where diagnostic facilities are freely available, thus introducing bias into estimation of prevalence. In the USA blacks and whites are equally affected.

Infective agents

A viral aetiology has been suggested but evidence is very limited. Cytomegalovirus was identified in the gastric mucosa of two children with Menetrier's disease[84, 87] and parainfluenza virus isolated from the nasopharynx of a 6-year-old boy 6 weeks after presentation[62]. There are no reports suggesting a viral aetiology in adults. Histoplasmosis of the stomach produce rugal hypertrophy with radiological features similar to Menetrier's but with diagnostic appearances on gastric biopsy[45]. Other infections may also produce gastric rugal hypertrophy (*see Table 6.2*).

Immunological factors

One of the most popular theories for the aetiology of Menetrier's disease is that it represents a hypersensitivity response to dietary or other antigens. In Scharschmidt's review[125], the possible relationship to hypersensitivity reactions was stressed[31, 47, 88, 130].

In the childhood form of the disease an acute onset, the presence of eosinophilia in 11 out of 13 reported cases and self-limiting course supports the 'hypersensitivity' hypothesis, and childhood Menetrier's disease has even been regarded as a variant of eosinophilic gastroenteritis[131]. In one adult case symptoms began shortly after the ingestion of crab meat[88], and the same patient was allergic to ^{51}Cr albumin. Another adult with a history of unexplained urticaria developed symptoms following ingestion of indomethacin for arthritis and these led to a diagnosis of Menetrier's disease[86]. Unfortunately, there are no reports of IgE levels or formal challenge tests, and eosinophilia is not a feature of the disease in most patients.

Hansen[59] measured the number of immunoglobulin-containing cells of different classes in the gastric mucosa from six patients with the disease. The number of IgM-producing cells was markedly increased but serum levels of IgM and other immunoglobulins and production of secretory immunoglobulins were normal. A possible role for IgM in the pathogenesis of the disorder was suggested, and the difference between Menetrier's disease and chronic atrophic gastritis where IgA and IgA plasma cell numbers are increased, was stressed. Studies of plasma immunoglobulin turnovers in 10 patients[66] showed a particularly rapid fractional catabolic rate for IgM, suggesting utilization of IgM in the gastric mucosa or loss into the gastric lumen in excess of other immunoglobulins. However, Krag[81] detected IgA, but no IgM or IgG in gastric juice from one patient, so that the mechanism of the apparent increased turnover of IgM and the significance of the increased number of IgM plasma cells in the gastric mucosa needs further evaluation. Complement studies are confined to a single case report[80], where cold activation of the classical complement pathway with asthma and eosinophilia (which persisted after gastric resection) were found.

An increased incidence of food antibodies[8] in Menetrier's disease has already been referred to, and results almost certainly from the increased gastric permeability to dietary antigens, disappearing when the disease progressed to atrophic gastritis. In one patient[8] parietal cell antibodies were initially positive, but later negative, suggesting that these were secondary to mucosal damage rather than playing a primary role in mucosal damage or progression to atrophic gastritis. Autoantibodies to DNA, smooth muscle, mitochondria and parietal cells were negative in the one patient[26], smooth muscle and intrinsic factor antibodies negative throughout the course of the disease in another[8], and parietal cell and intrinsic factor antibodies absent in another patient[47].

Gordon, Schaefer and Finkel[54] studied delayed hypersensitivity reactions to prick tests with mumps, *Candida* and BCG which showed no reactions. There are no further reports of anergy, and no *in vitro* studies of cell mediated immunity in Menetrier's disease. Granulomata were seen in the gastric mucosa obtained by suction biopsy in one patient[47] and in the surgically resected stomach from another patient[113], but are clearly the histological exception rather than the rule in this condition.

In summary, no firm conclusions can be drawn from the immunological data presented above other than the observations that the eosinophil may have a role in childhood Menetrier's disease; IgM may be important in mucosal response; increased mucosal permeability probably explains the findings of antibodies to dietary constituents; autoantibodies are uncommon and more work is required on the cellular immunology of this disorder.

Plasminogen activation

Though probably not of primary pathogenetic importance, the finding of increased plasminogen activation in gastric mucosal biopsies from patients with Menetrier's disease reported by Kondo[77,79], may be important in terms of the known effects of plasmin on vascular permeability and protein loss. The technique used by Kondo involves the preparation of three types of fibrin plates, standard, preheated (inactivated) and plates incorporating 0.1 per cent tranexamic acid as antiplasmin. Gastric mucosal biopsies are assayed on these plates by measuring the area of visible fibrinolysis developing around the biopsies as they autolyse, releasing the so-called tissue activator of plasminogen into the medium. Biopsies from normal controls produce 10–36 mm^2 of fibrinolysis on the standard plates compared to 46–120 mm^2 for biopsies from patients with Menetrier's disease. The increased fibrinolysis around patients' biopsies was inhibited by tranexamic acid. This *in vitro* test formed the basis for clinical trials of tranexamic acid (3 g daily) in patients, resulting in increased plasma albumin, reduced prominence of mucosal folds on barium meal and endoscopy (*see* p. 176 for details of therapeutic responses). Independent confirmation of the *in vitro* work and particularly of the *in vivo* responsiveness to antifibrinolytic activity is required, but for the present it remains an intriguing observation though its specificity for Menetrier's disease seems unlikely, since similar therapeutic responses are reported in Crohn's disease and lymphangiectasia[77].

Endocrine abnormalities

The increased cell turnover in the gastric mucosa of Menetrier's disease[24, 59] is reported to be greater than that in the Zollinger-Ellison syndrome[24] and it is tempting to ascribe the hyperplastic response to an unidentified endocrine abnormality. The major proliferative response would then appear to be in the mucous cell population since the proportion and number of specialized epithelial cells is often markedly reduced. The levels of gastrin and other hormones in Menetrier's disease have been discussed previously and give no indication that this disease is an endocrinopathy.

Conclusion

It seems that the hyperplastic mucosa of Menetrier's disease may be a response to either exogenous or endogenous stimuli, but the mechanism of the hyperplastic response and its relationship to the other hyperplastic disorders of the stomach remains obscure. In a single patient studied by the authors in some detail, none of the above aetiological factors could be implicated (*see* case report, p. 177).

Surgical treatment

There is widespread agreement that a full-thickness gastric biopsy obtained at laparotomy is necessary if endoscopic or suction biopsies fail to provide a firm histological diagnosis. However, the indications for gastric resection are limited to intractable symptoms, severe and persistent hypoproteinaemic oedema, bleeding, and the presence of, or a high risk of the presence of, carcinoma[43, 67, 85]. Although a majority of patients with the disease have a gastric resection[125], there has always been a view expressed that many cases, if not the majority, can be managed medically[9, 28, 100]. As evidence of spontaneous remissions and benefits from drug therapies accumulates, there is no longer justification for the view that a diagnosis of Menetrier's disease means that operation is virtually inevitable, a view that has often been expressed[4, 16, 75, 130].

Total gastrectomy

There is no doubt that total gastrectomy leads to relief of symptoms with cessation of gastric protein loss[3, 4, 23, 26, 35, 46, 53, 79, 93, 109, 113, 130, 132, 141, 155]; moreover the risk of developing a gastric carcinoma is removed[16]. Good technical results have been obtained with a Roux-en-Y oesophagojejunostomy with construction of a Hunt-Lawrence jejunal food pouch[130]. Oesophagantrostomy has been performed leaving the antrum as a food pouch[15], but as antral involvement is now well recognized[106] this operation would seem to be unwise.

Partial gastrectomy

Because of the operative mortality and morbidity as well as nutritional consequences of total gastrectomy, partial gastrectomies have been favoured in Menetrier's disease. Various types have been performed, Hofmeister[61]; Moynihan[56]; Billroth I[38, 60, 69, 113], Billroth II[52, 85, 113] and Polya[2, 69]. In many reports the type of partial gastrectomy is not specified[23, 35, 64, 68, 75, 86, 93, 109, 117]. In some instances local areas of Menetrier's disease have been excised[35]. The aim of partial gastric resection is to remove all the diseased stomach[64] and up to 80 per cent of the stomach may need to be removed[2], but this is not always technically possible so some patients have had diseased tissue in the gastric remnant[25, 56, 60, 69, 112]. In some of these patients, the remaining lesions may regress with return of serum proteins to normal[56, 60], but in others, symptoms persist and the disease progresses[25, 69], so that total gastrectomy may be indicated[25]. Another risk of leaving diseased stomach seems to be anastomotic leaks[63, 68, 117], which are probably the result of anastomoses involving diseased tissue[125]. With these risks it would seem advisable that when the removal of all diseased tissue is not possible, a total gastrectomy should be carried out. If all diseased stomach is removed by partial gastrectomy, then symptoms resolve and excessive protein loss from the stomach ceases. It has been stated that the disease will not recur if all diseased tissue has been removed[85]. However, there is one documented case of the appearance of typical Menetrier's disease in an apparently normal gastric remnant 6 years after a Billroth II gastrectomy for Menetrier's disease[52].

Results of gastric resection

Scharschmidt[125] reviewed the results of surgery in 80 patients operated on from his series of 120 cases. Twelve patients had a total gastrectomy, 67 patients had some form of partial gastrectomy, and one had an unspecified gastric resection. Follow-up information was available only for 42 partial and 10 total gastrectomy patients. There were seven postoperative deaths in the partial gastrectomy group: three due to anastomotic leak, two to generalized peritonitis, one to wound infection, intestinal obstruction and sepsis, and one to unspecified causes. There were no deaths in the total gastrectromy group, although there is a recent report of a death from pulmonary embolus following total gastrectomy for Menetrier's disease[17]. Long-term results are very difficult to assess but Scharschmidt[125] concluded that of 35 surviving partial gastrectomy patients on whom some follow-up information was available, 32 had satisfactory results and three had poor results, because of a marginal ulcer in one and recurrent symptoms in the other two, whereas of 10 surviving total gastrectomy patients, the one poor result was because of oesophagitis.

Vagotomy

As a consequence of a good short-term response to atropine, one patient had a proximal gastric vagotomy[121]. However, at 12 months after the operation, while her symptoms were better, her gastric protein loss, although reduced, was still excessive and the radiological appearances of her stomach were unchanged. One other patient had a vagotomy and pyloroplasty with no improvement in symptoms and later had a partial gastrectomy[113].

It is clear from the literature that if operation is indicated, the procedure of choice is total gastrectomy. Partial gastrectomy is a second best alternative and should be considered only if all the diseased stomach can be removed and if the anastomosis can be performed with normal gastric tissue. There seems to be no place for vagotomy in the treatment of Menetrier's disease.

Nonsurgical treatment

General measures and nutrition

Some patients may gain symptomatic relief from a bland diet and alkalies[43, 47, 90]. Nutrition is often impaired so the patient's nutritional status needs to be assessed. There is no evidence of maldigestion or malabsorption of fat or carbohydrate in most cases (*see above*), and nutrition is impaired because of a poor dietary intake secondary to gastric symptoms or because of protein loss from the stomach. While some of this protein is degraded and reabsorbed, the synthesis rate for proteins in the liver is usually already maximal, thus limiting the reutilization of the absorbed amino acids. Nevertheless, in spite of the theoretical objections, the basis of nutritional support remains a high-calorie, high-protein diet. However, patients cannot always tolerate it. Intravenous albumin infusions have been tried but while they alleviate the hypoproteinaemic oedema temporarily, they have no lasting effect on nutrition or the disease process[75]. If the patient is malnourished but unable to tolerate a high-calorie, high-protein diet, other forms of nutritional support may be indicated if the surgical option is not to be considered. Parenteral nutrition does not seem to be indicated in patients with a normal small intestine, but enteral feeding via a fine polyethylene nasojejunal tube could provide a very satisfactory alternative. Unfortunately, there are no reports of its use in Menetrier's disease in the literature to date. While nutritional support would seem to be important in the short term in an attempt to maintain the patient's nutritional status and to tide the patient over until symptoms settle, the stomach spontaneously improves, or until operation is performed, there is no evidence that high-calorie, high-protein diets alter the course of the disease[77].

Drugs

There are a number of claims that various drugs may alter the course of the disease, or diminish protein loss. However, for each report claiming benefit, there are others failing to show any effect. Virtually none of the drugs claiming to show benefit have been administered, stopped, and readministered to demonstrate improvement, relapse, and further improvement. Furthermore, many of the claims of successful drug treatment can be explained by spontaneous remission.

Anticholinergic and ganglion-blockers

Patients may gain symptomatic relief from anticholinergic drugs[43]. However, there are a number of reports of a decrease in gastric protein loss on long-term anticholinergic drugs. Gordon, Schaefer and Finkel[54] reported disappearance of oedema over 2 months and a normal serum albumin at 12 months with a decrease in gastric fold size after prolonged therapy with atropine 0.4 mg t.d.s. There was no relapse after stopping atropine. Smith and Powell[134] reported a decrease in gastric protein loss over 9 months of treatment with propantheline 105 mg per day in divided doses. The patient lost his oedema after 2 months of the therapy. There was no relapse during a follow-up period of 6 months after stopping the treatment. These authors concede that the improvement could have been due to spontaneous remission. There are other reports of success for long-term, unspecified anticholinergic drugs[25, 58, 82]. In contrast, others report no benefit with anticholinergics[77, 79] and with propantheline in particular[118]. More impressive are short-term studies which have demonstrated acute decreases in gastric protein loss with atropine[8, 82, 121]. However, Berenson's case responded only temporarily to atropine, and eventually remitted spontaneously with the development of gastric atrophy[8]. Similar acute decreases in gastric protein loss have been demonstrated with the ganglion-blockers, hexamethonium[66] and trimetaphan[121]. However, these drugs have not been used long term.

In conclusion, therefore, there is good evidence that anticholinergics can decrease gastric protein loss acutely and in the short term; however, convincing evidence of their benefit long term is not available. Nevertheless, if conservative therapy is indicated, they are worth a trial.

Fibrinolysis inhibitors

One Japanese group have reported dramatic improvements with the antiplasmin drug, tranexamic acid[77, 78, 79, 80]. The rationale for the therapy is their own observation that gastric mucosal fibrinolytic activity is increased in Menetrier's disease. They have reported seven cases in detail[77, 79]. All seven cases had increased gastric fibrinolytic activity which was inhibited *in vitro* and *in vivo* with tranexamic acid. Treatment with tranexamic acid, 3 g/day, for up to 4 months caused a rapid and persistent decrease in gastric protein loss and, in six, an improvement in gastric radiological and histological appearances. In three patients, placebo therapy for 6 weeks to 2 months, prior to tranexamic acid therapy, failed to alter the plasma proteins[79]. However, in four cases, there was no relapse on reintroduction of the placebo after successful tranexamic acid therapy[77, 79]. In one case after 15 months of tranexamic acid, during which the plasma protein improved but the stomach appearances remained unaltered, reintroduction of placebo caused a fall in plasma proteins. This patient proceeded to gastrectomy[79]. Gastric atrophy was found in the gastric biopsy of one of the patients during reintroduction of placebo after 4 months of tranexamic acid[79]. Therefore, the question must be asked whether some of these apparently successful treatments are not really the result of spontaneous remission. In the authors' own unpublished studies on one patient, they have also found increased gastric mucosal fibrinolytic activity, but a prolonged trial of tranexamic acid in this patient failed to show any benefit. It must be concluded that until others have shown the same dramatic effects as the Japanese workers, tranexamic acid remains unproved as a beneficial agent in Menetrier's disease.

Corticosteroids

There is one report of apparent benefit with large doses of prednisolone[157]. The patient, who also had ulcerative colitis, was treated with 60 mg/day reduced over 3 weeks to 20 mg/day. This dose

was continued for 6 months, after which the patient was maintained on
5–7.5 mg/day. However, improvement was slow, with normal plasma
proteins at 10 months and some improvement in gastric histology at 1
year. Others have reported no benefit with shorter courses of smaller
doses of prednisone, 15 mg/day for 5 weeks[47] and 20 mg/day for 4
weeks[54].

Cimetidine

There is one report of a decrease in gastric protein loss after 1 month's
therapy and by 4 months, the large gastric rugae had decreased in
size[81].

Irradiation

Gastric irradiation has been used in two cases of Menetrier's disease,
one with benefit[93] and one with no benefit whatsoever[3].

Case report

A 30-year-old woman was admitted to hospital on 16 September 1977.
She had first become ill while on a cruise to the Canary Islands and
now complained of malaise for 4 weeks, anorexia, nausea and
vomiting for 2 weeks and an intermittent low-grade pyrexia for 1
week. Examination revealed a thin but healthy-looking woman with a
temperature of 37.8 °C, there being no other abnormal physical signs.
Abnormal blood tests were a serum albumin of 36 g/l, alkaline
phosphatase of 54 u/l (N: 5–36) and SGOT of 122 u/l (N: 5–40). A
provisional diagnosis of resolving viral hepatitis was made and the
patient advised to rest at home.

On 31 October 1977, she was readmitted to the same hospital
complaining of persistent nausea, vomiting and fever. Serum albumin
was now 32 g/l, a barium meal revealed thickened gastric folds and
gastrosocopy showed features typical of Menetrier's disease. Over the
next 2 weeks there was rapid clinical deterioration; the serum albumin

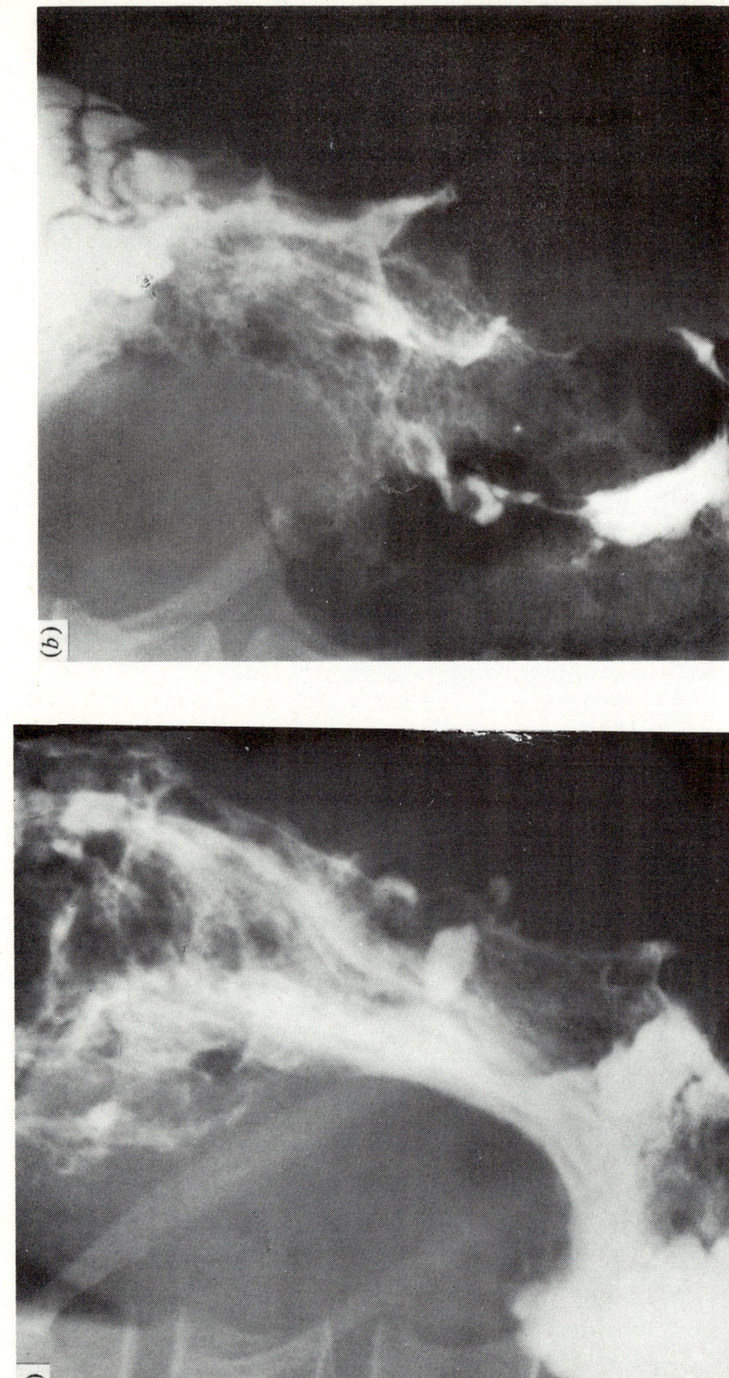

Figure 6.1a and b Barium meal showing large gastric folds some with polypoid appearance, poor coating with barium and apparent mucosal masses

fell to 22 g/l and peripheral oedema developed. Accordingly, she was transferred to Hammersmith Hospital for further assessment and consideration of gastric surgery.

The only new symptoms were moderately severe epigastric pain and weight loss of 12.7 kg (28 lb). The diagnosis was confirmed by repeat barium meal (*Figures 6.1a and b*); gastroscopy, which showed giant nondistensible gastric folds sparing the antrum, a haemorrhagic mucosa coated with tenacious mucus, and a circumferential ring of discrete polyps in the antrum; and a suction biopsy which showed typical histological features (*Figures 6.2 a, b, and c*). Gastric secretory studies showed complete achlorhydria, the pH of aspirated juice being 7. Plasma gastrin was moderately elevated at 65 pmol/l (N: less than 50). Plasma albumin was 27 g/l, IgG 4.1 g/l (N: 5–16, IgA 1.25 g/l (N: 1.25–4.25) and IgM 1.50 g/l (N: 0.5–1.80). Faecal ^{51}Cr excretion over 5 days was 7.75 per cent of the intravenous dose (N: 1–2 per cent) confirming gastrointestinal protein loss.

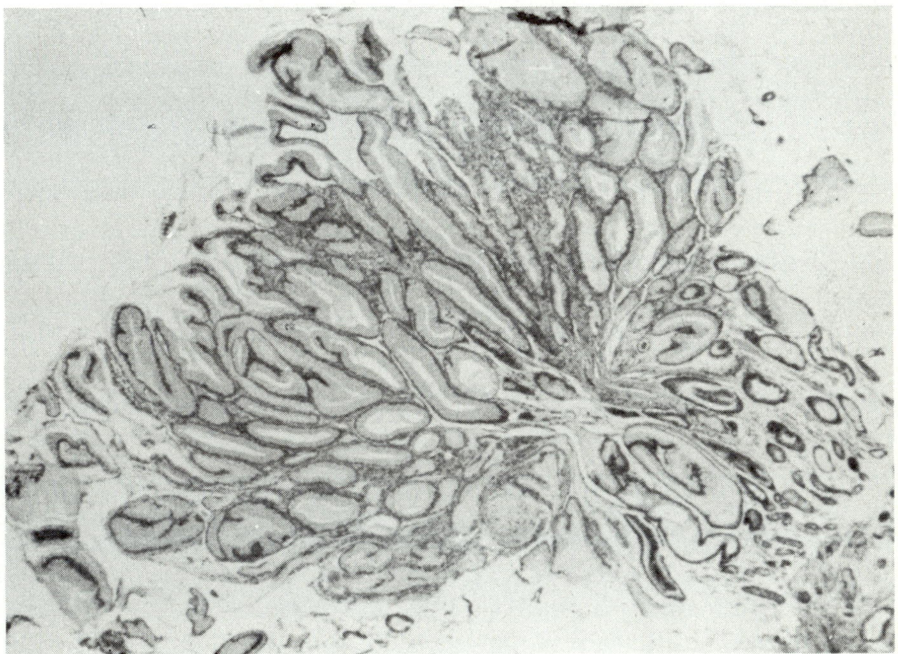

Figure 6.2a Low-power view showing increased numbers of mucus-producing cells in glands and cystic changes in deeper regions. Mucosa is thickened overall with elongation of gastric pits and glands

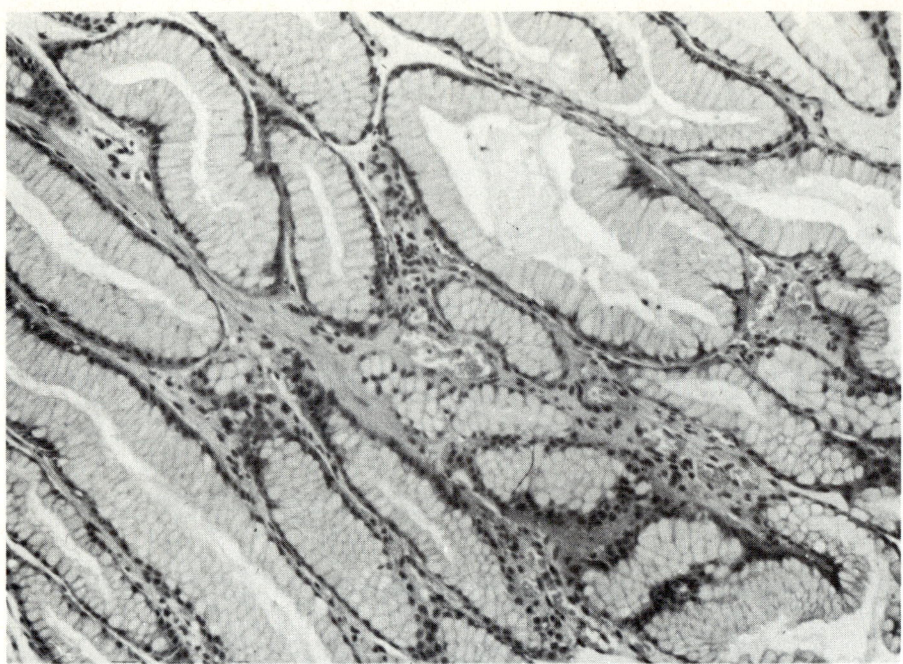

Figure 6.2b High-power view of mucous gland region. Smooth muscle fibres are visible extending through lamina propria between the glands. Only mild inflammatory infiltrate evident

No viruses were found in the gastric mucosa by electron microscopy or on culture, and immunocytochemistry showed normal numbers and distribution of endocrine cells in the gastric mucosa. Fibrinolytic activity[77] in gastric mucosal biopsies was increase, 1.55 ± 0.37 cm^2 (N: less than 0.45 cm^2) and was inhibited *in vitro* by tranexamic acid. A clinical trial of oral tranexamic acid (1 g t.d.s.) was undertaken for 6 weeks. Appetite improved slightly, vomiting was reduced to 1–2 times per day and there was less abdominal pain. Body weight increased by 1.8 kg (4 lb) during this trial. Repeat barium studies, gastroscopy and suction mucosal biopisies showed no change, serum albumin did not increase, and faecal ^{51}Cr excretion was actually greater at 21 per cent when repeated at 6 weeks. Fibrinolytic activity in gastric mucosa remained abnormally high 2.15 ± 0.49 cm^2 (N: less than 0.45 cm^2) and it was concluded that there had been no objective improvement with tranexamic acid.

Over the next 6 months she was treated empirically for nausea with chlorpromazine syrup 25 mg t.d.s. and remained reasonably well,

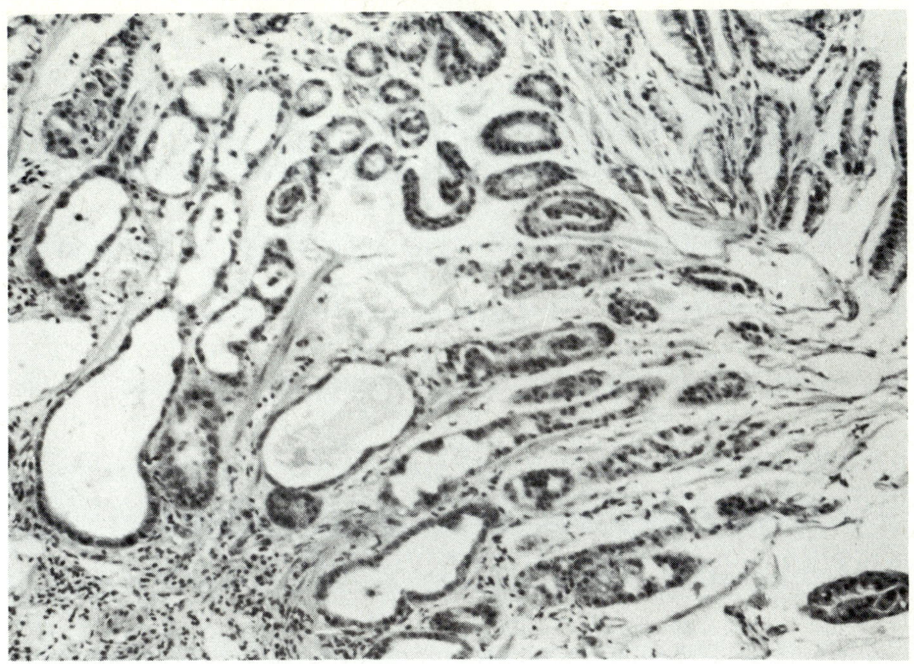

Figure 6.2c High-power view showing cystic dilatation of basal portions of glands

gained 3.2 kg (7 lb) in weight, ate normally and had evening nausea but no vomiting. She looked well and had mild epigastric tenderness and no peripheral oedema. An iron deficiency anaemia with an Hb of 8.7 g developed which responded to oral iron and the serum albumin varied between 25–29 g/l. Gastroscopy and biopsy showed no change at the end of this 6-month period. Although she had been amenorrhoeic from September 1977, normal menstruation returned by July 1978 and when reassessed in October 1978, she was symptom-free and in full-time work. Gastroscopy, however, showed persistence of the rugal hypertrophy and an increase in the number of antral polyps. In December 1978 she became pregnant, and a twin pregnancy was confirmed. Pregnancy was complicated by mild anorexia and nausea and iron deficiency anaemia treated by intravenous iron infusions. Serum albumin was maintained around 28 g/l and no oedema developed. Normal twins were delivered by caesarian section at 36 weeks gestation (23.7.79) because of a hand presentation of the first twin. One of the twins developed generalized oedema at 24 hours but this disappeared spontaneously, no apparent cause for this being established.

From 23 July 1979 until the present time, the patient has remained symptom-free.

Comment

This patient illustrates many of the typical features of Menetrier's disease. The onset of the disease was acute and the presence of fever and abnormal liver-function tests suggested a possible viral infection. However, no viral aetiology was demonstrated. In spite of gradual clinical improvement with return of menstruation and subsequent successful pregnancy, the gastroscopic features remain unchanged.

Conclusion

The clinical, radiological and pathological features of Menetrier's disease have been reviewed. The aetiology of this disorder is unknown and may be multifactorial. Conservative management remains an option providing clinical symptoms are mild. The risk of development of gastric carcinoma is probably 10 per cent after 10 years. This risk and the relatively low frequency of spontaneous remissions in adults with the disease means that many patients will require gastrectomy, which should probably take place early in those with severe unremitting symptoms, severe protein-losing gastropathy and malnutrition. It is almost 100 years since the first description of the disease appeared, and it is to be hoped that the application of modern diagnostic techniques will soon result in a clear understanding of the pathogenesis of this bizarre disorder.

References

1 ANDERRANT. H. B. Development and genetic characteristics of the adenomatous stomach lesions in strain I mice. *Public Health Reports*, **54,** 1851–1854 (1939)

2 BAKER, W. G., JR., KOLODNY, M., COLKER, J. L. and GOLDIN, H. Gastroscopy in Menetrier's disease. *Gastrointestinal Endoscopy*, **14,** 209–213 (1968)

3 BALFOUR, D. C., HIGHTOWER, N. C., GAMBILL, E. E., WAUGH, J. M. and DOCKERTY, M. B. Giant hypertrophy of the gastric rugae (Menetrier's disease) associated with severe hypoproteinaemia relieved by total gastrectomy. *Gastroenterology*, **16,** 773–781 (1950)

4 BARTLETT, J. P. and ADAMS, W. E. Generalised giant hypertrophic gastritis simulating neoplasm. *Archives of Surgery*, **60**, 543–558 (1950)

5 BECKER, V. and BRACKO, M. Villous adenoma of the rectum and Menetrier's disease in the same patient. *Zeitschrift für Gastroenterologie*, **9**, 514–521 (1971)

6 BELAICHE, J., MATUCHANSKY, C., ZITTOU, J., RAMBAUD, J. C., BERNIER, J. J. and CATTAN, D. 'Folate-losing gastropathy' and intestinal folate absorption in patients with Menetrier's disease (giant hypertrophic gastritis). *American Journal of Digestive Diseases*, **23**, 143–147 (1978)

7 BENEDICT, E. B. and MALLORY, T. B. Correlation of gastroscopic and pathological findings in gastritis. *Surgery, Gynecology and Obstetrics*, **76**, 129–135 (1943)

8 BERENSON, M. M., SANNELLA, J. and FRESTON, J. W. Menetrier's disease. Serial morphological, secretory and serological observations. *Gastroenterology*, **70**, 257–263 (1976)

9 BERGER, J. S., BUTZ, W. C. and GRAHAM, J. E. The problems of tumour simulating hypertrophic gastritis. *American Journal of Surgery*, **88**, 967–970 (1954)

10 BERMAN, J. and SPIEGEL, E. L. Menetrier's disease – case report with apparent spontaneous remission. *Gastrointestinal Endoscopy*, **15**, 230–234 (1969)

11 BERNARD, R., CARCASSONNE, M., GIRAUD, F., DELMONT, J., MAESTRAGGI, P., GRAN-JON, B. and GRATECOS, L. A. Menetrier's disease. Diabetes and cirrhosis in a fourteen-year-old child. *Pediatrie*, **25**, 787 (1970)

12 BONNE, C. and SANDGROUND, J. H. On the production of gastric tumours bordering on malignancy in Japanese monkeys through the agency of Nochtia nochti, a parasitic nematode. *American Journal of Cancer*, **37**, 173–185 (1939)

13 BRAMS, W. A. Plague-like adenoma of the stomach: its differential diagnosis and treatment. *Medical Clinics of North America*, **8**, 533–538 (1924)

14 BRASSINNE, A. Gastric clearance of serum albumin in normal man and in certain gastroduodenal disorders. *Gut*, **15**, 194–199 (1974)

15 BRDLIK, O. B. Giant hypertrophy of the gastric mucosa (Menetrier's disease): a survey of the literature and report of a case. *Journal of American Osteopath Association*, **76**, 198–203 (1976)

16 BRITISH MEDICAL JOURNAL. Editorial: Menetrier's disease. *British Medical Journal*, **1**, 150 (1979)

17 BROCHERIOU, C., BOUCHON, J. P., SQALLI, S. and CHOMETTE, G. Menetrier's giant hypertrophic gastritis. Histochemical and electron microscope study (author's translation). *Anatomie et Cytologie Pathologique*, **24**, 269–274 (1976)

18 BROOKS, A. M., ISENBERG, J. and GOLDSTEIN, H. Giant thickening of gastric mucosa with acid hypersecretion and protein losing enteropathy. *Gastroenterology*, **58**, 73–79 (1970)

19 BROWN, H. W. and RIAHI, M. Menetrier's disease or giant hypertrophic gastritis. A report of 4 cases with review of the literature. *International Surgery*, **45**, 403–409 (1966)

20 BROWNSTEIN, D. G., STRANDBERG, J. D., MONTALI, R. J., BUSH, M. and FORTNER, J. Cryptosporidium in snakes with hypertrophic gastritis. *Veterinary Pathology*, **14**, 606–617 (1977)

21 BRUNN, H. and PEARL, F. Diffuse gastric polyposis-adeno-papillomatosis gastrica. *Surgery, Gynecology and Obstetrics*, **43**, 559–598 (1926)

22 BURNS, B. and GAY, B. B. Menetrier's disease of the stomach in children. *American Journal of Roentgenology*, **106**, 300–306 (1968)

23 BUTZ, W. C. Giant hypertrophic gastritis. A report of 14 cases. *Gastroenterology*, **39**, 183–190 (1960)

24 CASTRUP, H. J. Regeneration des Magen-und-Darm Schleinhaut. *Fortschritte der Medizin*, **97**, 877–880 (1979)

25 CATANZARO, C., WEEKS, C. B. and KAFKA, R. M. Chronic hypertrophic gastritis. Report of 2 cases in siblings. *American Journal of Gastroenterology*, **37**, 525–536 (1962)

26 CHAMBOURLIER, P., PIN, G., TREFFOT, M. J., SCHEINER, C., REGNIER, F., AUSSILHOU, D. and MONGIN, M. Syndromes oedémateux révélateurs d'une maladie de Ménétrièr. *Semaine des hopitaux de Paris*, **55**, 684–688 (1979)

27 CHARLES, R. W., MOSS, A. J., KUNZ, W. and SEGAL, H. L. Gastric secretory derangement in Menetrier's disease. Report of 2 cases. *American Journal of Digestive Diseases*, **8**, 191–199 (1963)

28 CHOKAS, W. V., CONNOR, D. H. and INNES, R. C. Giant hypertrophy of the gastric mucosa, hypoproteinaemia and oedema (Menetrier's disease). *American Journal of Medicine*, **27**, 125–131 (1959)

29 CHRISTOPHER, F. Malignant diffuse gastric polyposis. *Annals of Surgery*, **106**, 139–142 (1937)

30 CHUSID, E. L., HIRSCH, R. L. and COLCHER, H. Spectrum of hypertrophic gastropathy. *Archives of Internal Medicine*, **114**, 621–628 (1964)

31 CITRIN, Y., STERLING, K. and HALSTED, J. A. The mechanism of hypoproteinaemia associated with giant hypertrophy of the gastric mucosa. *New England Journal of Medicine*, **257**, 906–912 (1957)

32 COLE, L. G. Hypertrophic gastritis. *Medical Clinics of North America*, **17**, 1–39 (1933)

33 DAVENPORT, H. W., WARNER, N. A. and CODE, C. F. Functional significance of the gastric mucosal barrier to sodium. *Gastroenterology*, **47**, 142–152 (1964)

34 DAVENPORT, H. W. Protein-losing gastropathy produced by sulfhydryl reagents. *Gastroenterology*, **60**, 870–879 (1971)

35 DAVIS, J. M., GRAY, G. F. and THORBJARNSON, B. A clinico-pathologic study of six cases. *Annals of Surgery*, **185**, 456–461 (1977)

36 DEGNAN, T. J. Idiopathic hypoproteinaemia. *Journal of Pediatrics*, **51**, 448–452 (1957)

37 DEMOLE, M., RUDLER, J. C., WIDGREN, S. and FILLIEZ, B. Giant hypertrophic gastritis (Menetrier's disease) with malignant histiocytic lymphoma. *Praxis*, **62**, 794–797 (1973)

38 DICKINSON, R. J. and AXON, A. T. R. Haematemesis in Menetrier's disease. *Postgraduate Medical Journal*, **55**, 751–752 (1979)

39 DOLAN, P. T. and SHERMAN, P. H. Tumoral hypertrophy of the gastric mucosa: a case report and summary of the findings. *American Journal of Digestive Diseases*, **19**, 171–175 (1952)

40 DWIGHT, K. Benign hypertrophy of the stomach and linitis plastica. *Annals of Surgery*, **85**, 683–697 (1927)

41 ECKHOFF, N. L. Gastric mucosal hypertrophy causing intussusception and acute pyloric obstruction. *Guy's Hospital Reports*, **92**, 38–43 (1943)

42 FASEL, J., BESSON, A., LOUP, P. and FONTOLLIET, C. Is Menetrier's disease a precancerosis? *Zeitschrift für Gastroenterologie*, **16**, 688–689 (1978)

43 FEIBER, S. S. Hypertrophic gastritis. Report of 2 cases and analysis of 50 pathologically verified cases from the literature. *Gastroenterology*, **28**, 39–69 (1955)

44 FERRARI, A., MEZZEDIMI, R. and CAVALLERO, M. Serum gastrin in various diseases of the digestive system. *Minerva Medicine*, **67**, 3881–3892 (1976)

45 FISHER, J. R. and SANOWSKI, R. A. Disseminated histoplasmosis producing hypertrophic gastric folds. *American Journal of Digestive Diseases*, **23**, 282–285 (1978)

46 FORRESTER-WOOD, W. R. Giant hypertrophic gastritis: survey of the literature and record of case treated surgically. *British Journal of Surgery*, **37**, 278–282 (1950)

47 FRANK, B. W. and KERN, F. JR. Menetrier's disease. Spontaneous metamorphosis of giant hypertrophy of the gastric mucosa to atrophic gastritis. *Gastroenterology*, **53**, 953–960 (1967)

48 GAMES, A. D., HANK, W. A., OWENS, F. J. and BROWN, C. H. Hypertrophic gastropathy and carcinoma of the stomach. *Gastrointestinal Endoscopy*, **12**, 29–33 (1966)

49 GAVA, L. and DEL FAVERO, E. Cancerization of gastric polyps. Observations on 4 cases. *Minerva Chirurgica*, **25**, 817–829 (1970)

50 GILLETT, R. Giant hypertrophic gastritis. *Lancet*, **2**, 1012–1013 (1956)

51 GLASS, G. B. J. and ISHIMORI, A. Passage of serum albumin into the stomach. Its detection by paper electrophoresis of gastric juice in protein losing gastropathies. *American Journal of Digestive Diseases*, **6**, 103–133 (1961)

52 GOLD, B. M. and MEYERS, M. A. Progression of Menetrier's disease with postoperative gastrojejunal intussusception. *Gastroenterology*, **73**, 583–586 (1977)

53 GOODALE, F. and SNIFFEN, R. C. Mucosal hypertrophy of the stomach. Report of a case. *New England Journal of Medicine*, **249**, 1105–1107 (1953)

54 GORDON, M. N., SCHAEFER, E. J. and FINKEL, M. Treatment of protein losing gastropathy with atropine. *American Journal of Gastroenterology*, **66**, 535–539 (1976)

55 GOTBAUM, I. Menetrier's disease: review of the literature and report of a case. *Journal of American Osteopathologic Association*, **69**, 472–477 (1970)

56 GRIME, R. T. and WHITEHEAD, D. R. Giant hypertrophic gastritis simulating malignant disease. *British Journal of Surgery*, **39**, 244–246 (1952)

57 HALSTEAD, C. H., ROBLES, E. A. and MEZEY, E. Intestinal malabsorption in folate deficient alcoholics. *Gastroenterology*, **64**, 526–532 (1973)

58 HAMMER, B. and GLOOR, F. Erosive exudative gastropathy: reversible Menetrier's disease? *Zeitschrift für Gastroenterologie*, **15**, 634–635 (1977)

59 HANSEN, O. H., JENSEN, K. B., LARSEN, J. K. and SOLTOFT, J. Gastric mucosal cell proliferation and immunoglobulin-containing cells in Menetrier's disease. *Digestion*, **16**, 293–298 (1977)

60 HANSSON, R., LUNDH, G. and SKOLD, G. Giant hypertrophic gastritis treated with gastric resection. *Acta Chirurgica Scandinavica*, **129**, 113–122 (1965)

61 HARRIS, C. M. Hypertrophic gastritis simulating carcinoma. *American Journal of Surgery*, **68**, 261–265 (1945)

62 HERSKOVIC, T., SPIRO, H. M. and GRYBOSKI, J. D. Acute transient gastrointestinal protein loss. *Pediatrics*, **41**, 818–821 (1968)

63 HINKEL, C. L. Hypertrophic gastritis simulating intramural tumors of the stomach. *American Journal of Roentgenology*, **53**, 20–27 (1945)

64 IIDA, F., SATO, A., KOIKE, Y. and MATSUDA, K. Surgical and pathologic aspects of protein losing gastropathy. *Surgery, Gynecology and Obstetrics*, **147**, 33–37 (1978)

65 IVEY, K. J. and CLIFTON, J. A. Ionic movement across the gastric mucosa of man: reproducibility and effect of intravenous atropine. *Journal of Laboratory and Clinical Medicine*, **78**, 753–764 (1971)

66 JARNUM, S. and JENSEN, K. B. Plasma protein turnover (albumin, transferrin, IgG, IgM) in Menetrier's disease (giant hypertrophic gastritis): evidence of non-selective protein loss. *Gut*, **13**, 128–137 (1972)

67 JEFFRIES, G. H. and SLEISENGER, M. H. Abnormal enteric loss of plasma protein in gastrointestinal diseases. *Surgical Clinics of North America*, **42**, 1125–1133 (1962)

68 JOHNSON, H. D. and STANSFIELD, A. Giant rugal hypertrophy of the stomach. *British Journal of Surgery*, **44**, 517–520 (1957)

69 JONES, E. A., YOUNG, W. B., MORSON, B. C. and DAWSON, A. M. A study of six patients with hypertrophy of the gastric mucosa with particular reference to albumin metabolism. *Gut*, **13**, 270–277 (1972)

70 JUBB, K. V. F. and KENNEDY, P. C. *Pathology of Domestic Animals*, 2nd edition, New York, Academic Press (1963)

71 KADLEC, G., GOODWIN, R., FELLOWS, R. and ANDREWS, B. Menetrier's disease in children. *Southern Medical Journal*, **72**, 33–36 (1976)

72 KANIN, H. J. Multiple gastric ulcers associated with Menetrier's disease. *Gastrointestinal Endoscopy*, **14**, 154–155 (1968)

73 KATZKA, I., GLICKEN, J. and SECKLER, J. Concentration of gastric juice protein in a patient with Menetrier's disease. Report of a case. *American Journal of Digestive Diseases*, **12**, 98–103 (1967)

75 KENNEY, F. D., DOCKERTY, M. B. and WAUGH, J. M. Giant hypertrophy of gastric mucosa: a clinical and pathological study. *Cancer*, **7**, 671–681 (1954)

76 KENRICK, K. G. and WALKER-SMITH, J. A. Immunoglobulins and dietary protein antibodies in childhood coeliac disease. *Gut,*, **11**, 635–640 (1970)

77 KONDO, M., BAMBA, T., HOSOKAWA, K., HOSADA, S., KAWAKI, K. and MASUDA, M. Tissue plasminogen activator in the pathogenesis of protein losing gastroenteropathy. *Gastroenterology*, **70**, 1045–1047 (1976)

78 KONDO, M., HOSOKAWA, K. and MASUDA, M. Treatment of protein-losing gastroenteropathy. *British Medical Journal*, **2**, 40 (1975)

79 KONDO, M., IKEZAKI, M., KATO, H. and MASUDA, M. Anti-fibrinolytic therapy of giant hypertrophic gastritis (Menetrier's disease). *Scandinavian Journal of Gastroenterology*, **13**, 851–856 (1978)

80 KONDO, M., NISHIBORI, H., IKEZAKI, M., TAKEMURA, S. and MASUDA, M. A case of Menetrier's disease associated with protein-losing gastropathy and abnormal serum complement profile. *Gastroenterologia Japonica*, **13**, 297–302 (1978)

81 KRAG, E., FREDERIKSEN, H. J., OLSEN, N. and HENRIKSEN, J. H. Cimetidine treatment of protein-losing gastropathy (Menetrier's disease). A clinical and pathophysiological study. *Scandinavian Journal of Gastroenterology*, **13**, 636–639 (1978)

82 KREJS, G. J., HORICA, C., BENES, I. and BLUM, A. L. Modified CR^{51} chromium-albumin test for the differential diagnosis of exudative gastropathies and enteropathies. *Schweizerische Medizinische Wochenschrift*, **105**, 1135–1137 (1975)

83 KRUININGEN, H. J. Giant hypertrophic gastritis of Basenji dogs. *Veterinary Pathology*, **14**, 19–28 (1977)

84 LACHMAN, R. S., MARTIN, D. J. and VAWTER, G. F. Thick gastric folds in childhood. *American Journal of Roentgenology*, **112**, 83–92 (1971)

85 LENNER, V., STAHLSCHMIDT, M., WAGNER, R. and NEHER, M. Pathology, clinical appearance and therapy of Menetrier's disease (author's translation). *Medizinische Klinik*, **72**, 319–325 (1977)

86 LEONARD, P. Hypertrophic giant fold gastropathy. Diagnostic and physiopathological considerations. *Acta Gastroenterologica Belgica*, **32**, 315 –335 (1969)

87 LEONIDAS, J. C., BEATTY, E. C. and WENNER, H. A. Menetrier's disease and cytomegalovirus infections in childhood. *American Journal of Diseases of Children*, **126**, 806–808 (1973)

88 LESSER, P. B., FALCHUK, K. R., SINGER, M. and ISSELBACHER, K. J. Menetrier's disease. Report of a case with transient and reversible findings. *Gastroenterology*, **68**, 1598–1601 (1975)

89 LEV, R. and BRUS, I. Morphologic and histochemical demonstration of protein in gastric surface epithelium in protein losing gastropathies. *American Journal of Digestive Diseases*, **16**, 589–598 (1971)

90 LIGHTDALE, C. J. and BISORDI, W. Menetrier's disease and adenocarcinoma of the pancreas. *American Journal of Gastroenterology*, **64**, 467–471 (1975)

91 LUSHBAUGH, C. C. Experimental hyperplastic gastritis and gastric polyposis in monkeys. *Journal of National Cancer Institute*, **7**, 313–320 (1947)

92 MAHMOOD, L., ALI, N. and NASH, E. C. Menetrier's disease. Report of a case with review of the literature. *Medical Annals of the District of Columbia*, **39**, 433–436 (1970)

93 MAIMON, S. N., BARTLETT, J. P. and HUMPHREYS, E. M. Giant hypertrophic gastritis. *Gastroenterology*, **8**, 397 (1947)

94 MARTIN, F. P., DEBRAY, C. and LAMBLING, A. Etude anatomique de la gastrite hypertrophique géante. *Acta Gastroenterologica Belgica*, **25**, 514–520 (1962)

95 MARTUL, E. V., INGLESIAS, J. L. V., MARDOMINGO, J. C. and RUVIRA, J. V. Hypertrophic-hyperplastic (Menetrier's disease) gastropathy associated with superficial gastric carcinoma. *Revista Española de las Enfermedades del Aparato Digestivo*, **54**, 173–179 (1978)

96 MATZNER, M. J., RAAB, A. P. and SPEAR, P. W. Benign giant gastric rugae complicated by submucosal gastric carcinoma. *Gastroenterology*, **18**, 296 –302 (1951)

97 McDONALD, W. C. and RUBIN, C. E. Gastric biopsy – a critical evaluation. *Gastroenterology*, **53**, 143–170 (1967)

98 MENETRIER, P. Des polyadenomes gastriques et de leurs rapports avec le cancer de l'estomac. *Archives de Physiologie et de Normale Pathologie*, **1**, 32–55; 236–262 (1888)

99 MILLS, G. P. Multiple polyps of the stomach (gastritis polyposa) with report of a case. *British Journal of Surgery*, **10**, 226–231 (1922)

100 MORAN, J. M. and BEAL, J. M. Giant hypertrophic gastritis. *American Journal of Surgery*, **98**, 584–592 (1959)

101 MUNRO, D. R. Route of protein loss during a model of protein losing gastropathy in dogs. *Gastroenterology*, **66**, 960–972, (1974)

102 NAIR, K. P. C. and DAMODARAM, S. Chronic hypertrophic gastritis in equines. *Indian Journal of Animal Health*, **8**, 137–139 (1969)

103 NARALAWA, S., NAITO, Y., TSUKAMOTO, Y. and AICHI, M. A case of giant rugae of the stomach with protein-loss (Menetrier's disease). *Stomach and Intestine (Tokyo)*, **13**, 1055–1060 (1978)

104 NEWMAN, C. L., MCCLURE, J. P. and BENTLEY, J. F. Menetrier's syndrome in children. *Acta Paediatrica Scandinavica*, **65**, 753–755 (1976)

105 NOMURA, M., HERABAYASHI, H., KIYAMA, T. and TAKEKARA, Y. A case of early gastric cancer associated with Menetrier's disease. *Stomach and Intestine (Tokyo)*, **7,** 83–85 (1972)

106 OLMSTED, W. W., COOPER, P. H. and MADEWELL, J. E. Involvement of the gastric antrum in Menetrier's disease. *American Journal of Roentgenology*, **126,** 524–529 (1976)

107 OVERHOLT, B. F. and JEFFRIES, G. H. Hypertrophic hypersecretory protein losing gastropathy. *Gastroenterology*, **58**, 80–87 (1970)

108 PALMER, E. D. Gastritis: a re-evaluation. *Medicine (Baltimore)*, **33**, 199–290 (1954)

109 PALUMBO, L. T., RUGTIV, G. M. and CROSS, K. R. Giant hypertrophic gastritis: its surgical and pathological significance. *Annals of Surgery*, **134**, 259–267 (1951)

110 PEAR, E. G. and HERSCH, R. Hypertrophic gastritis with malignant deterioration and metastases to bone. *American Journal of Gastroenterology*, **42,** 280–284 (1964)

111 PITTMAN, F. C., HARRIS, R. C. and BARKER, H. G. Transient edema and hypoproteinaemia. Possible Menetrier's disease. *American Journal of Diseases of Children*, **108**, 189–197 (1964)

111aPITTMANN, F. E. Transient Menetrier's disease. *Gastroenterology*, **70**, 147 (1976)

112 POPPER, H. L., GAWRON, W. W. and EISENSTAEDT, W. F. A case of Menetrier's disease. Giant hypertrophy of gastric mucosa. *International Surgery*, **45,** 77 (1966)

113 RAOTMA, H., ANGERVALL, L., DAHL, I. and DOTEVALL, G. Clinical and morphological studies of giant hypertrophic gastritis (Menetrier's disease). *Acta Medica Scandinavica*, **195**, 247–252 (1974)

114 REESE, D. F., HODGSON, J. R. and DOCKERTY, M. B. Giant hypertrophy of the gastric mucosa (Menetrier's disease): a correlation of the roentgenologic, pathologic, and clinical findings. *American Journal of Roentgenology*, **88,** 619–626 (1962)

115 REGAN, P. T., PHILLIPS, S. F. and DIMAGNO, E. P. Pancreatic insufficiency and Menetrier's disease. *American Journal of Digestive Diseases*, **23**, 759–762 (1978)

116 RICKETTS, W. E., KIRSNER, J. B. and PALMER, W. L. Large, otherwise normal gastric rugae simulating tumor of the stomach. A report of three cases. *Gastroenterology*, **8**, 123–130 (1947)

117 RIEGEL, N., DEL VECCHIO, A. and GILLSON, V. H. Menetrier's disease. A case report and brief literature review. *American Journal of Gastroenterology*, **53**, 264–271 (1970)

118 ROBERTS, H. J. V. Giant rugal hypertrophy of the stomach with protein loss and response to drug therapy (abstract). *Gut*, **11,** 980 (1970)

119 ROESCH, W. Endoscopic diagnosis and treatment in diseases predisposing to cancer and in early gastric carcinoma. *Der Chirurg,*, **49**, 473–478 (1978)

120 RUBIN, R. G. and FINK, H. Giant hypertrophy of the gastric mucosa associated with carcinoma of the stomach. *American Journal of Gastroenterology*, **47,** 379–388 (1967)

121 RUSSELL, I. J., SMITH, J., DOZOIS, R. R., WAHNER, H. W. and BARTHOLOMEW, L. G. Menetrier's disease. Effect of medical and surgical vagotomy. *Mayo Clinic Proceedings*, **52**, 91–96 (1977)

122 SANBERG, D. H. Hypertrophic gastropathy (Menetrier's disease in childhood). *Journal of Pediatrics*, **78,** 866–868 (1971)

123 SANNER, C. J., SALTZMAN, D. A. and MUELLER, J. C. Polypoid gastritis: report of a case associated with gastric adenocarcinoma and review of the literature. *American Journal of Digestive Diseases*, **23**, 19s–24s (1978)

124 SARRAZIN, A., SIMON, J., BOUSQUET, O., PAILLAS, J. and MONOD-BROCA, P. A case of Menetrier's disease with a microscopic carcinoid tumour of the stomach. *Archives Françaises des Maladies de l'Appareil Digestif*, **60**, 331–336 (1971)

125 SCHARSCHMIDT, B. F. The natural history of hypertrophic gastropathy (Menetrier's disease). *American Journal of Medicine*, **63**, 644–652 (1977)

126 SCHINDLER, R. *Gastritis*, New York, Grune and Stratton (1947)

127 SCHINDLER, R. On hypertrophic glandular gastritis, hypertrophic gastropathy and parietal cell mass. *Gastroenterology*, **45**, 77–83 (1963)

128 SCHINDLER, R. Menetrier's disease – giant fold gastritis. *Gastrointestinal Endoscopy*, **15,** 206–207 (1969)

129 SCHRODER, J. S. Protein losing gastroenteropathy: case report of Menetrier's disease and suggested aetiology. *Southern Medical Journal*, **54**, 249–252 (1961)

130 SCOTT, H. W., JR., SHULL, H. J., LAW, D. W., BURKO, H. and PAGE, D. L. Surgical management of Menetrier's disease with protein losing gastropathy. *Annals of Surgery*, **181**, 765–777 (1975)

131 SEAMAN, W. Non-neoplastic diseases of the stomach. In *Alimentary Tract Roentgenology*, edited by A. R. Margulis and H. J. Burhenne, 622–624. St. Louis, USA, C. V. Mosby Co (1973)

132 SINGH, A. K., CUMARASWAMY, R. C. and CORNIS, B. Diffuse hypertrophy of gastric mucosa (Menetrier's disease) and iron deficiency anaemia. *Gut*, **10,** 735–737 (1969)

133 SIURALA, M., VARIS, K. and WILJASALO, M. Studies of patients with atrophic gastritis. A 10 to 15-year follow-up. *Scandinavian Journal of Gastroenterology*, **1**, 40–48 (1966)

134 SMITH, R. L. and POWELL, D. W. Prolonged treatment of Menetrier's disease with an oral anticholinergic drug. *Gastroenterology*, **74**, 903–906 (1978)

135 SPELLBERG, M. A. and BAKER, L. Gastritis: its clinical significance with special emphasis on the tumour-simulating variety. *Medical Clinics of North America*, **37**, 41–61 (1953)

136 STAMATAKIS, J. D. Menetrier's disease and carcinoma of stomach. *Proceedings of Royal Society of Medicine*, **69**, 264–265 (1976)

137 STEIGMANN, F., HYMAN, S. and KANNAPEL, W. L. Large gastric rugae: benign or malignant. *Gastroenterology*, **33**, 72–84 (1957)

138 STEMPIEN, S. J., DAGRADI, A. E., REINGOLD, I. M., HEISKEL, C. L., GOODMAN, J. R., BLOOM, A. and WEEVER, D. S. Hypertrophic hypersecretory gastropathy. Analysis of 15 cases and a review of the pertinent literature. *American Journal of Digestive Diseases*, **9**, 471–493 (1964)

139 STOSIEK, P., EBERMANN, W. and VARGA, A. Simultaneous occurrence of Menetrier's disease, Dieulafoy's disease and early carcinoma of the stomach (case report). *Deutsche Zeitschrift für Verdauungs-und Stoffwechselkrankheiten*, **37**, 247–253 (1977)

140 STRICKLAND, R. G. and MACKAY, I. R. A reappraisal of the nature and significance of chronic atrophic gastritis. *American Journal of Digestive Diseases*, **18**, 426–440 (1973)

141 STRODE, J. E. Giant hypertrophy of gastric mucosa (hypertrophic gastritis). *Surgery*, **41**, 236–247 (1957)

142 SUSSMAN, H. M., WEINGARTEN, B. and MOSSBERG, S. M. Localised gastric mucosal hypertrophy simulating tumor. *American Journal of Digestive Diseases*, **10**, 710–718 (1965)

143 SYC, S., HERBA, Z. and KONDRAK, R. Co-existence of Menetrier's disease with early form of mucinogenic carcinoma. *Wiadomosci Lekarskie*, **28**, 51–54 (1975)

144 TACQUET, A. and LUEZ, J. Co-existence de cancer de la grande courbure et de gastrite cérébriforme. *Archives Françaises des Maladies de l'Appareil Digestif*, **45**, 405–409 (1956)

145 TEXTER, E. C., LEGERTON, C. W., REEVES, R. J., SMITH, A. G. and RUFFIN, J. M. Co-existent carcinoma of the stomach and hypertrophic gastritis. Report of a case with review of the literature. *Gastroenterology*, **24**, 579–586 (1953)

146 TISCHENKO, M. A. and BUTOV, Y. L. Chronic hypertrophic glandular gastritis and stomach cancer. *Arkhiv Patologii*, **37**, 23–29 (1975)

147 TRINCHET, J. C., BEAUGRAND, M., CHAMPAULT, G., MANOUX, A. and FERRIER, J. P. Giant hypertrophic gastritis (Menetrier's disease) and gastric ulcer. *Medecine et Chirurgie Digestives*, **7**, 493–494 (1978)

148 VAN DER GAAG, I., HAPPE, R. P. and WOLVEKAMP, W. T. A boxer dog with chronic hypertrophic gastritis resembling Menetrier's disease in man. *Veterinary Pathology*, **13**, 172–185 (1976)

149 VAN LOEWENTHAL, M., STEINITZ, H. and FRIEDLANDER, E. Gastritis hypertrophica gigantea und Magenkarzinom. *Gastroenterologia*, **93**, 133–144 (1960)

150 WALDMANN, T. A., STEINFELD, J. L., DUTCHER, T. F., DAVIDSON, J. D. and GORDON, R. S., JR. The role of the gastrointestinal system in 'idiopathic hypoproteinaemia'. *Gastroenterology*, **41**, 197–207 (1961)

151 WALDMANN, T. A. Protein-losing enteropathy. *Gastroenterology*, **50**, 422–443 (1966)

152 WALDMANN, T. A., WOCHNER, R. D. and STROBER, W. The role of the gastrointestinal tract in plasma protein metabolism: studies with ^{51}Cr albumin. *American Journal of Medicine*, **46**, 275–285 (1969)

153 WEAVER, G. A. and KLEINMAN, M. S. Gastric polyposis due to multiple hyperplastic adenomatous polyps. *American Journal of Digestive Diseases*, **23**, 346–352 (1978)

154 WHITEHEAD, R. Mucosal biopsy of the gastrointestinal tract. 2nd edition, 52–56 London, Saunders (1979)

155 WILLIAMS, E. Giant hypertrophic gastritis with haemorrhage requiring emergency gastrectomy. *Lancet*, **1**, 363–364 (1956)

156 WILLIAMS, S. M., HARNED, R. K. and SETTLES, R. H. Adenocarcinoma of the stomach in association with Menetrier's disease. *Gastrointestinal Radiology*, **3**, 387–390 (1978)

157 WINNEY, R. J., GILMOUR, H. M. and MATTHEWS, J. D. Prednisolone in giant hypertrophic gastritis (Menetrier's disease). *American Journal of Digestive Diseases*, **21**, 337–339 (1976)

158 ZOLLINGER, R. M. and CRAIG, T. V. Ulcerogenic tumors of the pancreas. *American Journal of Surgery*, **90**, 424 (1960)

7
Medical therapy of peptic ulcer disease

Lawrence R. Schiller and Mark Feldman

Introduction

Seventy-five years ago, peptic ulcer disease was treated with rest, dietary restrictions, gastric alkalinization, anticholinergics, bismuth subnitrate and electrical discharges[236]. The aims of therapy were to rest the stomach and to modify gastric secretions and thus effect a cure. Objective evidence of the efficacy of these treatments was not available, since radiology was in its infancy and endoscopy was not yet feasible. Today, many of these old remedies and strategies linger. Now, however, objective data have been accumulated which enable us to judge the efficacy, toxicity and cost of at least some of these older therapies. In addition, new therapeutic strategies and agents have been and are now being developed and tested. This chapter will review what is known about currently advocated nonsurgical treatments for peptic ulcer disease and those treatments being developed for the future.

A problem in the assessment of therapy for peptic ulcer is the high spontaneous healing rate when patients are treated with what are thought to be inactive placebos[115]. For instance, 20 ambulatory patients with chronic gastric ulcer were treated with daily subcutaneous injections of sterile water. They took no medications, were on no special diet and continued to smoke cigarettes as before. Their pain disappeared and all but one of the ulcers healed in 4–8 weeks, as quickly as a comparison group given the then standard treatment[108]. A more recent study claimed healing rates on placebo of 83 percent for gastric ulcers and 73 percent for duodenal ulcers after 6 weeks of 'treatment'[255]. Such high rates of healing with placebo are uncommon[115], but emphasize that placebo-controlled studies are necessary to prove that a particular treatment is effective. Now that several agents have been shown to be more effective in healing ulcers than placebo, comparisons with these standard agents are also meaningful. Whenever possible, the authors refer to placebo-controlled or standard therapy-controlled studies in this review.

Nonpharmacologic therapy

Psychotherapy

Many physicians and patients believe that periods of emotional stress often precede the development of a peptic ulcer. It seems logical, then, to apply psychotherapy in the management of these patients. However, psychotherapy is usually ignored as a therapeutic modality in treating patients with peptic ulcer, for several reasons. First, there are no convincing data, based upon controlled clinical trials, that psychotherapy is more effective than no therapy in healing ulcers or in preventing ulcer recurrences. In contrast, other forms of ulcer therapy (e.g. antacids, cimetidine) are of proven effectiveness. Second, psychotherapy, when performed by a psychiatrist, is expensive and time-consuming. Finally, many general physicians, internists, gastroenterologists, and surgeons do not take a careful psychosocial history and, therefore, stressful aspects of the patient's life may not be uncovered by the physician. Moreover, general physicians are often not trained in or familiar with psychotherapeutic techniques.

Most physicians who recommend psychotherapy for ulcer patients emphasize that this can be accomplished easily by the general physician[96, 246]. They suggest that the physician seek precipitating factors, look for temporal relationships between life events and symptom onset, and be generally supportive. As mentioned above, there is no evidence that such an approach improves ulcer healing. However, the information learned by the physician concerning the patient's life style, family, job, and financial condition may help the physician to understand his or her patient better and to plan therapy optimally.

In a recent study[254], four groups of duodenal ulcer patients were treated with a placebo by four different physicians. There were considerable differences between responses in the four groups. For example, patients treated with placebo by one physician had pain for an average of only 3.5 days, whereas a group of age- and sex-matched duodenal ulcer patients treated concurrently, but by another physician, had pain for an average of 12 days, a significant difference. This suggests that something that physicians do when treating ulcer patients influences the response to therapy. Although this study does not prove that psychotherapy is beneficial in peptic ulcer, it suggests that at least certain physicians can obtain desirable results by simply talking to the patient.

Hospitalization

Two studies[78, 125] suggest that hospital admission accelerates the healing of gastric ulcers. The explanation offered for this phenomenon is that removal of the patient from pressures at work or at home and institution of a vigorous 'antiulcer' regimen in hospital speed healing. Another explanation might be the placebo effect; the hospitalized patient may feel that his complaints are receiving more attention in hospital than they would were he an outpatient. Whatever the reason, the relevance of these older studies in an era when drug therapy provides effective control of gastric acidity is uncertain. A recent study of patients with gastric ulcer[89] showed no difference in healing between hospitalized patients and outpatients. Although lack of random assignment to inhospital or outpatient management weakens the conclusion of this report, we must view hospitalization as an unproven adjunct to current pharmacotherapy of gastric ulcer. The role of hospitalization in the management of duodenal ulcer has not been tested.

Because of these reasons and because of the expense involved, we do not advocate routine hospitalization of responsible patients with uncomplicated peptic ulcer. If the patient's symptoms do not subside promptly on an outpatient regimen, then hospitalization should be considered to assure compliance with the prescribed regimen before categorizing that patient's ulcer as 'intractable'. Hospitalization should be routine when acute bleeding or gastric outlet obstruction complicates the patient's course.

Diet therapy

Modification of the diet has been held to be helpful in the treatment of peptic ulcer for so long that it has become embedded in the popular mythology surrounding the disease. Most ulcer patients will ask for dietary advice if the physician does not prescribe it on his own initiative. The effect of this expectation is that dietary advice is still given to many patients with peptic ulcer[194, 289], even though scientific evidence of effectiveness is lacking and even though professional dieticians concede that most of the usual recommendations should not be made[4].

The rationale for diet therapy is that specific alterations in the intake of food might accelerate healing of an ulcer by reducing gastric acidity, decreasing gastric motility, and eliminating exposure of the mucosa to damaging agents[247]. These goals are supposed to be accomplished by altering the timing and size of meals, the consistency of the ingested food and the composition of the diet so that supposedly beneficial foods (such as milk and other 'bland' foods) are increased at the expense of potentially harmful foods (acid citrus juices, spices, coffee and alcohol).

While there is an appealing logic about this rationale, we must wonder about its application, since diet therapy has not improved the healing of peptic ulcers in controlled trials[45, 79, 166, 276]. This paradox between what is logical and what is observed is probably due to the fact that the changes made in the diet, in general, rarely produce the desired effect. For instance, although the frequent provision of food might be expected to raise intragastric pH because of the buffer capacity of food, frequent feedings have little effect on mean intragastric acidity[8, 210]. This probably results from the more continuous stimulation of gastric acid secretion provoked by this pattern of eating. Similarly, although mechanical abrasion of the ulcer by a coarse diet might be thought to delay healing, changes in the consistency of the diet produced no effect on the healing of uncomplicated experimental ulcers in rabbits[90]. However, healing was slower if a suture was present in the ulcer base and the rabbit was fed a coarse diet. The recommendation for a soft diet in ulcer patients hangs by that thread.

Another area in which the expectations of diet therapy are not met when tested is the selection of foods for the diet. While foods vary widely as stimulants of acid secretion[251], ulcer diets do not select foods that cause little acid secretion. Instead, foods are categorized as 'bland', or not, by appearance or taste. This has led to illogical recommendations. For example, milk, probably the most frequently recommended food in ulcer diets, is a strong stimulant of acid secretion[85, 134, 251] and is not a particularly good neutralizing agent[155, 174], so that gastric acidity is actually raised by regular ingestion of milk[31]. In contrast, citrus juices[74, 117] and spices[253, 256], both usually proscribed in ulcer diets, have little deleterious effect on the stomach or on gastric acidity. Thus, it should come as no surprise that 24-hour intragastric acidity profiles were not different among two ulcer diets and a free choice diet[173].

Ulcer diets also usually eliminate coffee, other caffeine-containing beverages, and alcohol. These recommendations stem from the thought that these substances are gastric secretagogues. While caffeine will stimulate gastric secretion somewhat[248], stimulation of acid secretion by coffee is mainly due to factors other than caffeine[60]. Thus advising ulcer patients to drink decaffeinated coffee is without firm support. Similarly, while ethanol can stimulate gastric acid secretion when given intravenously[128] and may release gastrin when placed in an antral pouch[294], the limited information available suggests that oral alcohol does not release gastrin in humans and may inhibit acid output[64]. In fact, one study of duodenal ulcer healing suggests that moderate consumption of alcohol speeds the healing of ulcer[260].

Extensive alteration of the diet may be hazardous. In one autopsy study[42], myocardial infarction was significantly increased among patients on a diet stressing prolonged, increased intake of milk. Other complications, such as milk-alkali syndrome may follow zealous adherence to a 'therapeutic' diet[95].

What then is appropriate dietary advice for the patient with peptic ulcer? In an era when food-stimulated acid secretion can be effectively blocked with drugs[233, 237, 239] and gastric acidity can be lowered throughout the day and night with these agents[222, 232], there seems to be little point to complicating the life of the ulcer patient with complex dietary advice. In order to reduce stimulation of nocturnal acid secretion, bedtime snacks should be avoided[95]. Other than this, however, little seems to be of benefit. We should follow Inglefinger's advice to 'let the ulcer patient enjoy his food'[131] and concentrate, instead, on areas of therapy that will meet with greater success.

Stopping cigarette smoking

Cigarette smoking has been linked to the occurrence of both duodenal and gastric ulcers in many studies[2, 81, 100, 142, 201, 218, 275], although some dissenting opinions have also been voiced[18, 139, 225]. However, it is unclear whether smoking tobacco *per se* predisposes to peptic ulcer or if the association occurs because patients who have ulcers also tend to smoke.

One question of therapeutic importance is whether smoking cigarettes affects ulcer healing. One placebo-controlled study of the effect of cimetidine on duodenal ulcer found no difference between smokers and nonsmokers in ulcer healing, regardless of treatment[126]. In a placebo-controlled study of an intensive antacid regimen in duodenal ulcer, placebo-treated smokers were less likely to have ulcer healing than nonsmokers, but antacid-treated smokers did not have significantly less healing than nonsmokers[224]. A third study, in which patients with duodenal ulcer were divided into smokers and nonsmokers and then randomized to standard cimetidine or potent antacid regimens, showed that fewer smokers healed their ulcers in 6 weeks than nonsmokers, even though both groups received identical treatment with effective agents[159]. Taken together, these studies suggest that continued cigarette smoking adversely affects ulcer healing under certain circumstances, but this conclusion cannot be regarded as firm.

A question of perhaps greater import is whether or not stopping smoking will assist in the healing or prevention of ulcers. Early studies[20, 112] indicated that some ulcer patients improved only after stopping smoking. In contrast, one retrospective study[125] could not show that stopping smoking exerted a beneficial effect on ulcer healing as measured radiographically at 3 weeks. However, two other studies show that cessation of cigarette smoking favourably affects the healing of peptic ulcers[81, 260]. In one of these studies[260], continued smoking favored relapse of duodenal ulcer disease during a one-year period after initial healing.

In light of these studies and in consideration of the general health hazards of tobacco, patients with ulcers are advised to stop smoking, if possible, or to reduce their consumption of cigarettes if they cannot stop.

Avoidance of 'ulcerogenic' drugs

That certain drugs damage gastrointestinal mucosa no longer seems to be a matter of controversy[65]. However, the question of which drugs have this propensity is moot. Aspirin seems to be the major culprit, both because of its widespread use and its potency as a harmful agent, but other nonsteroidal, anti-inflammatory agents are suspect[65]. Reserpine and corticosteroids, once thought to lead frequently to peptic ulceration, now appear less perilous[62, 65, 278], although high-dose corticosteroid therapy still may place the patient at risk[62, 217].

The other moot question is whether continued ingestion of ulcerogenic drugs delays the healing of peptic ulcer if adequate ulcer therapy is given at the same time. A preliminary study of 16 patients with aspirin-associated gastric ulcer suggests that small (less than 1 cm in diameter) ulcers will heal with antacids even while aspirin is continued, but larger ulcers will not heal if aspirin is continued even if antacids are combined with cimetidine[214]. This study must be confirmed in a larger group of patients before it can be accepted as valid. Whether or not cimetidine or antacids can prevent drug-related mucosal injury is uncertain although experiments in rats[185, 186] and humans[182] suggest the possibility of protection. Another group of agents being investigated for prophylactic and potentially therapeutic use in drug-induced ulcer are prostaglandins[145].

In the absence of clear-cut data, and with only limited information on potential drug–drug interactions, one should probably view most drugs used by the ulcer patient with suspicion. Agents necessary to the health and well-being of the patient should be continued in the lowest effective dose. Aspirin should be eliminated or replaced, if absolutely necessary, with other (possibly less ulcerogenic) anti-inflammatory agents. It is necessary to inform the patient that many over-the-counter drugs contain aspirin (*see* lists[13, 171]) and urge them to refrain from taking such medications. While this approach is arbitrary, the authors feel that it has merit in the absence of better information regarding the safety of continued use of allegedly 'ulcerogenic' drugs.

Pharmacological therapy

Drugs that decrease acid secretion

Current dogma holds that peptic ulcer results when the aggressive action of acid and pepsin overwhelms those factors preserving mucosal integrity. Based on this concept, logical therapy for peptic ulcer disease would consist of reducing the aggressive action of acid and pepsin or strengthening mucosal defense or both. Reducing acid secretion would presumably help ulcers heal by two mechanisms: (1) direct acid injury would be reduced as the concentration of acid in luminal contents is decreased, and (2) pepsin-mediated proteolysis would be inhibited as gastric acidity is reduced. This latter effect would be most marked at an intraluminal pH above 4.5, at which point the peptic activity of gastric juice drops sharply[226].

This concept has been strengthened by the demonstration that the marked reduction in acid secretion produced by histamine H_2-receptor antagonists is followed by accelerated healing of duodenal ulcer. Whether more complete inhibition of acid secretion than that available with the currently available histamine antagonist, cimetidine, would result in greater healing rates remains to be established.

This section will review what is known about ulcer treatment with drugs which reduce acid secretion: anticholinergics, histamine H_2-receptor antagonists and several newer experimental drugs.

Anticholinergics

These were the first, and, for a long time, the only agents known to decrease gastric acid secretion. Both natural and synthetic anticholinergics have been extensively investigated but, in spite of several hundred published studies, anticholinergics have to be classified as unproven for the treatment of peptic ulcer disease[137, 167].

Anticholinergic agents inhibit basal or nocturnal acid secretion by approximately 50 to 60 percent[9, 17, 83, 140, 200]. Food-stimulated acid secretion is reduced somewhat less, by approximately 30 to 40 percent[28, 91, 237]. While these changes in acid secretion have been regularly observed, an effect on gastric acidity has been less regularly demonstrated. In some studies, anticholinergics have significantly reduced postprandial gastric acidity[28, 200] while in others the reduction was marginal[61, 197] or not found[172, 231].

At one time, it was thought that prolonged anticholinergic therapy might have some long-lasting or permanent effect on gastric acid secretion, a 'medical vagotomy'. No such effect was seen in several studies[152, 212, 283]: basal and stimulated acid outputs were similar before and after long-term therapy. Moreover, direct comparison of acid secretion during chronic therapy with an anticholinergic to that after vagotomy showed the anticholinergic to have less effect on acid secretion than surgical vagotomy[140].

So far, all these agents have been lumped under the heading 'anticholinergics'. Are there differences between these drugs? Controversy prevails in this area also. Certainly, potency varies from agent to agent and, accordingly, the milligram dose is different from drug to drug. However, claims of greater gastric specificity of effect may be unwarranted. When several anticholinergics were given in doses that just failed to produce intolerable side-effects (the 'optimal effective dose'), all those agents tested affected basal and stimulated acid secretion to a similar degree[83]. However, another study reported that one anticholinergic, poldine, was more effective than atropine in suppressing postprandial gastric acidity[200]. Careful comparisons of several of these agents are needed to settle this question.

The method of selecting a dose of anticholinergic drug is also controversial. Since the work of Sun[267], the general recommendation has been to adjust the dose to a level just below the dose at which marked side effects developed (optimal effective dose). It was thought that these near-toxic doses were needed to adequately suppress gastric acid secretion[132]. It has recently been shown that a standard 15 mg dose of propantheline inhibited postprandial acid secretion by as much as an 'optimal effective dose' of this drug averaging 45 mg[91]. However, most recent clinical studies have employed the individually titrated 'optimal effective dose', so that the clinical effectiveness of the alternative standard dose regimen has not been tested.

Given the finding that anticholinergic drugs reduce acid secretion, how effective are they in the treatment of peptic ulcer disease? Two studies suggest that anticholinergics accelerate the healing of duodenal[119] and gastric[22] ulcers. One study claims that anticholinergic drugs hasten the resolution of ulcer dyspepsia[5]. The only study with anticholinergics utilizing endoscopy to assess healing showed a trend (but not a statistically significant difference) in favor of healing in 30 duodenal ulcer patients when a nighttime dose of an anticholinergic (rather than placebo) was combined with daytime antacids[39]. Another study suggested no benefit in ulcer healing with anticholinergics[172]. It should be pointed out that large-scale, placebo-controlled endoscopic studies, such as those done to evaluate cimetidine, have not been done with anticholinergics.

Thus, in spite of clear suppression of acid secretion, the effect of anticholinergics as single agents on ulcer healing seems marginal at best[137, 167]. This may be because anticholinergics do not inhibit acid secretion enough or, perhaps, because anticholinergics have other effects which offset the effectiveness of the reduction in gastric acid production (such as decreasing pancreatic secretion[86]).

Anticholinergics have a variety of dose-related side effects and contraindications that limit their usefulness. These agents cannot be used in patients with narrow-angle glaucoma or obstructive uropathy, and must be used with caution in elderly patients and patients with cardiac disease.

Anticholinergics have a limited role in ulcer therapy. They should not be used as the primary or sole agent for healing an ulcer. They are now second-line drugs (behind cimetidine) for the prevention of recurrence (*see* 'Prophylaxis of peptic ulcer' p. 218–220). Indications for use in peptic ulcer disease include persistent (especially nocturnal) pain during cimetidine treatment and situations like the Zollinger-Ellison syndrome, in which anticholinergics in combination with cimetidine may provide greater inhibition of acid secretion than cimetidine alone[191].

Histamine H_2-receptor antagonists

The most effective drugs for reducing acid secretion are the histamine H_2-receptor antagonists (H_2-blockers). In less than 10 years they have gone from synthesis in the laboratory to a major, if not yet fully defined, role in ulcer therapy.

H_2-blockers, unlike the classic antihistamines (H_1-blockers), inhibit the stimulating effect of histamine on acid secretion in a dose-dependent, competitive manner[33]. They have also been found to inhibit acid secretion in response to other exogenous stimulants: pentagastrin[33] and caffeine[50]. More importantly for ulcer therapy, H_2-blockers also inhibit basal or nocturnal acid secretion[124, 177] as well as acid secretion following ingestion of a meal[124, 233, 237, 239]. When tested against the other major category of antisecretory agents, the anticholinergics, H_2-blockers provided significantly greater inhibition of food-stimulated acid secretion[124, 237]. Inhibition of acid secretion by H_2-blockers resulted in significant decreases in gastric acidity throughout the day and night[222, 231, 232]. Thus, these agents held promise for the treatment of peptic ulcer.

This promise has been fulfilled most completely for duodenal ulcer[291, 296]. An early open trial[118] was encouraging and a series of double-blind, placebo-controlled studies done outside the USA have shown cimetidine to be superior to placebo in the healing of duodenal ulcer[11, 35, 36, 110, 126, 127]. Endoscopic healing rates of 80–90 percent were found in the cimetidine-treated groups and 25–40 percent in the placebo-treated groups over 4–6 weeks. In contrast to these clear results, a large USA study showed a significant difference in favor of cimetidine only after 2 weeks of therapy but not at 4 or 6 weeks[30]. This anomalous result has been attributed to *ad libitum* use of potent antacids for relief of dyspepsia in both placebo and cimetidine groups[291] since the failure to reach statistical significance was not because of a low healing rate on cimetidine (76 percent at 6 weeks) but because of a high 'placebo' healing rate (63 percent). When compared to an intensive antacid regimen previously shown to accelerate duodenal ulcer healing[224], cimetidine yielded similar healing rates to antacids[136]. It should be noted in this last trial that antacid therapy was complicated by diarrhea in 27 percent of the study group while cimetidine therapy had no such side effects. From these studies, it appears that cimetidine is effective in the treatment of duodenal ulcer in doses ranging from 800–1600 mg/day. However, not all duodenal ulcers will heal with cimetidine[296].

The situation with gastric ulcers is less clear because fewer studies have been performed, but the gastric ulcer studies paralleled the duodenal ulcer experience[99]. As with duodenal ulcers, an early open trial was encouraging[230]. Again, European double-blind, placebo-controlled studies[10, 102, 258] have indicated that ulcer healing occurs significantly more often with cimetidine than with placebo. One study in the USA which compared cimetidine to placebo[87] was unable to show a statistically significant benefit with cimetidine, even though there was a tendency towards accelerated healing with cimetidine. Once again, unrestricted use of potent antacids may have confounded the results. Another study[89] compared cimetidine treatment to an antacid regimen and to a combination of antacids and cimetidine. No placebo control group was included in this study. No difference was found among any of the treatment groups, so we do not know if they are equally good or equally bad at healing gastric ulcer. Using the European studies as support, it is likely that cimetidine is helpful in gastric ulcer but more large placebo-controlled studies will be needed to support this contention.

Cimetidine may be useful in the treatment of ulcers recurring after gastric surgery[93], even when peak acid output is relatively low[129]. However, another report suggests that cimetidine is of little help in postoperative ulcers[154]. Further studies are needed to assess the use of cimetidine in this situation.

The use of histamine H_2-receptor antagonists in the prevention of peptic ulceration will be discussed later in this chapter.

Cimetidine has been remarkably safe and free of side effects. Metiamide, its predecessor, was removed from use because of the occurrence of neutropenia. While neutropenia usually has been attributed to the thiourea side chain of metiamide (not present in cimetidine), neutropenia has been reported with cimetidine[66, 69, 138, 146, 156, 178, 228, 277] and has resulted in one death[54]. Thrombocytopenia[138, 192] and autoimmune hemolytic anemia[249] have also been described.

Histamine H_2-receptors may have regulatory effects on leukocytes. Histamine inhibits neutrophil lysosomal enzyme release[47], production of migration inhibitory factor[244], and T-cell mediated cytolysis[227]. All these effects can be blocked by H_2-receptor antagonists but not by H_1-blockers. Thus, treatment with cimetidine might affect leukocyte function and delayed hypersensitivity. One group has demonstrated enhancement of skin delayed hypersensitivity with cimetidine treatment[7]. In addition, there is one report of rapid rejection of renal allografts soon after two children were given cimetidine[235]. Others have noted no change in several immunological parameters in patients during short-term cimetidine therapy[193], although the possibility that such changes might occur with prolonged therapy remains moot[168].

Antiandrogenic effects are another potentially serious group of side effects. Cimetidine blunts gonadotrophin release[280] and cimetidine also stimulates a rapid rise in serum prolactin levels[52]. Decreased sperm counts (but not to abnormally low levels)[280] and decreased libido and impotence[220, 292] have been reported. Cimetidine therapy has been associated with gynecomastia[73, 120] and galactorrhea[19]. Gynecomastia occurs in less than 1 in 200 duodenal ulcer patients treated with cimetidine, but may occur in as many as 1 in 25 patients with Zollinger-Ellison syndrome receiving chronic cimetidine therapy[190].

Other major concerns with cimetidine have been possible long-term effects on acid secretion and gastric carcinogenesis. 'Acid rebound' – greater acid secretion after stopping therapy than before starting treatment – was a theoretical possibility after the prolonged suppression of acid secretion with H_2-blockers. Careful assessment of patients before and after cimetidine therapy has not supported this concept[291]. Gastric carcinoma has been reported in patients after cimetidine treatment[88]. However, the time course of these tumors and the circumstances of their discovery make it highly unlikely that the drug was involved, even though chemical transformation of cimetidine *in vivo* theoretically might yield potentially carcinogenic products such as nitroso-cimetidine[88].

A series of minor side effects have been reported. Mental confusion[71, 114, 243], neuromuscular irritability[109], ileus[287], diarrhea[94], bradycardia[143], hypotension[183], abnormal liver tests[35, 273], hepatitis[282], skin rashes[160], exfoliative dermatitis[297] and acute hypersensitivity[72] have all been noted in patients treated with cimetidine. While interstitial nephritis has rarely been reported[190], elevation of serum creatinine (usually within the normal range) is common and has been noted since the early clinical studies with cimetidine[35, 118]. Studies of renal function before and during administration of cimetidine[164] suggest that this minor elevation in serum creatinine is not due to decreased glomerular filtration but rather to altered tubular handling of creatinine. Although this list of possible side effects is imposing, we must remember that clinically important side effects are quite rare with cimetidine[190].

A new generation of histamine H_2-receptor antagonists is being developed. Two of these drugs, ranitidine[82, 158, 176, 221, 293] and tiotidine[238, 264] appear to be more potent and long lasting than cimetidine. Ranitidine 150 or 200 mg twice a day suppresses 24-hour gastric acidity more than does cimetidine in a dose of 200 mg with meals and 400 mg at bedtime (i.e. 4 times a day)[285]. These new agents have different ring structures than cimetidine and may not share some of the extragastric effects of cimetidine. For instance, ranitidine does not raise serum prolactin levels when given intravenously[82]. Thus, these agents may not only be more potent and long-lasting inhibitors of gastric acid secretion, allowing a more convenient twice-a-day dose schedule, but may also have fewer side effects than cimetidine.

Cimetidine has earned an important place in ulcer therapy. In general, it is the authors' first choice for duodenal ulcer therapy because, in comparison with an intensive antacid regimen, it is as effective[136], it is no more expensive, and it is more convenient for the patient. They also use cimetidine in gastric ulcer patients, but with less enthusiasm, pending the results of further trials.

Tricyclic antidepressants and related drugs
Psychoactive agents have had an uncertain place in ulcer therapy. Phenobarbital, although widely used as a sedative in ulcer patients, was shown in a controlled trial to have no effect on the course of chronic duodenal ulcer[276]. Another sedative, diazepam, was found to modestly reduce basal, but not stimulated, acid secretion[23, 32] but no clinical trials of its effect in ulcer healing have been reported.

Because 'masked depression' was thought to play an important role in duodenal ulcer disease, a double-blind trial of a tricyclic antidepressant, trimipramine, was done in duodenal ulcer patients[116]. Both an index of depression and the ulcer disease improved. The effect of this drug on gastric acid secretion was also studied. A 100 mg dose 3 hours before the study reduced basal acid secretion by 57 percent and histalog-stimulated secretion by 15 percent[206]. Pentagastrin-stimulated acid secretion was also inhibited, but insulin-stimulated acid secretion was not reduced[38].

Trimipramine probably has anticholinergic properties, since dry mouth and difficulty with micturition are side effects, but it is unclear whether this is the mechanism by which this drug reduces gastric acid secretion[206]. Recent investigations suggest that tricyclics are strong histamine H_2-antagonists in the central nervous system[113, 147]. Whether tricyclics interact with H_2-receptors on the parietal cell and inhibit acid secretion by this mechanism is uncertain[265]. Tricyclics also inhibit norepinephrine uptake by presynaptic neurons and may reduce acid secretion by enhancing adrenergic effects in the stomach[175].

Whatever the mechanism of acid reduction, several relatively small controlled studies suggest that tricyclic agents accelerate the healing of peptic ulcer[207]. Both duodenal[211, 290] and gastric[279] ulcers heal more often with 4 weeks of trimipramine (50 mg at bedtime) than with 4 weeks of placebo. Healing rates ranged from 60 to 100 percent with the active agent in these studies. Side effects (dryness of the mouth, blurred vision, difficulty voiding, tiredness) were noted most often during the first few days of therapy[211]. Other tricyclic antidepressants have been tested in peptic ulcer disease. Doxepin also may speed healing[184]. However, butriptyline in combination with antacid was no more effective than antacid alone[187].

Another tricyclic agent, although not an antidepressant, is pirenzepine. This drug has a structure similar to the tricyclic antidepressants but has ionizable side chains that render it hydrophilic. Accordingly, it does not cross the blood-brain barrier and has no central actions[55]. In addition, pirenzepine does not have atropine-like effects on the heart or the smooth muscle of the urinary bladder or gut. It does modestly inhibit salivary secretion[55]. Like the tricyclic antidepressants, pirenzepine inhibits basal and pentagastrin-stimulated gastric acid secretion but also inhibits insulin-stimulated gastric acid secretion[27, 141, 263].

Pirenzepine also seems to be effective in treating peptic ulcer[55]. Several trials have compared pirenzepine in various doses to placebo in duodenal ulcer. When given in doses of 100 or 150 mg per day, pirenzepine produced healing in 70–90 percent of cases, signficantly better than placebo[15, 75, 202, 216]. Lesser doses tended to improve symptoms but healing rates were not improved significantly[14, 105]. In another study, pirenzepine 150 mg/day was compared to cimetidine 1 g/day and placebo in 55 duodenal ulcer patients[26]. Symptoms improved equally with both active drugs and healing after 1 month was similar: 71 percent in the pirenzepine group and 82 percent in the cimetidine group. Gastric ulcer patients have also been treated with pirenzepine. Symptoms and healing with pirenzepine were significantly better than with placebo after 6 weeks of treatment[203]. Pirenzepine (75 mg/day for 4 weeks or 75 mg/day for 1 week and then 50 mg/day for 3 weeks) appeared to be as good as carbenoxolone in gastric ulcer healing in two small studies[105, 216] but not in another study[16]. Pirenzepine was tolerated better than carbenoxolone in all of these studies. Side effects are infrequent with pirenzepine but include diplopia and dryness of the mouth[75].

Pirenzepine and other tricyclic compounds may find application in peptic ulcer therapy since healing rates with these drugs are comparable to those with standard therapy. However, large trials are needed to confirm their efficacy before widespread use can be encouraged.

Prostaglandins

These agents are among the more potent inhibitors of gastric acid secretion. In addition, they have other characteristics that make them intriguing candidates for ulcer therapy.

The most widely investigated prostaglandin family for ulcer therapy is the PGE_2 group including the natural moiety and several methylated derivatives. Natural PGE_2 inhibits gastric acid secretion when given intravenously[209] but is ineffective when given orally[148], presumably because it is rapidly degraded in the stomach. Four methylated derivatives have been developed to be more resistant to degradation and have been tested for acid reducing potential. They are 15(S)-15 and 15(R)-15 methyl prostaglandin E_2 methyl ester, 16,16 dimethyl PGE_2, and 16,16 dimethyl PGE_2 methyl ester. These agents inhibit both basal and pentagastrin-stimulated gastric acid secretion in a dose-dependent manner when given orally[148, 149, 157, 213, 242]. Basal and even pentagastrin-stimulated acid secretion can be virtually eliminated for hours in some subjects with appropriately high doses[144, 148, 242]. These agents also reduce peptone and food-stimulated gastric acid, gastrin and pepsin secretion[133, 144, 157, 223].

The methylated derivatives of PGE_2 differ in potency, stability and side effects[144, 223]. For instance, the 15(S)- form is the most effective at reducing acid secretion when given orally but is less stable at room temperature. The 15(R)- form is more stable but must epimerize in an acid environment to the 15(S)- form to be an effective gastric acid inhibitor[223]. Side effects, mostly related to increased motility, such as cramps and diarrhea, occur with larger doses, particularly with the potent 15 (S)- form and the somewhat less potent 16,16 dimethylated forms[133, 149, 157, 223].

In addition to reducing gastric acid secretion, prostaglandins seem to bolster those factors preserving mucosal integrity. Minute doses of prostaglandins (much lower than required to inhibit acid secretion) protect rat gastric mucosa from the injurious topical effects of absolute alcohol, strong acid or base, hypertonic saline and even thermal injury[241]. Such actions have been termed 'cytoprotection'[240] and their mechanism, like that of prostaglandin-induced acid inhibition[84], is unknown but may involve prostaglandin-stimulated bicarbonate and mucus secretion. It is known that application of a PGE_2 analogue leads to prompt secretion of mucus by the gastric mucosa[104], mirrored by an increase in the mucosal output of N-acetyl neuraminic acid[144].

Only a few clinical trials of prostaglandin in peptic ulcer disease have been reported. A small study of 10 gastric ulcer patients showed that $150\,\mu g$ of 15(R)-15 methyl prostaglandin E_2 methyl ester every 6 hours led to complete healing in three and considerable healing in six patients over 2 weeks. The corresponding control group had only two of nine patients in either of those categories, a statistically significant difference[103]. Another study of 77 peptic ulcer patients showed that 15(S)-15 methyl PGE_2 methyl ester significantly decreased gastric acid secretion and shortened the time necessary for ulcer healing[106]. A preliminary report of a multicenter trial of 105 patients[281] claimed that 15(R)-15 methyl PGE_2 significantly accelerated the healing of duodenal ulcer, producing a healing rate of 63 percent over 4 weeks compared with 39 percent in the placebo-treated group. Diarrhea was noted in nine of 51 prostaglandin-treated patients. These early reports are encouraging and suggest that prostaglandins may eventually become part of the therapeutic armamentarium against peptic ulcer.

Sulpiride
This agent, a hypothalamic neuroleptic chemically related to metoclopramide, has multiple actions on gastric motility, blood flow, gastrin release and gastric acid secretion[12, 49, 161]. Specifically, the gastrin and gastric acid responses to a beef-extract meal are reduced by pretreatment with this drug[49]. Early studies with this drug suggested that it was superior to placebo in healing peptic ulcers[12]. However, a recent endoscopic study of 101 patients with duodenal ulcer could not

demonstrate a significant difference between sulpiride and and placebo in complete healing rate[162], although a 4-week course of the drug significantly reduced ulcer size when compared with placebo. In addition to healing established ulcer, it has been claimed that sulpiride prevents stress ulceration[12, 122]. Further trials are needed before this agent can be recommeneded for ulcer therapy or prevention.

Other drugs which reduce acid secretion

Three other types of agents reduce acid secretion and may find some role in ulcer treatment eventually. The first of these are the adrenergic agents. The β_2 agonist, terbutaline, reduces food-stimulated acid secretion by as much as 75 percent in dogs with Heidenhain pouches, perhaps by a direct action on parietal cells[270]. A sympathomimetic, spasmolytic drug, nolinium bromide, has been found to reduce pentagastrin-stimulated gastric acid secretion by 30 percent in patients with duodenal ulcer[163]. The second type of drug which has been found to reduce acid secretion is the opiate antagonist, naloxone. This agent has been found to reduce both basal (by 65 percent) and food-stimulated (by 35 percent) acid secretion in humans[92]. The third group of agents that is under development is the substituted benzimidazoles. These substances are very potent, long-acting inhibitors of gastric acid secretion[215]. They are neither anticholinergic agents nor H_2-blockers but rather appear to work within the parietal cell to block secretion of hydrogen ion. Whether any of these categories of drugs will be developed to the point of application in ulcer therapy remains to be seen; so far no clinical trials have been reported.

Drugs that neutralize secreted acid (antacids)

Antacids reduce gastric acidity by neutralizing hydrochloric acid. In the fasting stomach, antacids reduce acidity for 30 minutes or less because they empty from the stomach rapidly. However, when taken after a meal, some antacids can reduce gastric acidity and peptic activity for several hours[97]. *Figure 7.1* shows the effects of Maalox (an aluminum hydroxide-magnesium hydroxide antacid) and Phosphaljel (an aluminum phosphate antacid) on the mean gastric acidity (*left*) and pH (*right*) in 11 patients with duodenal ulcer. Sixty ml of medication (or water as a control) were given an hour after a steak meal.

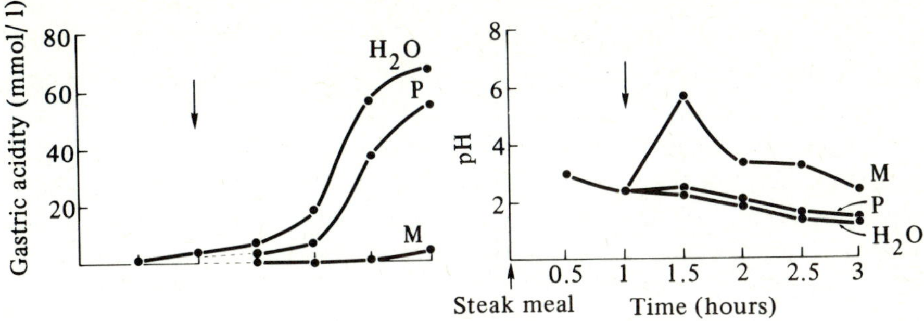

Figure 7.1 Mean gastric acidity (*left*) and pH (*right*) following a steak meal in 11 patients with duodenal ulcer. One hour after the meal either 60 ml of H_2O or antacid (Phosphaljel, P, or Maalox, M,) were ingested (arrows). (After Fordtran, Morawski and Richardson[98])

Phosphaljel reduced gastric acidity only slightly, whereas Maalox kept acidity low for 3 hours. Gastric pH ranged between 1 and 3 (a pH range ideal for peptic activity) with water and with Phosphaljel. On the other hand, Maalox led to much higher pH levels (above 4.5, peptic activity is minimal). Thus, antacids differ markedly in their ability to reduce gastric acidity and peptic activity.

It would be difficult to measure the effects of each commercially available antacid on gastric acidity in large numbers of patients. However, in 1973 Fordtran, Morawski, and Richardson[98] observed that the ability of an antacid to reduce gastric acidity *in vivo* is closely correlated with the ability of that antacid to titrate 0.1 N-HCl to pH 3.0 *in vitro*. Using their *in vitro* technique, these workers tested neutralizing capabilities of large numbers of liquid antacids. Potency varied almost 20-fold: from 6 to 105 mmol neutralizing capacity per 15 ml dose. Subsequent testing also revealed that commercially available antacid tablets are much less potent than liquids.

Therefore, the ability of an antacid to reduce postprandial gastric acidity is a function of its neutralizing capability and the time of administration in relation to a meal. A third variable is the maximum acid secretory capacity of the patient being treated. Much less antacid is required to reduce acidity to near zero in hyposecretors (e.g. some patients with gastric ulcer) than in hypersecretors (such as some duodenal ulcer patients)[98]. Antacids also vary in sodium content, taste, and cost[135]. These differences should also be considered when prescribing antacids for a particular patient.

Hollander and Harlan[130] published in 1973 the first placebo-controlled double-blind trial of antacids in 50 patients with duodenal ulcer. Patients chewed either two Titralac tablets (containing calcium carbonate and glycine) or two inert placebo tablets. Each antacid tablet had an *in vitro* neutralizing capacity of 4.1 mmol. Therefore, antacid-treated subjects ingested 131 mmol/day (*Table 7.1*). Healing at 3 weeks was defined as greater than a two-thirds reduction in ulcer size on barium meal study. Using this criterion, ulcers healed in 24 of 27

Table 7.1 Comparison of antacid and placebo therapy in duodenal ulcer disease

Author	Antacid	Neutralizing capacity (mmol/day)	Healed ulcers Antacid %	Placebo%
Hollander and Harlan[130]	CaCO$_3$ Tablets	131	89	74
Peterson *et al.*[224]	Al(OH)$_3$, Mg(OH)$_2$ liquid	1008	78	45
Lam *et al.*[162]	Al(OH)$_3$, Mg(OH)$_2$ tablets	175	77	33

*$P < 0.005$ vs placebo.

(89 percent) antacid-treated patients and in 17 of 23 (74 percent) placebo-treated patients ($P = 0.2$). Thus, although there was a trend in favor of antacids, the high healing rate in the placebo group precluded statistical significance.

Peterson *et al.*[224] treated two groups of duodenal ulcer patients; one group received a potent liquid antacid similar to Mylanta-II in a 30 ml dose administered 1 and 3 hours after meals and at bedtime (1008 mmol/day) and the other group received a liquid placebo also seven times per day. Both groups were permitted antacid tablets (Mylanta-II) as needed for ulcer symptoms. Ulcer healing rates, measured by fiberoptic duodenoscopy after 4 weeks, were 78 percent in antacid-treated patients compared to 45 percent in the placebo-treated group ($P < 0.005$, *Table 7.1*). However, two of every three antacid-treated patients had to be switched to an alternate aluminum hydroxide antacid because of bothersome diarrhea, whereas only one in five in the placebo group complained of diarrhea.

Recently, Lam *et al.*[162] treated Chinese patients with duodenal ulcer for 4 weeks with either two placebo or two magnesium hydroxide-aluminum hydroxide tablets, chewed 1 and 3 hours after meals and at bedtime. Two antacid tablets provided 25 mmol *in vitro* neutralizing capacity. Therefore, antacid-treated patients ingested 175 mmol/day (*Table 7.1*), less than 20 percent of the amount of antacid in Peterson's study. These workers found endoscopic healing in 77 percent of antacid-treated patients, compared to 33 percent of placebo-treated patients ($P < 0.005$). These results are remarkably similar to those in Peterson's study. Importantly, however, only two of 26 antacid-treated patients in Lam's study developed diarrhea.

It is tempting to conclude from Lam's study that much lower antacid doses than used by Peterson are effective in duodenal ulcer. However, Lam's Chinese patients had a maximum acid output of around 20 mmol/h, as compared to a mean value of around 40 mmol/h in American duodenal ulcer patients. Since the ability of a given dose of antacid to reduce gastric acidity is inversely proportional to the patient's maximum secretory capacity[98], it is perhaps not proper to think of Lam's regimen as a low-dose regimen.

At present, although there is evidence to suggest that low-dose antacid regimens may be effective in duodenal ulcer disease, further studies are needed to determine whether low-dose regimens are as effective as high-dose regimens. If this is borne out by future clinical trials, side effects and cost of antacid therapy can be substantially reduced and, perhaps, compliance to medication increased.

Neither Hollander and Harlan[130], Peterson *et al*[224], nor Lam *et al*.[162] found that antacids were superior to placebo for symptom relief, although all found a trend in that direction. Sturdevant *et al*.[266] also found no significant differences between liquid antacid and placebo in relieving ulcer pain. However, Lorber, Stelzer and Mayer[180] found that a liquid antacid was more effective than saline when administered through a nasogastric tube for an episode of ulcer pain. Whether antacids relieve ulcer pain is unproven. This is somewhat puzzling since most physicians consider relief with antacids a classic component to the ulcer pain syndrome.

Gastric ulcer patients, unlike duodenal ulcer patients, tend to secrete less than normal amounts of gastric acid. However, since benign gastric ulcer rarely occurs in an achlorhydric stomach, it is reasonable to try to reduce gastric acidity and peptic activity in patients with gastric ulcer.

There have been four controlled trials of antacids in gastric ulcer. The earliest, by Doll *et al*.[80] in 1956, found that sodium bicarbonate added to a continuous intragastric milk drip did not increase radiologic ulcer healing above the incidence in a large group of gastric ulcer patients not given the milk-alkali drip.

In 1969, Baume and Hunt[21] reported their results in 28 patients with gastric ulcer. Fifteen received five aluminum hydroxide tablets per day. These tablets had virtually no acid-neutralizing capacity. Thirteen other patients received one teaspoon (50 mmol) of calcium carbonate powder per hour during waking hours (around 800 mmol/day). During a 3-week period, ulcer size on barium studies decreased by an average of 56 percent in the group receiving the 'inert' aluminum hydroxide and by only 29 percent in the potent calcium carbonate-treated group. Therefore, they found no evidence that antacids in high doses accelerated gastric ulcer healing.

In 1973, Hollander and Harlan[130] treated 16 gastric ulcer patients, half with calcium carbonate tablets (131 mmol day) and half with placebo tablets. After 4 weeks, they found 'healing' (greater than two-thirds decrease in size on gastroscopy and barium meal studies) in all eight antacid-treated patients, and in only four of eight placebo-treated patients ($P = 0.04$). They also found that pain relief was more common in the antacid-treated than the placebo-treated patients ($P = 0.03$).

Most recently, Butler and Gersh[48] treated 29 patients with gastric ulcer for 3 weeks. Fifteen received 30 ml of a liquid aluminum hydroxide-magnesium hydroxide antacid every 2 hours while awake, and 13 patients received liquid placebo. A greater than two-thirds reduction in size, assessed endoscopically, was seen in 11 of 15 (73 percent) in the antacid group and in 10 of 13 (77 percent) in the placebo group, an insignificant difference.

Thus, the three larger series found no evidence that antacids facilitate gastric ulcer healing, whereas the smaller study found a 'statistically' significant difference ($P = 0.04$). At present, the role of antacids in the management of gastric ulcer is unclear.

Altered stool frequency represents the most common side effect of antacid therapy, especially when high-dose regimens are used. In general, magnesium-containing antacids cause diarrhea, whereas aluminum-containing antacids cause constipation. Many preparations contain both magnesium and aluminum hydroxide, the net effect on stool frequency being variable. In most patients, the change in stool frequency is of little consequence and, in some, the mild cathartic action of these compounds is somewhat pleasant. In other patients, however, diarrhea becomes bothersome and patients will choose to decrease the dose of antacid or to discontinue medication. Some physicians prescribe two antacids, a magnesium-containing antacid and an aluminum hydroxide preparation, explaining to patients how to titrate stool frequency by alternating one antacid with the other. This process may be confusing and cumbersome for some patients, but most can learn by 'trial and error'. Since these side effects are dose-related, smaller doses of antacid will lead to less alteration of bowel habits than will high doses.

Sodium-containing antacids react with HCl to form NaCl, which is absorbed. In some patients, especially those with impaired renal function, this can contribute to fluid retention. The sodium content of commercially available antacids varies widely[135] and should be taken into consideration in patients with congestive heart failure, renal disease, cirrhosis, and hypertension. Calcium-containing antacids react with HCl to form $CaCl_2$. Although most of this $CaCl_2$ soon reacts with pancreatic bicarbonate to form insoluble $CaCO_3$, about 10 percent of the $CaCl_2$ is absorbed. Ingestion of large amounts of calcium-containing antacids can lead to hypercalcemia, especially in the presence of renal dysfunction (*see below*). Magnesium is also absorbed in small amounts (5–10 percent). Hypermagnesemia is rare, however, because of renal magnesium excretion. Even in patients with renal failure, hypermagnesemia usually does not occur because intestinal magnesium absorption is impaired in these patients[41]. Aluminum is also absorbed in significant quantities and in patients with renal failure can accumulate in plasma and in tissue (brain, bone, muscle)[1]. Aluminum hydroxide antacids are often used in uremic patients to bind phosphate. There is some evidence in experimental animals and man that aluminum is toxic to the central nervous system[1, 24, 68]. Since parathormone increases aluminum absorption in animals, it is possible that renal failure patients with secondary hyperparathyroidism absorb excessive dietary aluminum, even in the absence of aluminum-containing antacid therapy[272].

Aluminum-containing antacids, by forming insoluble aluminum phosphate salts, decrease phosphate absorption. In patients with normal renal function and therefore without hyperphosphatemia, aluminum hydroxide can lead to hypophosphatemia, hypophosphaturia, and hypercalcuria. Symptoms of phosphate depletion include anorexia, malaise and muscle weakness. If severe and prolonged, phosphate depletion can lead to metabolic bone disease (osteomalacia, osteoporosis)[261]. Since aluminum also binds fluoride ions in the gut, it is possible that metabolic bone disease is partly related to impaired fluoride absorption.

HCl secreted by the stomach is normally neutralized by pancreatic bicarbonate or absorbed in the upper small intestine, resulting in no net gain or loss of acid from the body. When antacid is administered, HCl is neutralized. Unless the chloride salt of the cation (e.g. $CaCl_2$) can then react with pancreatic bicarbonate, neutralization of HCl will result in a net gain of bicarbonate and tend to produce alkalosis. Since $CaCl_2$, $MgCl_2$, and $AlCl_3$ all react with pancreatic bicarbonate, alkalosis produced by calcium, magnesium, and aluminum antacids is minimal. On the other hand, sodium-containing antacids such as sodium bicarbonate react irreversibly with HCl, producing NaCl. This salt does not react with pancreatic bicarbonate and thus sodium-containing antacids can lead to alkalosis, especially in the presence of impaired renal function.

Milk-alkali syndrome is characterized by hypercalcemia, azotemia and, usually, alkalosis. The syndrome is caused by high calcium intake (milk, $CaCO_3$) combined with a factor which tends to cause alkalosis (vomiting, $NaHCO_3$ ingestion)[196].

At present antacids are of proven efficacy in the treatment of active duodenal ulcer. A potent liquid antacid 30 ml, 1 and 3 hours after meals should be prescribed for at least 4 weeks. This regimen is as effective as cimetidine 1200 mg daily[136]. Although smaller doses of antacids (liquids or tablets) may be as effective, there is not yet enough data in non-Chinese duodenal ulcer patients to recommend reduced dosages. There is also no evidence that chronic antacid therapy prevents duodenal ulcer recurrences. Thus, it is customary to restart full-dose antacid therapy when symptoms recur.

There is little evidence that antacids are effective in benign gastric ulcer. However, it is known that moderately high doses of liquid antacids (15 ml 1 and 3-h p.c. and h.s.) are as effective as cimetidine 1200 mg per day[89]. Moreover, antacids alone are as effective as cimetidine plus antacids[89]. It is the prediction of the authors that, in the near future, clinical trials will prove that antacids are helpful in healing gastric ulcer, and therefore they recommend antacids in treating these patients. Since the optimal antacid dosage for patients with gastric ulcer is unknown, and since non healing will usually result in surgery, at present the authors recommend frequent doses of a potent liquid antacid for at least 6 weeks.

Drugs that increase mucosal resistance, coating agents, miscellaneous agents

The factors that are responsible for mucosal resistance to damage by gastric juice and those factors that allow an ulcer crater to re-epithelialize and heal are undefined at present. Nevertheless, several agents are thought to accelerate the healing of peptic ulcers by increasing mucosal resistance or by physically coating the ulcer crater, protecting it from gastric juice. In this section, we shall review these drugs and several others that may favorably effect ulcer healing by other mechanisms.

Carbenoxolone

Licorice extracts were incorporated in a variety of old remedies for dyspepsia. However, it was not until Doll *et al.*[77] observed that the licorice derivative, carbenoxolone, could accelerate the healing of gastric ulcer that scientific interest in these compounds was stimulated. Since that time, many mechanisms have been advanced to account for the beneficial response of ulcers to carbenoxolone. Carbenoxolone enhances gastric mucus production by stimulating the addition of sugar residues to the protein moieties of mucus, thus accelerating glycoprotein synthesis[219]. In addition, carbenoxolone increases the life-span of gastric epithelial cells[219], strengthens the mucosal barrier to hydrogen ion back-diffusion[286], inhibits gastric juice peptic activity[25, 123], and increases circulating secretin[245] and aldosterone[219] levels. Carbenoxolone has anti-inflammatory properties and uncouples oxidative phosphorylation[219]. Which of these actions, if any, is responsible for the beneficial clinical effect in peptic ulcer is unknown[286].

In the study of Doll *et al.*[77], 37 percent of the gastric ulcers in the carbenoxolone group healed as opposed to 5 percent in the placebo group. Later placebo-controlled studies have shown gastric ulcer healing rates of from 36 to 64 percent with carbenoxolone[59, 76, 107, 199, 286] and most, but not all, of these have shown a significant difference in healing rates in favor of carbenoxolone over placebo. A recent direct comparison of carbenoxolone and cimetidine in gastric ulcer patients did not show a significant difference in healing rates between these drugs[271]. Thus, while not unanimous, most studies show carbenoxolone to be effective in gastric ulcer.

An early study[44] of carbenoxolone in duodenal ulcer showed an acceleration in ulcer healing soon after treatment began but no difference from placebo after 12 weeks of therapy. Symptoms were not noticeably improved by carbenoxolone. Later studies, using an encapsulated form of the drug designed to be released in the duodenum, showed significantly better healing rates than with placebo[6, 70, 208, 250, 298]. Healing rates with carbenoxolone ranged from 60 to 81 percent in these studies. Carbenoxolone thus appears to be of benefit in patients with duodenal ulcers.

Carbenoxolone therapy is frequently complicated by side effects due to excessive mineralocorticoid activity: fluid retention, hypertension and hypokalemia. These effects appear to be dose-related and occur in 12–50 percent of patients treated with this agent[286]. They are usually mild but may require administration of diuretics and/or potassium supplements. Rarely, the drug will have to be discontinued because of the severity of side effects. If carbenoxolone is to be used, the patient must be monitored with frequent weights, blood pressure determinations and serum potassium levels.

In view of the high frequency of side effects compared to cimetidine – a drug that is equally effective[271] – the authors do not recommend carbenoxolone for routine use in peptic ulcer disease.

Colloidal bismuth compounds

These agents, given in liquid form, coat the gastric mucosa[179] and, in an acid environment, form a protective protein-bismuth complex with the necrotic tissue at the site of a peptic ulcer[43]. These drugs are not antacids in the usual sense, but may have antipeptic activity[43].

Tri-potassium di-citratobismuthate (De-nol) has been the most widely tested of these compounds. Remarkably, every trial in which an adequate number of subjects was studied has shown colloidal bismuth compounds to be superior to placebo in the healing of gastric[40, 170, 288] and duodenal[63, 67, 204, 205, 229, 252, 257] ulcer. Healing rates of up to 90 percent have been reported with bismuth with no side effects of importance[179]. Bismuth-containing antacids do not appear to have this favorable effect on ulcer healing.

Colloidal bismuth compounds precipitate out of gastric juice and are no longer active as the intragastric pH is raised. Accordingly, they should not be used in combination with agents that markedly reduce intragastric acidity, such as antacids[43]. They should not be used in patients with renal failure for fear that bismuth might accumulate in the body. Patients should be warned that bismuth compounds may turn their stools black and also that the drug has an unpleasant, ammonia-like odor. In spite of these minor inconveniences, bismuth appears to be a safe and effective treatment for peptic ulcer. Colloidal bismuth compounds are not yet available in the United States.

Sucralfate

Another agent with mucosal-coating properties is sucralfate[29]. The drug is formed by combining sucrose sulfate and an aluminum salt. It is insoluble in water but is partially soluble in dilute acid solutions and in such solutions partially breaks down into its components. It has only weak acid-neutralizing properties, and, like colloidial bismuth compounds, is thought to form a chemical complex with the material in the ulcer crater, forming a barrier to further acid-peptic attack[29]. It may also have antipeptic properties. Sucralfate is not absorbed from the gastrointestinal tract and does not have any known systemic effects[29].

One placebo-controlled multicenter trial of sucralfate[195] in 215 duodenal ulcer patients found healing rates which were significantly better after 2 and 4 weeks of sucralfate than after placebo. After 4 weeks, 76 percent of ulcers in patients treated with sucralfate had healed as opposed to 65 percent in the placebo-treated group ($P <$ 0.05). The relatively high placebo response may have been due to the free use of antacids in this study. No significant side effects were noted. If these results can be confirmed, sucralfate may find application in ulcer therapy.

Miscellaneous drugs

A small controlled trial suggested that zinc sulfate 220 mg three time a day for 3 weeks, hastened the healing of gastric ulcer[101]. Zinc may work by increasing gastric mucus production[56]. Further studies of its effectiveness are needed.

Another agent recommended for peptic ulcer is the antipeptic agent, amylopectin (Depepsen)[268], a sulfated polysaccharide. Therapy with this agent has been claimed to accelerate healing[53, 179] and prevent recurrence[269] of ulcers. Others have found it to have no beneficial effect clinically[58].

Stilbestrol therapy yielded good short and long-term results in duodenal ulcer in one study[276]. It accelerated healing and prevented recurrence. In contrast, another study could not demonstrate a statistically significant response in patients with gastric ulcer[76]. The role of estrogens in peptic ulcer therapy, if any, is uncertain.

Combination therapy

Most of the effective antiulcer drugs mentioned above heal 60–90 percent of ulcers within 4 to 8 weeks when given alone. Since these drugs are thought to work by different mechanisms (inhibition of secretion, neutralization of acid, bolstered mucosal defenses), it seems logical to combine two or more of these agents in an attempt to heal a greater percentage of ulcers with a single course of treatment. For instance, better results might occur if an antisecretory drug were combined with an antacid. The number of such combinations is large. Data are available on a few such combinations and certain theoretical considerations need to be addressed.

The combination of cimetidine and potent antacids is one such regimen. The logic behind this combination is faultless. Cimetidine, by virtue of its antisecretory properties, substantially reduces acid output, thus making acid neutralization by antacid that much easier. Such a regimen does, in fact, reduce gastric acidity during the day substantially better than cimetidine alone[222]. However, when subjected to clinical trial, a combination of cimetidine and antacid did not heal significantly more gastric ulcers than either agent alone[89].

Combination of an H_2-blocker and an anticholinergic additively reduces gastric acid secretion[91, 237]. Curiously though, 24-hour intra-gastric acidity is not further reduced beyond that reduction due to cimetidine alone[222, 231]. Clinical evaluation of this combination has not been reported except for isolated cases of Zollinger-Ellison syndrome in which anticholinergics may make cimetidine therapy more effective[191].

Certain factors have to be taken into consideration when planning combination therapy. First, side effects from either of the agents may occur. Second, drug–drug interactions have to be considered. For instance, while certain antacids (e.g. Rennie, Aludrox) do not effect cimetidine absorption[46], another antacid preparation (Mylanta II) appears to impair cimetidine bioavailability[262]. It is uncertain, how-ever, if this results in decreased clinical effectiveness. Third, more complex drug regimens may be more difficult for patients to comply with and are more expensive.

Combination therapy should be considered in patients whose ulcers are resistant to a standard single-agent regimen, but there is little published data to help the practitioner decide which agents to com-bine. The authors do not advocate combination therapy for ordinary ulcer cases.

Prophylaxis of peptic ulcer

The prevention of peptic ulceration becomes an important considera-tion in two situations. The first is the prevention of *recurrence* in the patient who has already had one or more episodes of ulcer. The second is the prevention of *occurrence* in the critically ill patient who is liable to get 'stress' ulcers or in the patient taking ulcerogenic drugs (*see* p. 197–198 for discussion of ulcerogenic drugs).

Peptic ulcer disease, both duodenal and gastric, tends to be a chronic, relapsing disorder[3, 34, 169]. The likelihood of recurrence is not related to the size, location or time required for healing of the previous ulcer[169]. Ulcer recurrence cannot be predicted with precision nor can patients at especially high risk be identified at present (other than patients with Zollinger-Ellison syndrome). No medical therapy has been shown to alter the risk of recurrence once the therapy is discontinued. Therefore, to minimize ulcer recurrence, prophylactic therapy would have to be given to almost every ulcer patient for extended periods of time, perhaps for life.

Of the drugs available for ulcer therapy, only two have been studied in depth as prophylactic agents: the anticholinergics and cimetidine. As with ulcer-healing studies, long-term treatment with anticholinergics in full doses has met with mixed results in ulcer prevention. Some studies have noted significant benefit[22, 267, 269, 283], and others have found no benefit[58, 153, 197, 274]. In contrast, cimetidine 400 mg once or twice a day has been very successful in preventing duodenal ulcer relapse[34, 37, 51, 57, 111, 126] and shows promise in preventing gastric ulcer relapse[295]. These studies show that 70–80 percent of patients with duodenal ulcer can be maintained free of ulcer recurrence for 6 to 12 months in contrast to only 10–30 percent of placebo-treated patients. Because of the marginal effectiveness of anticholinergics and the clear-cut effectiveness of cimetidine, cimetidine is preferred when attempting to prevent ulcer recurrence.

The question of who should receive such prophylaxis and for how long is moot. The side effects of long-term therapy are not yet fully defined. Therefore, maintenance therapy is limited to those individuals who have complicated ulcer disease, who are poor surgical risks (or who refuse surgery) or for whom an ulcer recurrence would be a severe disability. These criteria may be broadened as further experience with long-term cimetidine is reported. When the patient does not fit into one of the above categories, the authors prefer to treat the patient promptly as the recurrences occur, rather than prophylactically.

The prevention of the occurrence of peptic ulcer in patients at great risk is another matter. Although the cause of stress ulceration is unknown[198], elevation of intragastric pH by antacids[121, 189, 234, 259] or possibly by cimetidine[181] is associated with less gastrointestinal bleeding and better outcomes. Antacid appears to be superior to cimetidine in preventing stress-induced bleeding. In situations where antacids[181] or cimetidine[188, 234] have failed to decrease bleeding events in critically ill patients, the drugs have not been given with sufficient frequency to elevate intragastric pH above certain arbitrary pH levels (ranging from 3.5 to 5.0). Sulpiride has also been used to prevent stress ulcer[12, 122] but it is unclear how this effect is mediated and how effective sulpiride is in comparison with vigorous efforts to elevate intragastric pH.

Medical therapy of peptic ulcer complications

Peptic ulcer can be complicated by perforation, obstruction, or bleeding. Although surgery is usually required for management of perforation[284], medical therapy is often tried first in the other complications.

Obstruction is due either to edema or scarring at the site of active or previous peptic ulcer disease. Patients who have gastric outlet obstruction, manifested by vomiting or gastric distention, need gastric decompression by nasogastric intubation and aspiration. Nutritional support by parenteral feeding and careful electrolyte replacement should be provided during the period without oral intake, especially if prolonged. If an active ulcer is present or suspected (as it almost always is), therapy with cimetidine is appropriate since it can be given parenterally. Antacid therapy may be helpful once the obstruction is relieved and nasogastric aspiration is no longer required. Often, acute obstruction due to active ulceration will respond to medical treatment and operative intervention will not be needed. In contrast, chronic obstruction due to scarring will usually require surgical management.

Gastrointestinal bleeding is a frequent and sometimes life-threatening complication of peptic ulcer. In certain instances, bleeding may be the first symptom of ulcer. The keystone of management is the maintenance of blood volume by adequate fluid and blood administration[165]. There is little or no evidence that other treatments, such as iced saline lavage, topical coagulants, systemic vasoconstrictors, or ulcer therapy with cimetidine or antacids will stop or prevent bleeding. New treatments of acute bleeding, such as somatostatin infusions[150] or laser photocoagulation appear promising, but must be regarded as experimental therapy for now. Lacking evidence in favor of one treatment over another, the authors rely on a treatment plan that appears logical to them. They advise that patients with gastrointestinal bleeding should be treated intensively with both cimetidine 1200–1800 mg/day and potent antacids hourly as required to maintain intragastric pH above 5 or 6. The rationale for this advice is that the activity of pepsin, a proteolytic enzyme that might adversely affect clot stability, is markedly reduced above pH 4.5[226]. Recurrent hemorrhage while pH is elevated on this regimen is an indication for surgical management in most cases.

Summary

Several safe and effective treatments for peptic ulcer are available today. The authors' current recommendations are summarized in *Table 7.2*. Additional agents with novel modes of action are being developed and new strategies for dealing with the peptic ulcer patient

Table 7.2 Recommendations for the therapy of uncomplicated peptic ulcer

---

Nonpharmacological therapy

    In every patient:

(1) Informal psychotherapy: let the patient discuss his anxieties and problems
(2) Diet therapy: avoid bedtime snacks and foods that produce symptoms; otherwise a regular diet
(3) Cigarette smoking: should be eliminated or reduced
(4) Ulcerogenic drugs: review and discontinue aspirin-containing drugs, if possible

Pharmacological therapy

    Use one of the following agents of proven value for 4–6 weeks:

(1) Cimetidine: 4 times a day; 800–1200 mg daily
(2) Potent antacids: 1 and 3 hours after meals and at bedtime
(3) Colloidial bismuth (De-Nol)*: 5 ml in 15 ml water, 1 hour before meals and at bedtime
(4) Carbenoxolone*: 200–300 mg daily for 1 week then 150–200 mg daily

    If symptoms persist or if the ulcer has not healed, consider:

(1) A longer period of treatment with the same single agent
(2) Combination therapy, e.g. antacids *and* cimetidine
(3) Surgery

Prophylactic therapy

    In situations where ulcer recurrence poses special problems:

    Cimetidine: 400 mg at bedtime or twice a day

---

*Not available in the United States

are under investigation. Such activity suggests that the medical therapy of ulcer will be as different in 10 years' time as today's therapy differs from that of a decade ago.

References

1 ALFREY, A. C., LEGENDRE, G. R. and KAEHNY, W. D. The dialysis encephalopathy syndrome. Possible aluminum intoxication. *New England Journal of Medicine*, **294**, 184–188 (1973)

2 ALP, M. H., COURT, J. H. and KERR GRANT, A. Personality pattern and emotional stress in the genesis of peptic ulcer. *Gut*, **11**, 773–777 (1970)

3 ALTHAUSEN, T. L. Prevention of recurrences in peptic ulcers. *Annals of Internal Medicine*, **30**, 544–559 (1949)

4 AMERICAN DIETETIC ASSOCIATION. Position paper on bland diet in the treatment of chronic duodenal ulcer disease. *Journal of the American Dietetic Association*, **59**, 244 (1971)

5 AMURE, B. O. Anticholinergic drugs in the management of duodenal ulcer. *Practitioner*, **195,** 335–339 (1965)

6 ARCHAMBAULT, A., FARLEY, A., GOSSELIN, D. and BIRKETT, J. P. A Canadian multi-centre double-blind study of the use of Duogastrone for the treatment of duodenal ulcer. Chapter 9 in *Peptic Ulcer Healing: Recent Studies on Carbenoxolone*, edited by F. A. Jones, M. J. S. Langman and R. D. Mann, 95–100. Baltimore, University Park Press (1978)

7 AVELLA, J., MADGEN, J. E., BINDER, H. J. and ASKENASE, P. W. Effect of histamine H_2-receptor antagonists on delayed hypersensitivity. *Lancet*, **1**, 624–626 (1978)

8 BABOURIS, N., FLETCHER, J. and LENNARD-JONES, J. E. Effect of different foods on the acidity of the gastric contents in patients with duodenal ulcer: Part II. Effect of varying the size and frequency of meals. *Gut*, **6,** 118–120 (1965)

9 BACHRACH, W. H. Anticholinergic drugs. Survey of the literature and some experimental observations. *American Journal of Digestive Diseases*, **3,** 743–799 (1958)

10 BADER, J. P., MORIN, T., BERNIER, J. J., BERTRAND, J., BETOURNE, C., GASTARD, J., LAMBERG, R., RIBERT, A., SARLES, H. and TOULET, J. Treatment of gastric ulcer by cimetidine. A multicentre trial. Chapter 26 in *Cimetidine: Proceedings of the Second International Symposium on Histamine H_2-Receptor Antagonists*, edited by W. R. Burland and M. Simkins, 287–292. Amsterdam, Excerpta Medica (1976)

11 BANK, S., BARBEZAT, G. O., NOVIS, B. H., OUTIM, L., ODES, H. S., HELMAN, C., NARUNSKY, L., DUYS, P. J. and MARKS, I. N. Histamine H_2-receptor antagonists in the treatment of duodenal ulcers. *South African Medical Journal*, **50,** 1718–1785 (1976)

12 BANK, S. and MARKS, I. N. Evaluation of new drugs for peptic ulcer. *Clinics in Gastroenterology*, **2**, 379–395 (1973)

13 BANKS, C. N. and BARON, J. H. Drugs containing aspirin. *Lancet*, **1,** 1165 (1964)

14 BARBARA, L., BELSASSO, E., BIANCHI-PORRO, G., BLASI, A., CAENAZZO, E., CHIERICHETTI, S. M., DIFEBO, G., DIMARIO, F., FARINI, R., GIORGI-CONCIATO, M., GROSSI, E., MANGIAMELI, A., MIGLIOLI, M., NACCARATO, R. and PETRILLO, M. Pirenzepine in duodenal ulcer. A multicentre double-blind controlled clinical trial. First of two parts. *Scandinavian Journal of Gastroenterology*, **14** (Supplement 57), 11–15 (1979)

15 BARBARA, L., BELSASSO, E., BIANCHI-PORRO, G., BLASI, A., CAENAZZO, E., DIFEBO, G., DIMARIO, F., FARINI, R., GIORGI-CONCIATO, M., MANGIAMELI, A., MIGLIOLI, M., NACCARATO, R. and PETRILLO, M. Pirenzepine in duodenal ulcer. A multicentre double-blind controlled clinical trial. Second of two parts. *Scandinavian Journal of Gastroenterology*, **14** (Supplement 57), 17–19 (1979)

16 BARBARA, L., BELSASSO, E., BLASI, A., CAENAZZO, E., DIFEBO, G., DIMARIO, F., GIORGI-CONCIATO, M., MARLETTA, F., MIGLIOLI, M., PETRILLO, M., SALVAGNINI, M. and SCALABRIN, G. Pirenzepine and carbenoxolone in gastric ulcer. Preliminary results of a multicentre double-blind controlled clinical trial. *Scandinavian Journal of Gastroenterology*, **14** (Supplement 57), 21–24 (1979)

17 BARMAN, M. L. and LARSON, R. K. The effect of glycopyrrolate on nocturnal gastric secretion in peptic ulcer patients. *American Journal of Medical Sciences*, **246**, 325–328 (1963)

18 BARNETT, C. W. Tobacco smoking as a factor in the production of peptic ulcer and gastric neurosis. *Boston Medical and Surgical Journal*, **197**, 457–459 (1927)

19 BATESON, M. C., BROWNING, M. C. K. and MACCONNACHIE, A. Galactorrhoea with cimetidine. *Lancet*, **2**, 247 (1977)

20 BATTERMAN, R. C. and EHRENFELD, I. The influence of smoking upon the management of the peptic ulcer individual. *Gastroenterology*, **12**, 575–585 (1949)

21 BAUME, P. E. and HUNT, J. H. Failure of potent antacid therapy to hasten healing in chronic gastric ulcers. *Australasian Annals of Medicine*, **18**, 113–116 (1969)

22 BAUME, P. E., HUNT, J. H. and PIPER, D. W. Glycopyrronium bromide in the treatment of chronic gastric ulcer. *Gastroenterology*, **63**, 399–406 (1972)

23 BENNETT, P. N., DAVIES, P., FRIGO, G. M., WEERASINGHE, W. M. T. and LENNARD-JONES, J. E. Effect of diazepam on unstimulated and on stimulated gastric secretion. *Scandinavian Journal of Gastroenterology*, **10**, 101–103 (1975)

24 BERLYNE, G. M., YAGIL, R., BEN-ARI, J., WEINBERGER, G., KNOPF, E. and DANOVITCH, G. M. Aluminum toxicity in rats. *Lancet*, **1**, 564–568 (1972)

25 BERSTAD, A. Inhibition of peptic activity in man by carbenoxolone sodium. *Scandinavian Journal of Gastroenterology*, **7**, 129–135 (1972)

26 BIANCHI-PORRO., PETRILLO, M., LAZZARONI, M., DALMONTE, P. R., D'IMPERIO, N. and GIULIANI-PICCARI, G. Pirenzepine versus cimetidine in the treatment of duodenal ulcer. An interim report of a double-blind trial. *Scandinavian Journal of Gastroenterology*, **14** (Supplement 57), 59–62 (1979)

27 BIANCHI-PORRO, B., PRADA, A., PETRILLO, M. and GROSSI, M. Inhibition of pentagastrin and insulin-stimulated gastric secretion by pirenzepine in healthy and duodenal ulcer subjects. *Scandinavian Journal of Gastroenterology*, **14** (Supplement 57), 63–67 (1979)

28 BIEBERDORF, F. A., WALSH, J. H. and FORDTRAN, J. S. Effect of optimum therapeutic dose of poldine on acid secretion, gastric acidity, gastric emptying, and serum gastrin concentration. *Gastroenterology*, **68**, 50–57 (1975)

29 BIGHLEY, L. D. and GIESING, D. Sucralfate: A new concept in ulcer therapy. Chapter 12 in *Peptic Ulcer Disease: An Update*. 307–319. New York, Biomedical Information Corporation Publications (1979)

30 BINDER, H. J., COCCO, A., CROSSLEY, R. J., FINKELSTEIN, W., FONT, R., FRIEDMAN, G., GROARKE, J., HUGHES, W., JOHNSON, A. F., MCGUIGAN, J. E., SUMMERS, R., VLAHCEVIC, R., WILSON, E. C. and WINSHIP, D. H. Cimetidine in the treatment of duodenal ulcer. A multicentre double-blind study. *Gastroenterology*, **78**, 380–388 (1978)

31 BINGLE, J. P. and LENNARD-JONES, J. E. Some factors in the assessment of gastric antisecretory drugs by a sampling technique. *Gut*, **1**, 337–344 (1960)

32 BIRNBAUM, D., KARMELI, F. and TEFERA, M. The effect of diazepam on human gastric secretion. *Gut*, **12**, 616–618 (1971)

33 BLACK, J. W., DUNCAN, W. A. M., DURANT, C. J., GANELLIN, C. R. and PARSONS, E. M. Definition and antagonisms of histamine H_2-receptors. *Nature*, **236**, 385–390 (1972)

34 BLACKWOOD, W. S., MAUDGAL, D. P. and NORTHFIELD, T. C. Prevention by bedtime cimetidine of duodenal ulcer relapse. *Lancet*, **1**, 626–627 (1978)

35 BLACKWOOD, W. S., MAUDGAL, D. P., PICKARD, R. G., LAWRENCE, D., and NORTHFIELD, T. C. Cimetidine in duodenal ulcer: Controlled trial. *Lancet*, **2**, 174–176 (1976)

36 BODEMAR, G. and WALAN, A. Cimetidine in the treatment of active duodenal and prepyloric ulcers. *Lancet*, **2**, 161–164 (1976)

37 BODEMAR, G. and WALAN, A. Maintenance treatment of recurrent peptic ulcer by cimetidine. *Lancet*, **1**, 403–407 (1978)

38 BOHMANN, T., SCHRUMPF, E. and MYREN, J. The effect of trimipramine (Surmontil) on gastric secretion and the serum gastrin release in healthy young students. *Scandinavian Journal of Gastroenterology*, **12** (Supplement 43), 7–17 (1977)

39 BOWERS, J., FORBES, J. and FRESTON, J. Effect of night time anisotropine methyl bromide on duodenal ulcer healing. *Gastroenterology*, **72**, 1032 (1977)

40 BOYES, B. E., WOOLF, I. L., WILSON, R. Y., COWLEY, D. J. and DYMOCK, I. W. Effective treatment of gastric ulceration with a bismuth preparation (DeNol). *Gut*, **15**, 833 (1974)

41 BRANNAN, P. G., VERGNE-MARINI, P., PAK, C. Y. C., HULL, A. R. and FORDTRAN, J. S. Magnesium absorption in the human small intestine. Results in normal subjects, patients with chronic renal disease and patients with absorptive hypercalciuria. *Journal of Clinical Investigation*, **57**, 1412–1418 (1976)

42 BRIGGS, R. D., RUBENBERG, M. L., O'NEAL, R. M., THOMAS, W. A. and HARTROFT, W. S. Myocardial infarction in patients treated with Sippy and other high-milk diets. *Circulation*, **21**, 538–542 (1960)

43 BROGDEN, R. N., PINDER, R. M., SAWYER, P. R., SPEIGHT, T. M. and AVERY, G. S. Tri-potassium di-citrato bismuthate: A report of its pharmacological properties and therapeutic efficacy in peptic ulcer. *Drugs*, **12**(6), 401–411 (1976)

44 BROWN, P. SALMON, P. R., THIEN-HTUT AND READ, A. E. Double-blind trial of carbenoxolone sodium capsules in duodenal ulcer therapy, based on endoscopic diagnosis and follow-up. *British Medical Journal*, **3**, 661–664 (1972)

45 BUCHMAN, E., KAUNG, D. T., DOLAN, K. and KREPP, R. N. Unrestricted diet in the treatment of duodenal ulcer. *Gastroenterology*, **56**, 1016–1020 (1969)

46 BURLAND, W. L., DARKIN, D. W. and MILLS, M. W. Effect of antacids on absorption of cimetidine (letter). *Lancet*, **2**, 965 (1976)

47 BUSSE, W. W. and SOSMAN, J. Histamine inhibition of neutrophil lysosomal enzyme release: An H_2 histamine receptor response. *Science*, **194**, 737 (1976)

48 BUTLER, M. L. and GERSH, H. Antacid vs placebo in hospitalized gastric ulcer patients: A controlled therapeutic study. *American Journal of Digestive Diseases*, **20**, 803–807 (1975)

49 CALDARA, ROMUSSI, M. and FERRARI, C. Inhibition of gastrin secretion by sulpiride treatment in duodenal ulcer patients. *Gastroenterology*, **74**, 221–223 (1978)

50 CANO, R., ISENBERG, J. I. and GROSSMAN, M. I. Cimetidine inhibits caffeine-stimulated gastric acid secretion in man. *Gastroenterology*, **70**, 1055–1057 (1976)

51 CARGILL, J. M., PEDEN, N., SAUNDERS, J. H. B. and WORMSLEY, K. G. Very long-term treatment of peptic ulcer with cimetidine. *Lancet*, **2**, 1113–1115 (1978)

52 CARLSON, H. E. and IPPOLITI, A. F. Cimetidine, an H_2-antihistamine, stimulates prolactin secretion in man. *Journal of Clinical Endocrinology and Metabolism*, **45**, 367 (1977)

53 CAYER, D. and RUFFIN, J. M. Effect of depepsen in the treatment of peptic ulcer. *Annals of the New York Academy of Science*, **140**, 744–746 (1967)

54 CHANG, H. K. and MORRISON, S. L. Bone-marrow suppression associated with cimetidine. *Annals of Internal Medicine*, **91**, 580 (1979)

55 CHIERICHETTI, S. M., GAETANI, M. and PETRIN, G. Pirenzepine in peptic ulcer. Introduction to clinical trials reports. *Scandinavian Journal of Gastroenterology*, **14** (Supplement 57), 7–10 (1979)

56 CHO, C. H. and OGLE, C. W. Does increased gastric mucus play a role in the ulcer-protecting effects of zinc sulphate? *Experientia*, **34**, 90–91 (1978)

57 CLARK, C. G. The influence of cimetidine on current surgical treatment of peptic ulceration. *British Journal of Clinical Practice*, **33**, 216–219 (1979)

58 COCKING, J. B. A trial of amylopectin sulfate (SN-263) and propantheline bromide in the long-term treatment of chronic duodenal ulcer. *Gastroenterology*, **62**, 6–10 (1972)

59 COCKING, J. B. and MACCAIG, J. N. Effect of low dosage of carbenoxolone sodium on gastric ulcer healing and acid secretion. *Gut,,* **10**, 219–225 (1969)

60 COHEN, S. and BARTH, G. H. Gastric acid secretion and lower esophageal sphincter pressure in response to coffee and caffeine. *New England Journal of Medicine*, **293**, 897–899 (1975)

61 COLLYNS, A. H. and FORDTRAN, J. S. Controlled analysis of antacids and anticholinergics in modifying gastric acidity and peptic activity after steak in patients with duodenal ulcer. *Gastroenterology*, **48**, 812 (1965)

62 CONN, H. O. and BLITZER, B. L. Nonassociation of adrenocorticosteroid therapy and peptic ulcer. *New England Journal of Medicine*, **294**, 473–479 (1976)

63 CONNON, J. J. De-Nol, an effective drug in the therapy of duodenal ulceration. *Irish Medical Journal*, **70**, 206 (1977)

64 COOKE, A. R. Ethanol and gastric function. *Gastroenterology*, **62**, 501–502 (1972)

65 COOKE, A. Drug damage to the gastroduodenum, Chapter 47 in *Gastrointestinal Disease: Pathophysiology, Diagnosis, Management*, edited by M. H. Sleisenger and J. S. Fordtran, 807–826. Philadelphia, W. B. Saunders Company (1978)

66 CORBETT, C. L. and HOLDSWORTH, C. D. Fever, abdominal pain and leukopenia during treatment with cimetidine. *British Medical Journal*, **1**, 753–754 (1978)

67 COUGHLIN, M. B. The effect of tripotassium dicitrato-bismuthate (De-Nol) on the healing of chronic duodenal ulcers. *Medical Journal of Australia*, **1**, 294–298 (1977)

68 CRAPPER, D. R., KRISHNAN, S. S. and DALTON, A. J. Brain aluminum distribution in Alzheimer's disease and experimental neurofibrillary degeneration. *Science*, **180**, 511–513 (1973)

69 CRAVEN, E. R. and WHITTINGTON, J. M. Agranulocytosis four months after cimetidine therapy. *Lancet*, **2**, 294 (1977)

70 DAVIES, W. A. and REED, P. I. Controlled trial of duogastrone in duodenal ulcer. *Gut*, **18**, 78–83 (1977)

71 DELANEY, J. C. and RAVEY, M. Cimetidine and mental confusion. *Lancet*, **2**, 512 (1977)

72 DELAUNOIS, L. Hypersensitivity to cimetidine. *New England Journal of Medicine*, **300**, 1216 (1979)

73 DELLE FAVE, G. F., TAMBURRANO, G., DE MAGISTRIS, L., NATOLI, C., SANTORO, M. L., CARRATU, R. and TORSOLI, A. Gynecomastia with cimetidine. *Lancet*, **1**, 1319 (1977)

74 DIMMLER, C., POWER, M. H. and ALVAREZ, W. C. The effect of orange juice on gastric acidity. *American Journal of Digestive Diseases*, **5**, 86–87 (1938)

75 D'IMPERIO, N., GIULIANI-PICCARI, G., LEPORE, A. M., SARTI, F. and DALMONTE, P. R. Pirenzepine in the treatment of duodenal ulcer. *Scandinavian Journal of Gastroenterology*, **14** (Supplement 57), 41–44 (1979)

76 DOLL, R., HILL, I. D. and HUTTON, C. F. Treatment of gastric ulcer with carbenoxolone sodium and oestrogens. *Gut*, **6**, 19–24 (1965)

77 DOLL, R., HILL, I. D., HUTTON, C. and UNDERWOOD, D. J. Clinical trial of a triterpenoid liquorice compound in gastric and duodenal ulcer. *Lancet*, **2**, 793–796 (1962)

78 DOLL, R. and PYGOTT, F. Factors influencing the rate of healing of gastric ulcers. Admission to hospital, phenobarbitone and ascorbic acid. *Lancet*, **1**, 171–175 (1952)

79 DOLL, R., FRIEDLANDER, P. and PYGOTT, F. Dietetic treatment of peptic ulcer. *Lancet*, **1**, 5–9 (1956)

80 DOLL, R., PRICE, A. V., PYGOTT, F. and SANDERSON, P. H. Continuous intragastric milk drip in treatment of uncomplicated gastric ulcer. *Lancet*, **1**, 70–73 (1956)

81 DOLL, R., JONES, F. A. and PYGOTT, F. Effect of smoking on the production and maintenance of gastric and duodenal ulcers. *Lancet*, **1,** 657–662 (1958)

82 DOMSCHKE, W., LUX, G. and DOMSCHKE, S. Potent inhibition of gastric acid secretion by a new type of histamine H_2-receptor antagonist in man. *Gastroenterology*, **76,** 1123 (1979)

83 DOTEVALL, G., SCHRODER, G. and WALAN, A. Effect of poldine, glycopyrrolate and L-Hyosyamine on gastric secretion of acid in man. *Acta Medica Scandinavica*, **177,** 169–174 (1965)

84 DOUSA, T. P. and DOZOIS, R. R. Interrelationships between histamine, prostaglandins, and cyclic AMP in gastric secretion: A hypothesis. *Gastroenterology*, **73,** 904 (1977)

85 DOUTHWAITE, A. H. and HUNT, J. N. Continuous drip treatment of peptic ulcer. *Lancet*, **1,** 1019 (1950)

86 DREILING, D. A. and JANOWITZ, H. D. Inhibitory effect of new anticholinergics on the basal and secretin-stimulated pancreatic secretion in patients with and without pancreatic disease. *American Journal of Digestive Diseases*, **5,** 639–654 (1960)

87 DYCK, W. P., BELSITO, A., FLESHLER, B., LIEBERMANN, T. R., DICKINSON, P. B. and WOOD, J. M. Cimetidine and placebo in the treatment of benign gastric ulcer. A multicentre double blind study. *Gastroenterology*, **74,** 410–415 (1978)

88 ELDER, J. B., GANGULI, P. C. and GILLESPIE, J. E. Gastric cancer in patients who have taken cimetidine. *Lancet*, **2,** 245 (1979)

89 ENGLERT, E., JR., FRESTON, J. W., GRAHAM, D. Y., FINKELSTEIN, W., KRUSS, D. M., PRIEST, R. J., RASKIN, J. B., RHODES, J. B., ROGERS, A. I., WERGER, J., WILCOX, L. L. and CROSSLEY, R. J. Cimetidine, antacid and hospitalization in the treatment of benign gastric ulcer. *Gastroenterology*, **74,** 416–425 (1978)

90 FAULEY, G. B. and IVY, A. C. Experimental gastric ulcer: The effect of the consistency of the diet on healing. *Archives of Internal Medicine*, **46,** 524–532 (1930)

91 FELDMAN, M., RICHARDSON, C. T., PETERSON, W. L., WALSH, J. H. and FORDTRAN, J. S. Effect of low-dose propantheline on food-stimulated gastric acid secretion. Comparison with an 'optimal effective dose' and interaction with cimetidine. *New England Journal of Medicine*, **297,** 1427–1430 (1977)

92 FELDMAN, M., WALSH, J. H. and TAYLOR, I. L. Effect of naloxone and morphine on gastric acid secretion and on serum gastrin and pancreatic polypeptide concentrations in humans. *Gastroenterology*, **79,** 294–298 (1980)

93 FESTEN, H. P., LAMERS, C. B. H., DRIESSEN, W. M. M. and VAN TONGEREN, J. H. M. Cimetidine in anastomotic ulceration after partial gastrectomy. *Gastroenterology*, **77** (1), 83–85 (1979)

94 FIELD, R. and MEYER, G. W. Diarrhea from cimetidine. *New England Journal of Medicine*, **299,** 262 (1978)

95 FORDTRAN, J. S. Reduction of acidity by diet, antacids and anticholinergic agents. Chapter 57 in *Gastrointestinal Disease: Pathophysiology, Diagnosis, Management*, edited by M. H. Sleisenger and J. S. Fordtran, 718–742. Philadelphia, W. B. Saunders Company (1973)

96 FORDTRAN, J. S. Psychological factors in duodenal ulcer. *Practical Gastroenterology*, **3,** 24–31 (1979)

97 FORDTRAN, J. S. and COLLYNS, J. A. H. Antacid pharmacology in duodenal ulcer. Effect of antacids on postcibal gastric acidity and peptic activity. *New England Journal of Medicine*, **274,** 921–927 (1966)

98 FORDTRAN, J. S., MORAWSKI, S. G. and RICHARDSON, C. T. In vivo and in vitro evaluation of liquid antacids. *New England Journal of Medicine*, **288**, 923–928 (1973)

99 FRESTON, J. W. Cimetidine in the treatment of gastric ulcer. Review and commentary. *Gastroenterology*, **74**, 426–430 (1978)

100 FRIEDMAN, G. D., SIEGELAUB, A. B. and SELTZER, C. C. Cigarettes, alcohol and peptic ulcer. *New England Journal of Medicine*, **290**, 469–473 (1974)

101 FROMMER, D. J. The healing of gastric ulcers by zinc sulphate. *Medical Journal of Australia*, **2**, 793–796 (1975)

102 FROST, F., RAHBEK, I., RUNE, S. J., BIRGER-JENSEN, K., GUDMAND-HOYER, E., KRAG, E., RASK-MADSEN, J., WULFF, H. R., GARBOL, J., GOTLIE, B., JENSEN, K., HOJLUND, M. and NISSEN, L. R. Cimetidine in patients with gastric ulcer: A multicentre controlled trial. *British Medical Journal*, **2**, 795–797 (1977)

103 FUNG, W., KARIM, S. M. and TYE, C. Y. Effect of 15R 15 methyl prostaglandin E_2 methyl ester on healing of gastric ulcers. *Lancet*, **2**, 10–12 (1974)

104 FUNG, W., LEE, S. K. and KARIM, S. M. M. Effect of prostaglandin 15(R)15 methyl-E_2-methyl ester on the gastric mucosa in patients with peptic ulceration: Endoscopic and histological study. *Prostaglandins*, **5**, 465–472 (1974)

105 GASBARRINI, G., GIORGI-CONCIATO, M., D'ANCHINO, M., DiTOMMASO, B., PESA, O., SOLLECITO, A. and CIFANI, G. Pirenzepine in the treatment of benign gastro-duodenal diseases. A double blind controlled clinical trial. *Scandinavian Journal of Gastroenterology*, **14** (Supplement 57), 25–31 (1979)

106 GIBINSKI, K., RYBICKA, J., MIKOS, E. and NOWAK, A. Double-blind clinical trial on gastroduodenal ulcer healing with prostaglandin E_2 analogues. *Gut*, **18** (8), 636–639 (1977)

107 GILBERT, J. A. L. and BIRKETT, J. P. A placebo-controlled multicentre evaluation of Biogastrone in gastric ulcer. Chapter 5 in *Peptic Ulcer Healing: Recent Studies on Carbenoxolone*, edited by F. A. Jones, M. J. S. Langman and R. D. Mann, 51–58. Baltimore, University Park Press (1978)

108 GILL, A. M. Pain and the healing of peptic ulcers. *Lancet*, **1**, 291 (1947)

109 GRAVE, W., NADORP, J. H. S. M. and RUTTEN, J. J. M. H. Cimetidine and renal failure. *Lancet*, **2**, 719 (1977)

110 GRAY, G. R., MACKENZIE, I., SMITH, I. S., CREAN, G. P. and GILLESPIE, G. Oral cimetidine in severe duodenal ulceration: A double-blind controlled trial. *Lancet*, **1**, 4–7 (1977)

111 GRAY, G. R., SMITH, I. S., MACKENZIE, I. and GILLESPIE, G. Long-term cimetidine in the management of severe duodenal ulcer dyspepsia. *Gastroenterology*, **74**, 397–401 (1978)

112 GRAY, I. Tobacco smoking and gastric symptoms. *Annals of Internal Medicine*, **3**, 267–277 (1929)

113 GREEN, J. P. and MAAYANI, S. Tricyclic antidepressant drugs block histamine H_2 receptor in brain. *Nature*, **269**, 163–165 (1977)

114 GRIMSON, T. A. Reactions to cimetidine, *Lancet*, **1**, 858 (1977)

115 GUDJONSSON, B. and SPIRO, H. M. Response to placebos in ulcer disease. *American Journal of Medicine*, **65**, 399–402 (1978)

116 GULDAHL, M. The effect of trimipramine (Surmontil) on masked depression in patients with duodenal ulcer. A double-blind study. *Scandinavian Journal of Gastroenterology*, **12** (Supplement 43), 27–31 (1977)

117 HAGGARD, H. N. and GREENBERG, L. A. The influence of certain fruit juices on gastric function. *American Journal of Digestive Diseases*, **8,** 163–170 (1941)

118 HAGGIE, S. J., FERMONT, D. C. and WYLLIE, J. H. Treatment of duodenal ulcer with cimetidine. *Lancet*, **1,** 983–984 (1976)

119 HALL, A. A., HORNISHER, C. J. and WEEKS, R. E. The effect of Banthine on the disappearance time of duodenal ulcer craters. *Gastroenterology*, **18,** 197–200 (1951)

120 HALL, W. H. Breast changes in males on cimetidine. *New England Journal of Medicine*, **295,** 841 (1976)

121 HASTINGS, P. R., SKILLMAN, J. J., BUSHNELL, L. S. and SILEN, W. Antacid titration in the prevention of acute gastrointestinal bleeding. *New England Journal of Medicine*, **298,** 1041–1045 (1978)

122 HEINKELEIN, J. Prevention of stress ulcers with sulpiride. *La Semaine des hôpitaux* (Paris), **55,** 973–976 (May 1979)

123 HENMAN, F. D. Inhibition of peptic activity by carbenoxolone and glycyrrhetinic acid. *Gut*, **11,** 344–351 (1970)

124 HENN, R. M., ISENBERG, J. I., MAXWELL, V. and STURDEVANT, R. A. L. Inhibition of gastric acid secretion by cimetidine in patients with duodenal ulcer. *New England Journal of Medicine*, **293,** 371–375 (1975)

125 HERRMAN, R. P. and PIPER, D. W. Factors influencing the healing rate of chronic gastric ulcer. *American Journal of Digestive Diseases*, **18,** 1–6 (1973)

126 HETZEL, D., HANSKY, J., SHEARMAN, D. J. C., KORMAN, M. G., HECKER, R., TAGGART, G. J., JACKSON, R. and GABB, B. W. Cimetidine treatment of duodenal ulceration. *Gastroenterology*, **74,** 389–392 (1978)

127 HETZEL, D., TAGGART, G. J., HANSKY, J., HECKER, R. and SHEARMAN, D. J. C. Cimetidine in the treatment of duodenal ulcer. *Medical Journal of Australia*, **1,** 312–319 (1977)

128 HIRSCHOWITZ, B. I., POLLARD, H. M., HARTWELL, S. W., JR. and LONDON, J. The action of ethyl alcohol on gastric acid secretion. *Gastroenterology*, **30,** 244–253 (1956)

129 HOARE, A. M., JONES, E. L. and HAWKINS, C. F. Cimetidine for ulcers recurring after gastric surgery. *British Medical Journal*, **1,** 1325–1326 (20 May 1978)

130 HOLLANDER, D. and HARLAN, J. Antacids vs placebos in peptic ulcer therapy. A controlled double-blind investigation. *Journal of the American Medical Association*, **266,** 1181–1185 (1973)

131 INGELFINGER, F. J. Let the ulcer patient enjoy his food. In *Controversy in Internal Medicine*, edited by F. J. Ingelfinger, A. S. Relman and M. Finland, 171–179. Philadelphia, W. B. Saunders Company (1966)

132 INNES, I. R. and NICKERSON, M. Atropine, scopolamine and related antimuscarinic drugs. In *The Pharmacologic Basis of Therapeutics*, edited by L. S. Goodman and A. Gilman, 514–532. New York, MacMillan (1975)

133 IPPOLITI, A. F., ISENBERG, J. I., MAXWELL, V. and WALSH, J. H. The effect of 16,16-dimethyl prostaglandin E_2 on meal-stimulated gastric acid secretion and serum gastrin in duodenal ulcer patients. *Gastroenterology*, **70,** 488–491 (1976)

134 IPPOLITI, A. F., MAXWELL, V. and ISENBERG, J. I. The effect of various forms of milk on gastric acid secretion. Studies in patients with duodenal ulcer and normal subjects. *Annals of Internal Medicine*, **84,** 286–289 (1976)

135 IPPOLITI, A. and PETERSON, W. L. The pharmacology of peptic ulcer disease. *Clinics in Gastroenterology*, **8**, 53–67 (1979)

136 IPPOLITI, A. F., STURDEVANT, R. A. L., ISENBERG, J. I., BINDER, M., CAMACHO, R., CANO, R., COONEY, C., KLINE, M. M., KORETZ, R. L., MEYER, J. H., SAMLOFF, I. M., SCHWABE, A. D., STROM, E. D., VALENZUELA, J. E. and WINTROUB, R. H. Cimetidine versus intensive antacid therapy for duodenal ulcer. *Gastroenterology*, **74**, 393–395 (1978)

137 IVEY, K. J. Anticholinergics: Do they work in peptic ulcer? *Gastroenterology*, **68**, 154–166 (1975)

138 JAMES, C. and PROUT, B. J. Marrow suppression and intravenous cimetidine. *Lancet*, **1**, 987 (1978)

139 JAMIESON, R. A., ILLINGWORTH, C. F. W. and SCOTT, L. D. W. Tobacco and ulcer dyspepsia. *British Medical Journal*, **2**, 287–288 (1946)

140 JASKA, F. Inhibition of basal and pentagastrin-stimulated gastric acid secretion after treatment with benzilonium bromide and after selective proximal vagotomy. *Scandinavian Journal of Gastroenterology*, **12**, 695–699 (1977)

141 JAUP, B. H., STOCKBRUGGER, R. and DOTEVALL, F. The effect of pirenzepine on basal, pentagastrin- and insulin-stimulated gastric acid secretion in patients with peptic ulcer disease. *Scandinavian Journal of Gastroenterology*, **14**, 621–624 (1979)

142 JEDRYCHOWSKI, W. and POPIELA, T. Association between the occurrence of peptic ulcers and tobacco smoking. *Public Health*, **88**, 195–200 (1974)

143 JEFFREYS, D. B. and VALE, J. A. Cimetidine and bradycardia. *Lancet*, **1**, 828 (1978)

144 JOHANSSON, C. and KOLLBERG, B. Prostaglandin E_2 analogues–acid inhibitory and mucosal protective properties. *Scandinavian Journal of Gastroenterology*, **14** (Supplement 55), 126–128 (1979)

145 JOHANSSON, C., KOLLBERG, B., NORDEMAR, R., SAMUELSON, K. and BERGSTROM, S. Protective effect of prostaglandin E_2 in the gastrointestinal tract during indomethacin treatment of rheumatic diseases. *Gastroenterology*, **78**, 479–483 (1980)

146 JOHNSON, N. M., BLACK, A. E., HUGHES, A. S. B. and CLARKE, S. W. Leukopenia with cimetidine. *Lancet*, **2**, 1226 (1977)

147 KANOF, P. D. and GREENGARD, P. Brain histamine receptors as targets for antidepressant drugs. *Nature*, **272**, 329–333 (1978)

148 KARIM, S. M., CARTER, D. C., BHANA, D. and GANESAN, P. A. Effect of orally administered prostaglandin E_2 and its 15-methyl analogues on gastric secretion. *British Medical Journal*, **1**, 143–146 (1973)

149 KARIM, S. M., CARTER, D. C., BHANA, D. and GANESAN, P. A. The effect of orally and intravenously administered prostaglandin 16,16 dimethyl E_2 methyl ester on human gastric secretion. *Prostaglandins*, **4**, 71–83 (1973)

150 KAYASSEH, L., GYR, K., KELLER, U., STALDER, G. A., KELLER, U. and WALL, M. Somatostatin and cimetidine in peptic-ulcer haemorrhage. A randomized controlled trial. *Lancet*, **1**, 844–846 (1980)

151 KAYE, M. D. Anticholinergic drugs in duodenal ulcer. *Gastroenterology*, **62**, 502–504 (1972)

152 KAYE, M. D., BECK, P., RHODES, J. and SWEETRAN, P. M. Gastric acid secretion in patients with duodenal ulcer treated for one year with anticholinergic drugs. *Gut*, **10**, 774–778 (1969)

153 KAYE, M. D., RHODES, J., BECK, P., SWEETRAN, P. M., DAVIES, G. T. and EVANS, K. T. A controlled trial of glycopyrronium and L-hyoscyamine in the long-term treatment of duodenal ulcer. *Gut*, **11**, 559–566 (1970)

154 KENNEDY, T. Recurrent ulcer after vagotomy or gastrectomy treated with cimetidine. Chapter 6 in *Cimetidine. The Westminster Hospital Symposium*, edited by C. Wastell and P. Lance, 79–83. Edinburgh, Churchill Livingstone (1978)

155 KIRSNER, J. B. and PALMER, W. L. The effect of various antacids on the hydrogen ion concentration of the gastric contents. *American Journal of Digestive Diseases*, **7**, 85–93 (1940)

156 KLOTZ, S. A. and KAY, B. F. Cimetidine and agranulocytosis. *Annals of Internal Medicine*, **88**, 579–580 (1978)

157 KONTUREK, S. J., KWIECIEN. N., SWIERCZEK, J., OLESKY, J., SITO, E. and ROBERT, A. Comparison of methylated prostaglandin E_2 analogues given orally in the inhibition of gastric responses to pentagastrin and peptone meal in man. *Gastroenterology*, **70**, 683–687 (1976)

158 KONTUREK, S. J., OBTULOWICZ, W., KWIECIEN, N., SITO, E., MIKOS, E. and OLESKY, J. Comparison of ranitidine and cimetidine in the inhibition of histamine, sham-feeding, and meal-induced gastric secretion in duodenal ulcer patients. *Gut*, **21**, 181–186 (1980)

159 KORMAN, M. G., HANSKY, J., SCHMIDT, G. T., SHAW, R. G. and STEM, A. I. Cigarette smoking adversely influences the healing of duodenal ulcer treated with either cimetidine or high dose Mylanta II. *Gastroenterology*, **78**, 1199 (1980)

160 KRUSS, D. M. and LITTMAN, A. Safety of cimetidine. *Gastroenterology*, **74**, 478–482 (1978)

161 LAM, S. K. and LAI, C. L. Inhibition of sulpiride on the cephalic phase of gastric acid and gastrin secretion in duodenal ulcer patients. *Scandinavian Journal of Gastroenterology*, **11**, 27–31 (1976)

162 LAM, S. K., LAM, K. C., LAI, C. L., YEUNG, C. K., YAM, L. Y. C. and WONG, W. S. Treatment of duodenal ulcer with antacid and sulpiride. A double-blind controlled study. *Gastroenterology*, **76**, 315–322 (1979)

163 LARACH, J. R., DOZOIS, R. R. and MALAGELADA, J. R. Nolinium Bromide: A new antisecretory agent in duodenal ulcer. *Gastroenterology*, **78**, 1204 (1980)

164 LARSSON, R., BODEMAR, G. and KAGEDAL, B. The effect of cimetidine, a new histamine H_2-receptor antagonist on renal function. *Acta Medica Scandinavica*, **205**, 87–89 (1979)

165 LAW, D. H. and WATTS, H. D. Gastrointestinal bleeding. Chapter 11 in *Gastrointestinal Disease: Pathophysiology, Diagnosis, Management*, edited by M. H. Sleisenger and J. S. Fordtran, 217–240. Philadelphia, W. B. Saunders Company (1978)

166 LAWRENCE, J. S. Dietetic and other methods in the treatment of peptic ulcer. *Lancet*, **1**, 482–485 (1952)

167 LEADING ARTICLE: Anticholinergics and duodenal ulcer. *Lancet*, **2**, 1173 (1970)

168 LEADING ARTICLE: Cimetidine, publicity and safety. *Lancet*, **1**, 129 (1977)

169 LEADING ARTICLE: Preventing recurrence of ulcers. *British Medical Journal*, **2**, 1440 (1977)

170 LEE, S. P. and NICHOLSON, G. I. Increased healing of gastric and duodenal ulcers in a controlled trial using tripotassium dicitrato-bismuthate. *Medical Journal of Australia*, **1**, 808–812 (1977)

171 LEIST, E. R. and BANWELL, J. G. Products containing aspirin. *New England Journal of Medicine*, **291**, 710–712 (1974)

172 LENNARD-JONES, J. E. Experimental and clinical observations on poldine in treatment of duodenal ulcer. *British Medical Journal*, **1**, 1071–1076 (1961)

173 LENNARD-JONES, J. E. and BABOURIS, N. Effect of different foods on the acidity of the gastric contents in patients with duodenal ulcer: Part I. A comparison between two 'therapeutic' diets and freely-chosen meals. *Gut*, **6**, 113–117 (1965)

174 LENNARD-JONES, J. E., HART, J. C. D. and WILCOX, P. B. Acidity of gastric contents during nocturnal intragastric drip therapy in patients with duodenal ulcer. *Gut*, **6**, 274–278 (1965)

175 LIPPMAN, W. and SEETHALER, K. Effects of tandamine and pirandamine, selective blockers of biogenic amine uptake mechanisms, on gastric acid secretion and ulcer formation in the rat. *Life Sciences*, **20**, 1393–1400 (1977)

176 LOHRMANN, A., HOTZ, J., EYSSELEIN, V., SINGER, M. V. and GOEBELL, H. Effects of intraduodenal administration of ranitidine and cimetidine on secretion of gastric acid, pepsin, gastrin and pancreatic polypeptide in man. *Gastroenterology*, **78**, 1210 (1980)

177 LONGSTRETH, G. F., GO, V. L. W. and MALAGELADA, J. R. Cimetidine suppression of nocturnal gastric secretion in active duodenal ulcer. *New England Journal of Medicine*, **294**, 801–804 (1976)

178 LOPEZ-LUQUE, A., RODRIQUEZ-CUARTERO, A., PEREZ-GALVEZ, N., POMARES-MORA, J. and PENA-JANEZ, A. Cimetidine and bone marrow toxicity. *Lancet*, **1**, 444 (1978)

179 LORBER, S. H. Antipeptic agents, carbenoxolone and mucosal coating agents: Status report. Chapter 11 in *Peptic Ulcer Disease: An Update*, 295–304. New York, Biomedical Information Corporation Publications (1979)

180 LORBER, S. H., STELZER, F. A. and MAYER, E. M. Effect of antacid and placebo on pain of duodenal ulcer. *Gastroenterology*, **74**, 1058 (1978)

181 MACDOUGALL, B. R. D., BAILEY, R. J. and WILLIAMS, R. H_2-receptor antagonists and antacids in the prevention of acute gastrointestinal haemorrhage in fulminant hepatic failure: Two controlled trials. *Lancet*, **1**, 617–619 (1977)

182 MACKERCHNER, P. A., IVEY, K. J., BASKIN, U. N., KRAUSE, W. and JEFFREY, G. E. Effect of cimetidine on aspirin-induced human gastric mucosal damage. *Gastroenterology*, **70**, 912 (1976)

183 MAHON, W. A. and KOLTON, M. Hypotension after intravenous cimetidine. Lancet, **1**, 828 (1978)

184 MANGLA, J. C. and PEREIRA, M. Tricyclics in the treatment of peptic ulcer disease. *Gastroenterology*, **78**, 1215 (1980)

185 MANN, N. S. and SACHDER, A. J. Prevention of naproxen induced acute erosive gastritis by Mylanta II, metiamide and cimetidine. *Gastroenterology*, **70,** 914 (1976)

186 MANN, N. S. and SACHDER, A. J. Prevention of aspirin, ketoprofen and ibuprofen induced acute erosive gastritis by metiamide and cimetidine. *Gastroenterology*, **70,** 914 (1976)

187 MARKS, I. N. Healing of peptic ulcers on conventional antacid therapy with or without butriptyline. *South African Medical Journal*, **55**, 331–334 (3 March 1979)

188 MARTIN, L. F., STALOCH, D. K., SIMONOWITZ, D. A., DELLINGER, E. P. and MAX, M. H. Failure of cimetidine prophylaxis in the critically ill. *Archives of Surgery*, **114**, 492–496 (1979)

189 MCALHANY, J. C., CZAJA, A. J. and PRUITT, B. A. Antacid control of complications from acute gastro-duodenal disease after burns. *Journal of Trauma*, **16,** 645–649 (1976)

190 MCCARTHY, D. M. Peptic ulcer: Antacids or cimetidine? *Hospital Practice*, **14,** 52–64 (December 1979)

191 MCCARTHY, D. M. and HYMAN, P. E. Cholinergic influence on gastric acid secretion in the Zollinger-Ellison syndrome. *Gastroenterology*, **76,** 1198 (1979)

192 MCDANIEL, J. L. and STEIN, J. J. Thrombocytopenia with cimetidine therapy. *New England Journal of Medicine*, **300,** 864 (1979)

193 MCGREGOR, G. G. A., COCHRAN, A. J., OGG, L. J., GRAY, G. R., SMITH, I. S., GILLESPIE, G. and FORRESTER, J. Immunological and other laboratory studies of patients receiving short-term cimetidine therapy. *Lancet*, **1,** 122–123 (1977)

194 MCHARDY, G. G. Diet therapy: Perspective and current status. Chapter 8 in *Peptic Ulcer Healing: An Update*, 261–273. New York, Biomedical Information Corporation Publications (1979)

195 McHARDY, G. G. Role of sucralfate in duodenal ulcer disease: Account of a double-blind, randomized, multicenter, endoscopically controlled evaluation of ulcer response. Chapter 13 in *Peptic Ulcer Healing: An Update*, 321–330. New York, Biomedical Information Corporation Publications (1979)

196 MCMILLAN, D. E. and FREEMAN, R. B. The milk-alkali syndrome. A study of the acute disorder with comments on the chronic condition. *Medicine*, **44,** 485–501 (1965)

197 MELROSE, A. G. and PINKERTON, I. W. Clinical evaluation of poldine methosulphate. *British Medical Journal*, **1,** 1076–1078 (1961)

198 MENGUY, R. The prophylaxis of stress ulceration. *New England Journal of Medicine*, **302,** 461–462 (1980)

199 MIDDLETON, W. R. J., COOKE, A. R., STEPHEN, D. and SKYRING, A. P. Biogastrone in inpatient treatment of gastric ulcer. A double-blind study. *Lancet*, **1,** 1030–1032 (1965)

200 MITCHELL, R. D., HUNT, J. W. and GROSSMAN, M. I. Inhibition of basal and postprandial gastric secretion by poldine and atropine in patients with peptic ulcer. *Gastroenterology*, **43,** 400–406 (1962)

201 MONSON, R. R. Cigarette smoking and body form in peptic ulcer. *Gastroenterology*, **58,** 337–344 (1970)

202 MORELLI, A., NARDUCCI, F., PELLI, M. A. and SPADACINI, A. A double-blind, short-term clinical trial of pirenzepine in duodenal ulcer. *Scandinavian Journal of Gastroenterology*, **14** (Supplement 57), 45–49 (1979)

203 MORELLI, A., PELLI, A., NARDUCCI, F. and SPADACINI, A. Pirenzepine in the treatment of gastric ulcer. A double-blind short-term clinical trial. *Scandinavian Journal of Gastroenterology*, **14** (Supplement 57), 51–55 (1979)

204 MOSHAL, M. G. A bismuth-peptide complex in the treatment of duodenal ulceration. A double-blind duodenoscopic study. *South African Medical Journal*, **49**, 1157–1159 (1975)

205 MOSHAL, M. G. The treatment of duodenal ulcers with TDB: A duodenoscopic double-blind cross-over investigation. *Postgraduate Medical Journal*, **51** (Supplement 5), 36–39 (1975)

206 MYREN, J. and BERSTAD, A. The early effect of trimipramine (Surmontil) on gastric secretion in man. *Scandinavian Journal of Gastroenterology*, **10**, 817–819 (1975)

207 MYREN, J. and BERSTAD, A. Comments on the effects of carbenoxolone and trimipramine on peptic ulcer healing. *Scandinavian Journal of Gastroenterology*, **11** (Supplement 42), 159–161 (1976)

208 NAGY, G. S. An endoscopically-assessed and placebo-controlled study of the use of a positioned-release capsule of carbenoxolone in duodenal ulcer. Chapter 8 in *Peptic Ulcer Healing: Recent Studies on Carbenoxolone*, edited by F. A. Jones, M. J. S. Langman and R. D. Mann, 87–94. Baltimore, University Park Press (1978)

209 NEWMAN, A., DE MORAES-FILHO, J. P. P., PHILIPPAKOS, D. and MISIEWICZ, J. J. The effect of intravenous infusions of prostaglandins E_2 and $F_{2\alpha}$ on human gastric function. *Gut*, **16**, 272–276 (1975)

210 NICOL, B. M. Control of gastric acidity in gastric ulcer. *Lancet*, **2**, 881–884 (1939)

211 NITTER, L., JR., HARALDSSON, A., HOLCK, P., HOY, C., MUNTHE-KASS, J., MYRHOL, K. and PAULSEN, W. The effect of trimipramine on the healing of peptic ulcer. A double-blind study. Multicentre investigation–G.P. *Scandinavian Journal of Gastroenterology*, **12** (Supplement 43), 39–41 (1977)

212 NORGAARD, R. P., POLTER, D. E., WHEELER, J. W. and FORDTRAN, J. S. Effect of long-term anticholinergic therapy on gastric acid secretion, with observations on the serial measurement of peak histalog response. *Gastroenterology*, **58**, 750–755 (1970)

213 NYLANDER, B. and ANDERSSON, B. Gastric secretory inhibition induced by three methyl analogs of prostaglandin E_2 administered intragastrically to man. *Scandinavian Journal of Gastroenterology*, **9**, 751–758 (1974)

214 O'LAUGHLIN, J. C., SILVOSO, G. R. and IVEY, K. J. Effects of an H_2-blocker on gastric ulcers in patients taking aspirin: A double-blind study. *Gastroenterology*, **78**, 1230 (1980)

215 OLBE, L., BERGLINDH, T., ELANDER, B., HELANDER, H., FELLENIUS, E., SJOSTRAND, S. E., SUNDELL, G. and WALLMARK, B. Properties of a new class of gastric acid inhibitors. *Scandinavian Journal of Gastroenterology*, **14** (Supplement 55), 131–132 (1979)

216 OSELLADORE, D., CHIERICHETTI, S. M., NORBERTO, L. and VIBELLI, C. Pirenzepine

(LS 519) in severe duodenal ulcer and in gastric ulcer. A double-blind clinical trial. *Scandinavian Journal of Gastroenterology*, **14** (Supplement 57), 33–39 (1979)

217 OTTONELLO, G. A. Gastrointestinal complications of high-dose corticosteroid therapy in acute cerebrovascular patients. *Stroke*, **10**, 208–210 (1979)

218 PAFFENBARGER, R. S., WING, A. L. and HYDE, R. T. Chronic disease in former college students XIII. Early precursors of peptic ulcer. *American Journal of Epidemiology*, **100,** 307–315 (1974)

219 PARKE, D. V. Some recent advances in the pharmacology of carbenoxolone. Chapter 1 in *Peptic Ulcer Healing: Recent Studies on Carbenoxolone*, edited by F. A. Jones, M. J. S. Langman and R. D. Mann, 1–8, Baltimore, University Park Press (1978)

220 PEDEN, N. R., CARGILL, J. M., BROWNING, M. C. K., SAUNDERS, J. H. B. and WORMSLEY, K. G. Male sexual dysfunction during treatment with cimetidine. *British Medical Journal*, **1,** 659 (1979)

221 PEDEN, N. R., SAUNDERS, J. H. B. and WORMSLEY, K. G. Inhibition of pentagastrin-stimulated and nocturnal gastric secretion by ranitidine. *Lancet*, **1,** 690 –692 (1979)

222 PETERSON, W. L., BARNETT, C. , FELDMAN, M. and RICHARDSON, C. T. Reduction of twenty-four hour gastric acidity with combination drug therapy in patients with duodenal ulcer. *Gastroenterology*, **77,** 1015–1020 (1979)

223 PETERSON, W., FELDMAN, M., TAYLOR, I. and BREMER, M. The effect of 15(R)-15 methyl prostaglandin E_2 on meal-stimulated gastric acid secretion, serum gastrin and pancreatic polypeptide in duodenal ulcer patients. *Digestive Diseases and Sciences*, **24,** 381–384 (1979)

224 PETERSON, W. L., STURDEVANT, R. A. L., FRANKL, H. D., RICHARDSON, C. T., ISEN-BERG, J. I., ELASHOFF, J. D., SONES, J. Q., GROSS, R. A., McCALLUM, R. W. and FORDTRAN, J. S. Healing of duodenal ulcer with an antacid regimen. *New England Journal of Medicine*, **297,** 341–345 (1977)

225 PFIEFFER, C. J., FODOR, J. and GEIZEROVA, H. An epidemiologic study of the relationship of peptic ulcer disease in 50–54-year-old urban males with physical health and smoking factors. *Journal of Chronic Diseases*, **26,** 291–302 (1973)

226 PIPER, D. W. and FENTON, B. H. pH stability and activity curves of pepsin with special reference to their clinical importance, *Gut*, **6,** 506–508 (1965)

227 PLAUT, M., LICHTENSTEIN, L. M. and HENNEY, C. S. Properties of a subpopulation of T cells bearing histamine receptors. *Journal of Clinical Investigation*, **55,** 856–874 (1975)

228 POSSNET, D. N., STEIN, R. S., GRABER, S. E. and KRANTZ, S. B. Cimetidine-induced neutropenia, a possible dose-related phenomenon. *Archives of Internal Medicine*, **139,** 584–586 (1979)

229 POULANTZAS, J., POLYMEROPOULOS, P. S. and PAPASOMATIOUS, A. A double-blind evaluation of the effect of tri-potassium di-citrato bismuthate in peptic ulcer. *British Journal of Clinical Practice*, **32,** 147–148 (1978)

230 POUNDER, R. E., HUNT, R. H., STEKELMAN, M., MILTON-THOMPSON, G. J. and MIS-IEWICZ, J. J. Healing of gastric ulcer during treatment with cimetidine. *Lancet*, **1,** 337–338 (1976)

231 POUNDER, R. E., HUNT, R. H. and VINCENT, S. H. Twenty-four-hour intragastric acidity and nocturnal acid secretion in patients with duodenal ulcer during oral administration of cimetidine and atropine. *Gut*, **18**, 85–90 (1977)

232 POUNDER, R. E., WILLIAMS, J. G., MILTON-THOMPSON, G. J. and MISIEWICZ, J. J. Effect of cimetidine on 24-hour intragastric acidity in normal subjects. *Gut*, **17**, 133–138 (1976)

233 POUNDER, R. E., WILLIAMS, J. G., RUSSELL, R. C. G., MILTON-THOMPSON, G. J. and MISIEWICZ, J. J. Inhibition of food-stimulated gastric acid secretion by cimetidine. *Gut*, **17**, 161–168 (1976)

234 PRIEBE, H. J., SKILLMAN, J. J., BUSHNELL, L. S., LONG, P. C. and SILEN, W. Antacid versus cimetidine in preventing acute gastrointestinal bleeding. A randomized trial in 75 critically ill patients. *New England Journal of Medicine*, **302**, 426–430 (1980)

235 PRIMACK, W. A. Cimetidine and renal-allograft rejection. *Lancet*, **1**, 824–825 (1978)

236 REED, B. *Lectures to General Practitioners on the Diseases of the Stomach and Intestines*, 2nd edition, New York, E. B. Tract and Company (1907)

237 RICHARDSON, C. T., BAILEY, B. A. and WALSH, J. H. The effect of an H_2-receptor antagonist on food stimulated acid secretion, serum gastrin and gastric emptying in patients with duodenal ulcer. *Journal of Clinical Investigation*, **55**, 536–542 (1975)

238 RICHARDSON, C. T., FELDMAN, M. and FORDTRAN, J. S. A new long-acting H_2-receptor antagonist. *Gastroenterology*, **78**, 1243 (1980)

239 RICHARDSON, C. T., WALSH, J. H. and HICKS, M. I. The effect of cimetidine, a new histamine H_2-receptor antagonist on meal-stimulated acid secretion, serum gastrin and gastric emptying in patients with duodenal ulcer. *Gastroenterology*, **71**, 19–23 (1976)

240 ROBERT, A. Cytoprotection by prostaglandins. *Gastroenterology*, **77**, 761–767 (1979)

241 ROBERT, A., NEZAMIS, J. E., LANCASTER, C. and HANCHAR, A. J. Cytoprotection by prostaglandins in rats. Prevention of gastric necrosis produced by alcohol, HCl, NaOH, hypertonic NaCl, and thermal injury. *Gastroenterology*, **77**, 433–443 (1979)

242 ROBERT, A., NYLANDER, B. and ANDERSSON, S. Marked inhibition of gastric secretion by two prostaglandin analogs given orally to man. *Life Sciences*, **14**, 533–538 (1974)

243 ROBINSON, T. J. and MULLIGAN, T. O. Cimetidine and mental confusion. *Lancet*, **2**, 719 (1977)

244 ROCKLIN, R. E. Regulation of migration inhibitory factor (MIF) production by histamine receptor-bearing lymphocytes. *Federation Proceedings*, **34**, 977 (1975)

245 ROONEY, P. J., OAKLEY, C., STURROCK, R. D., DICK, W. C., HAYES, J. R. and BUCHANAN, K. D. Effect of carbenoxolone upon immunoreactive secretin in patients with rheumatoid arthritis. *Lancet*, **1**, 592–594 (1974)

246 ROTH, H. P. Psychotherapy and psychotherapeutic agents in the medical treatment of peptic ulcer. In *The Stomach Including Related Areas in the Esophagus and Duodenum*, 360–370. New York, Grune and Stratton (1967)

247 ROTH, J. L. A. The ulcer patient should watch his diet. In *Controversy in Internal Medicine*, edited by F. J. Ingelfinger, A. S. Relman and M. Finland, 161–170. Philadelphia, W. B. Saunders Company (1966)

248 ROTH, J. A. and IVY, A. C. The effect of caffeine upon gastric secretion in the dog, cat and man. *American Journal of Physiology*, **141**, 454–461 (1944)

249 ROTOLI, B., FORMISANO, S. and ALFINITO, F. Autoimmune haemolytic anaemia associated with cimetidine. *Lancet*, **2**, 583 (1979)

250 SAHEL, J. and SARLES, H. A multi-centre study of the endoscopically assessed efficacy of carbenoxolone sodium capsules in duodenal ulcer. Chapter 11 in *Peptic Ulcer Healing: Recent Studies on Carbenoxolone*, edited by F. A. Jones, M. J. S. Langman and R. D. Mann, 111–116. Baltimore, University Park Press (1978)

251 SAINT-HILAIRE, S., LAVERS, M. D., KENNEDY, J. and CODE, C. G. Gastric acid secretory value of different foods, *Gastroenterology*, **39**, 1–11 (1960)

252 SALMON, P. R., BROWN, P., WILLIAMS, R. and READ, A. E. Evaluation of colloidal bismuth (De-Nol) in the treatment of duodenal ulcer employing endoscopic selection and follow-up. *Gut*, **15**, 189–193 (1974)

253 SANCHEZ-PALOMERA, E. The action of spices on the acid gastric secretion, on the appetite and on the caloric intake. *Gastroenterology*, **18**, 254–268 (1951)

254 SARLES, H., CAMATTE, R. and SAHEL, J. A study of the variations in the response regarding duodenal ulcer when treated with placebo by different investigators. *Digestion*, **16**, 289–292 (1977)

255 SCHEURER, U., WITZEL, L., HALTER, F., KELLER, H. M., HUBER, R. and GALEAZZI, R. Gastric and duodenal ulcer healing under placebo treatment. *Gastroenterology*, **72**, 838–841 (1977)

256 SCHNEIDER, M. A., DELUCA, V., JR. and GRAY, S. J. Effect of spice ingestion on stomach. *American Journal of Gastroenterology*, **26**, 726–732 (1956)

257 SHREEVE, D. R. A double-blind study of tri-potassium di-citrato bismuthate in duodenal ulcer. *Postgraduate Medical Journal*, **51** (Supplement 5), 33–35 (1975)

258 SMITH, P. M., EDWARDS, J. L. and AUBREY, D. A. Gastric secretory studies and cimetidine treatment in gastric ulcers. Chapter 23 in *Cimetidine. The Westminster Hospital Symposium*, edited by C. Wastell and P. Lance, 258–272. Edinburgh, Churchill Livingstone (1978)

259 SOLEM, L. D., STRATE, R. G. and FISCHER, R. P. Antacid therapy and nutritional supplementation in the prevention of Curling's ulcer. *Surgery, Gynecology and Obstetrics*, **148**, 367–370 (1979)

260 SONNENBERG, A., SCHMID, P., MULLER-LISSNER, S. A., VOGEL, E. and BLUM, A. L. What makes duodenal ulcer heal and relapse? *Gastroenterology*, **78**, 1266 (1980)

261 SPENCER, H. and LENDER, M. Adverse effects of aluminum-containing antacids on mineral metabolism. *Gastroenterology*, **76**, 603–606 (1979)

262 STEINBERG, W. M. and LEWIS, J. H. Mylanta II inhibits the absorption of cimetidine. *Gastroenterology*, **78**, 1269 (1980)

263 STOCKBRUGGER, R., JAUP, B., HAMMER, R. and DOTEVALL, G. Inhibition of gastric acid secretion by pirenzepine (LS 519) in man. *Scandinavian Journal of Gastroenterology*, **14**, 615–620 (1979)

264 STRECKER, R., VALENZUELA, J. E. and DOUGLAS, A. P. Inhibition of nocturnal acid secretion by a new H_2-receptor antagonist (ICI 125,211) in duodenal ulcer patients. *Gastroenterology*, **78**, 1271 (1980)

265 STURDEVANT, R. A. L. Tricyclics and histamine H_2-receptors. *Gastroenterology*, **74**, 961–962 (1978)

266 STURDEVANT, R. A. L., ISENBERG, J. I., SECRIST, D. and ANSFIELD, J. Antacid and placebo produced similar pain relief in duodenal ulcer patients. *Gastroenterology*, **72**, 1–5 (1977)

267 SUN, D. C. H. Long-term anticholinergic therapy for prevention of recurrences in duodenal ulcer. *American Journal of Digestive Diseases*, **9**, 706–716 (1964)

268 SUN, D. C. H. Effect of a synthetic sulfated polysaccharide (SN-263) on gastric peptic activity in humans. *Annals of the New York Academy of Sciences*, **140**, 747–753 (1967)

269 SUN, D. C. and RYAN, M. L. A controlled study on the use of propantheline and amylopectin sulphate (SN-263) for recurrences in duodenal ulcer. *Gastroenterology*, **58**, 756–761 (1970)

270 SWIERCZEK, J. S., DEVITT, P. G., SUDDITH, R. L., RAYFORD, P. L. and THOMPSON, J. C. β_2-adrenergic action in gastric acid secretion and gastrin release in dogs. *Gastroenterology*, **78**, 1273 (1980)

271 TAYLOR, R. H., LAIDLOW, J. M., CHAPMAN, R. G., COLIN-JONES, D. G., GOLDING, P. L., HUNT, R. H., VINCENT, S. H., MILTON-THOMPSON, G. J. and MISIEWICZ, J. J. Double-blind trial comparing cimetidine with carbenoxolone in the treatment of benign gastric ulcer. *Gut*, **18**, 420A (1977)

272 THURSTON, H., GILMORE, G. R. and SWALES, J. D. Aluminum retention and toxicity in chronic renal failure. *Lancet*, **1**, 881–883 (1972)

273 TILLY, J. R., HITCH, D. C. and JAVITZ, N. B. Cimetidine cholestatic jaundice in children. *Journal of Surgical Research*, **24**, 384–387 (1978)

274 TREVINO, H. ANDERSON, J., DAVEY, P. G. and HENLEY, K. S. The effect of glycopyrrolate on the course of symptomatic duodenal ulcer. *American Journal of Digestive Diseases*, **12**, 983–987 (1967)

275 TROWELL, O. A. The relation of tobacco smoking to the incidence of chronic duodenal ulcer. *Lancet*, **1**, 808–809 (1934)

276 TRUELOVE, S. C. Stilboestrol, phenobarbitone and diet in chronic duodenal ulcer. *British Medical Journal*, **2**, 559–566 (1960)

277 UFBERG, M. H., BROOKS, C. M., BOSANAC, P. P. and KINTZEL, J. E. Transient neutropenia in a patient receiving cimetidine. *Gastroenterology*, **73**, 635–638 (1977)

278 URIBE, M., GO, V. L. M. and SUMMERSKILL, W. H. J. Peptic ulcer, prednisone and serum gastrin in chronic active liver disease. *New England Journal of Medicine*, **296**, 173 (1977)

279 VALNES, K., MYREN, J. and QVIGSTAD, T. Trimipramine in the treatment of gastric ulcer. *Scandinavian Journal of Gastroenterology*, **13**, 497–500 (1978)

280 VAN THIEL, D. H., GAVALER, J. S., SMITH, W. I. and PAUL, G. Hypothalamic-pituitary-gonadal dysfunction in men using cimetidine. *New England Journal of Medicine*, **300**, 1012–1015 (1979)

281 VANTRAPPEN, G., POPIELA, T., TYTGAT, D. N. J., LAMBERT, R. and ROBERT, A. A multicentre trial of 15(R)-15 methyl prostaglandin E_2 in duodenal ulcer. *Gastroenterology*, **78,** 1283 (1980)

282 VILLENEUVE, J. P. and WARNER, H. A. Cimetidine hepatitis. *Gastroenterology*, **77,** 143–144 (1979)

283 WALAN, A. Studies on peptic ulcer disease with special reference to the effect of L-hyoscyamine. *Acta Medica Scandinavica*, Supplement 516, 1–57 (1970)

284 WALKER, C. O. Complications of peptic ulcer disease and indications for surgery. Chapter 53 in *Gastrointestinal Disease: Pathophysiology, Diagnosis, Management*, edited by M. H. Sleisenger and J. S. Fordtran 914–931. Philadelphia, W. B. Saunders Company (1978)

285 WALT, R. P., PRICE, D., RAWLINGS, J., HUNT, R. H., MILTON-THOMPSON, G. J. and MISIEWICZ, J. J. The effect of ranitidine on twenty-four-hour intragastric acidity, nocturnal and food-stimulated acid secretion. *Gastroenterology*, **78,** 1286 (1980)

286 WATKINSON, G. Closing remarks: '10 years later'. In *Peptic Ulcer Healing: Recent Studies on Carbenoxolone*, edited by F. A. Jones, M. J. S. Langman and R. D. Mann, 135–147. Baltimore, University Park Press (1978)

287 WATSON, W. C., KUTTY, P. K. and COLCLEUGH, R. G. Does cimetidine cause ileus in the burned patient? *Lancet*, **2,** 720 (1977)

288 WEISS, G. and SERFONTEIN, W. J. The efficacy of a bismuth-protein-complex compound in the treatment of gastric and duodenal ulcers. *South African Medical Journal*, **45,** 467–470 (1971)

289 WELSH, J. D. Diet therapy of peptic ulcer disease. *Gastroenterology*, **72,** 740–745 (1977)

290 WETTERHUS, S., AUBERT, E., BERG, C. E., BJERKESET, T., HALVORSEN, L., HOVDENAK, N., MYREN, J., ROWLAND, M., SIGSTAD, H. and GULDAHL, M. The effect of trimipramine (Surmontil) on symptoms and healing of peptic ulcer. A double-blind study. *Scandinavian Journal of Gastroenterology*, **12** (Supplement 43), 33–38 (1977)

291 WINSHIP, D. Cimetidine in the treatment of duodenal ulcer: Review and commentary. *Gastroenterology*, **74,** 402–406 (1978)

292 WOLFE, M. M. Impotence on cimetidine treatment. *New England Journal of Medicine*, **300,** 94 (1979)

293 WOODINGS, E. P., DIXON, G. T., HARRISON, C., CAREY, P. and RICHARDS, D. A. Ranitidine–a new H_2-receptor antagonist. *Gut*, **21,** 187–191 (1980)

294 WOODWARD, E. R., ROBERTSON, C., RUTTENBERG, H. D. and SCHAPIRO, H. Alcohol as a gastric secretory stimulant. *Gastroenterology*, **32,** 727–737 (1957)

295 WULFF, H. R. and RUNE, S. J. A comparison of studies on the treatment of gastric ulceration with cimetidine. Chapter 25 in *Cimetidine. The Westminster Hospital Symposium*, edited by C. Wastell and P. Lance 281–288. Edinburgh, Churchill Livingstone (1978)

296 WYLLIE, J. H. Histamine H_2-receptor antagonist in treatment of peptic ulcer. *Postgraduate Medicine*, **63**(4), 91–96 (1978)

297 YANTIS, P. L., BRIDGES, M. E. and PITTMAN, F. E. Cimetidine-induced exfoliative dermatitis. *Digestive Diseases and Sciences*, **25,** 73–74 (1980)

298 YOUNG, G. P., ST. JOHN D. J. B. and COVENTRY, D. A. A double-masked endoscopic evaluation of carbenoxolone sodium in duodenal ulcer: Further evidence for a beneficial effect. Chapter 12 in *Peptic Ulcer Healing: Recent Studies on Carbenoxolone*, edited by F. A. Jones, M. J. S. Langman and R. D. Mann, 117–125. Baltimore, University Park Press (1978)

8
Motility disorders of the foregut

James Christensen

Introduction

Disorders of motility in the foregut have been recognized for a long time but they are still not carefully defined or understood. This chapter will review those disorders that are generally recognized and accepted as clinical entities in which disordered gut motility is primary. The emphasis will be on physiology, pathophysiology, and pathogenesis. Much of the evidence that exists in these matters comes from animal studies. In some cases, data are available from human studies, but many of these are fragmentary or indecisive because of the methodological limitations of the study of gastrointestinal motility in man.

Esophagus

Upper esophageal sphincter dysfunction

The upper esophageal sphincter is a term that is used to refer to a segment of the tubular gut that lies between the pharynx and the esophagus. This segment can be operationally distinguished from both the pharynx above and the esophagus below. The term has been used principally in association with the technique of esophageal manometry by which the upper esophageal sphincter is detected as a zone of elevated intraluminal pressure. This pressure represents the consequence of luminal occlusion. This pressure is maintained at a reasonably constant level at rest, up to 60 cm of water above atmosphere, but it falls to atmospheric pressure at the initiation of a swallow, resting pressure being restored after about one second or so. The closed lumen is readily appreciated endoscopically as well.

The muscular walls of this segment, 2–4 cm long in man, include the cricopharyngeus muscle and, possibly, some of the muscle of the adjacent pharynx and upper esophagus as well. It is generally accepted now that the maintained luminal closure at rest is a consequence of a sustained contraction of the striated musculature of the walls of the gut at this level and that the disappearance of the pressure during a swallow represents transient abolition of that contraction. In times past, however, both closure at rest and opening with a swallow were believed to be passive. Closure was attributed to the natural elasticity or to the structure of the wall, or to compression of the region by extra-esophageal tissues; opening was attributed to stretching of the organ through the laryngeal elevation that occurs in swallowing. Though such passive factors may indeed have some influence, it is generally accepted now that the major component of sphincteric function is active, being established by the special character of the neuromuscular apparatus of the gut wall.

Dysfunction of the upper esophageal sphincter produces oropharyngeal dysphagia, a sense of difficulty in swallowing that is perceived in the neck. It may be accompanied by aspiration of swallowed food or by nasopharyngeal reflux of swallowed liquids. It seems clear, though, that these symptoms cannot be attributable to sphincter dysfunction alone, for patients with such difficulties also have disordered function of the pharyngeal musculature.

Appropriate studies done in a variety of animals, but not in man, have established the basis for closure and opening of the upper esophageal sphincter. The electromyogram of the cricopharyngeus muscle shows continuous spike activity at rest[3, 5, 9, 37, 50, 71]. The upper esophageal muscle shows no such activity[2], but the inferior pharyngeal constrictor muscle does. The presence of continuous spike activity in these striated muscles indicates that they are in a tonically contracted state. Thus, it seems to be well established that sphincteric closure is due to a maintained tonic contraction of the striated muscle at this level.

This muscle has only one kind of innervation, a somatic type of innervation rather than an autonomic innervation. The somatic motor nerves pass from vagal nuclei by way of the vagi to end in motor end-plates like those of somatic striated muscle generally. There is no evidence for synaptic interruption of these vagal motor pathways.

There is a plexus of nerves about the distal pharynx into which vagal branches containing these motor nerves enter. There are no intramural plexuses at this level.

The closure of the upper esophagus sphincter that is maintained at rest represents a contraction of this striated muscle that is sustained by tonic discharge of these cholinergic motor nerves. Interruption of this tonic discharge occurs in swallowing, and this is the mechanism of relaxation of the muscle that allows opening of the upper esophageal sphincter[15, 29]. In swallowing there is a series of contractions and relaxations that involves the lingual, laryngeal, pharyngeal, and esophageal musculature. Relaxation of the upper esophageal sphincter is one of these actions occurring in a sequence that is ordered by the swallowing center of the brain stem. Thus, sphincter relaxation, a consequence of transient cessation of the tonic nerve discharge, is neurally determined in the swallowing center.

No specific symptoms or disorders represent upper esophageal sphincter dysfunction alone, for disorders of the sphincter always involve the pharyngeal musculature as well. These disorders can be primarily either neural or muscular in origin.

The commonest neural disorder that is associated with these symptoms is that due to vascular disease of the brain stem. When the posterior inferior cerebellar artery is obstructed, oropharyngeal dysphagia, reflecting death or dysfunction of that part of the brain stem where the swallowing center and nuclei are located, is sudden in onset and usually improves gradually. Poliomyelitis likewise produced oropharyngeal dysphagia through damage to the central nervous structures. Other neuropathic causes for such dysphagia are much less common. They include amyotrophic lateral sclerosis, Huntington's chorea, multiple sclerosis, and the miscellaneous causes of peripheral cranial neuropathy.

Diseases of striated muscle constitute the other causes for oropharyngeal dysphagia. These include myasthenia gravis (or the myasthenic syndrome), myotonic dystrophy, oculopharyngeal muscular dystrophy, and dermatomyositis-polymyositis.

Zenker's diverticulum, a full-thickness diverticulum arising from a point of weakness just above the upper esophageal sphincter, would certainly seem to be attributable to a disordered coordination of pharyngeal contraction and sphincteric relaxation. Indeed, evidence has been advanced to support the view that the upper esophageal sphincter contracts prematurely after swallowing-induced relaxation[31, 51], such contraction presumably leading to a transient, abnormally elevated pressure at that level. But others have not been able to confirm this abnormality. There are fundamental methodological problems in the study of this matter, related to the deficiences in the techniques by which the operation of the upper esophogeal sphincter can be studied. The first problem is that the sphincter is not radially symmetric. Rather, it is a crescentic slit, the shape being determined by the arc of the cricopharyngeus muscle. It follows that intraluminal pressure, as determined by manometry, varies according to the direction in which the sensing point of the intraluminal catheter is facing. Much lower pressures are detected when the sensing point faces one of the horns of the crescent than when it is facing the midpoint of either of the two arcs that define the crescent. A second problem is that the muscular tone is not uniform throughout the several centimeters of the sphincter length: it seems probable that some shift of the catheter along the axis of the tubular conduit occurs during swallowing. A third, and the most severely limiting problem, is that the rapidity with which the striated muscle contracts and relaxes is such that the usual manometric devices cannot follow the changes with precision because of damping in the fluid-filled elastic catheters. Thus, sufficiently accurate studies of the magnitude and the timing of sphincteric actions in swallowing in normal persons and in patients with Zenker's diverticulum remain to be done. An accurate measure of timing, of course, could be made using electromyographic recording from the sphincteric musculature, as has been done in animals. This has not been done in man.

The theory that sphincteric abnormalities cause Zenker's diverticulum, however, has influenced therapy, for the lesion is now being treated by surgical division of the cricopharyngeus and elevation, rather than resection, of the diverticulum itself. Anecdotal evidence that this is successful at least supports the theory of pathogenesis.

Diffuse esophageal spasm

This term is used for patients with a variety of symptoms and findings that, however, all seem to reflect abnormalities in the contractions of the part of the esophagus in which the walls are composed of smooth muscle, the distal half or so. The abnormality appears to be one in which the response of this part of the esophagus to a single swallow is changed from a single progressive contraction to one that is simultaneous along the smooth-muscled segment, or to one that occurs in no particular order from one level to another. This contraction may also be of higher amplitude than normal and of much longer duration, up to 30 seconds. Also, contractions may occur that are spontaneous (unrelated to a swallow) and repetitive. These abnormalities are often variably present. The dysphagia associated with the abnormal contractions is often precipitated by the drinking of hot or very cold liquids.

Little has been published on the pathology of the esophagus in diffuse esophageal spasm. There are reports of thickening of the muscle in the smooth-muscled parts of the esophagus, the distal two-thirds, but not all agree even on this point[30 34 35, 47]. The problem lies, in part, in inadequate understanding of the morphology of the normal esophageal smooth muscle. Since patients with this diagnosis are usually in middle-age or older, and since at least some features of the disorder seem to be very frequent in asymptomatic nonagenarians[74], the question of normal controls is critical in the definition of the entity, both clinically and pathologically. The same criticism can be made about another frequently cited report that degenerative changes were found in the vagus nerves of patients operated on for treatment of diffuse spasm[35]. The degenerated neurons were interpreted as being vagal afferents because of their number.

Loss of the progressive nature of swallowing-induced contraction in the smooth-muscled segment is the most prominent feature of diffuse esophageal spasm. If the basis for the progressive nature of this contraction were known, the genesis of esophageal spasm might be partially explained. The genesis and control of peristalsis in the smooth-muscled segment has received considerable attention recently. It is now widely accepted that the progressive nature of peristalsis in esophageal smooth muscle does not require organized sequences or firing of central nervous structures, as was once thought. Electrical stimulation of the distal end of the cut vagus excites a peristaltic sequence in the smooth-muscled part of the esophagus[28, 57]. Also, peristaltic or progressive contractions of the smooth muscle that are excited by local distention of the esophagus are not affected by vagotomy[49, 63, 64]. This, and much other evidence, indicates that the programming that establishes the progressive nature of the swallow-induced contraction of esophageal smooth muscle is not in the central nervous system but peripheral. That is, the mechanism lies within the wall of the esophagus. It would be natural to think that the programming occurs in the myenteric plexuses, and this has been proposed[27]. This idea has not, however, been sufficiently tested.

The theory that the programming occurs in the smooth muscle itself has been proposed as well[84], and considerable evidence exists to support it. The circular layer of smooth muscle from the esophageal body shows only one response to nerve stimulation, both vagal stimulation and stimulation of the intramural plexuses. This is a single brief contraction that follows well after the end of the period of electrical stimulation. There is a brief delay between the end of the stimulus and the onset of the contraction. This delay, or latency, is not constant at all levels of the smooth-muscled segment. Rather, it exists as a monotonic gradient, being shortest at the top of the smooth-muscled segment and longest at the bottom. It is this gradient that is proposed as the basis for the progressive nature of swallowing-induced contraction in esophageal smooth muscle.

According to this hypothesis[84], the nerves that excite the smooth muscle of the esophagus after a swallow are really inhibitory in nature (the inhibitory neurotransmitter being unknown). The nature of the neuromuscular interaction is such that the muscle, after the end of the period of inhibition, contracts in a rebound contraction. Because esophageal muscle shows no spontaneous contractions, the period of inhibition is not apparent, so that only the rebound contraction is seen. The gradient in latency of this rebound contraction makes it appear that the contraction is one that sweeps from the top of the smooth-muscled segment to the bottom.

If the basis for the progression of the contraction lies entirely in the muscle, then loss of the progression would be attributable to a disorder of the muscle rather than to nerve dysfunction. This is compatible with the histopathology that, although very limited, indicates changes in the smooth muscle but not in the intramural plexuses.

The latency gradient, if it is based in the muscle itself, should represent a gradient in some character of the muscle, and there is evidence for a gradient in the intracellular ionic composition of the muscle. There is a gradient in the potassium content of the muscle along the esophagus[25, 68, 70] and this may be reflected in a gradient in the electrical behavior of the muscle cell membranes[25]. It is still not clear exactly how this gradient is related to the gradient in the latency of the nerve-induced rebound contraction.

If diffuse esophageal spasm is a primary disease of smooth muscle, then why is this disease confined to the esophagus? The answer is that it may not be. The patients are often at or beyond middle-age when at least one other disorder occurs that is characterized by hypertrophy of gastrointestinal muscles, diverticulosis coli.

Achalasia

Like esophageal spasm, this too is a disease of the part of the esophagus that is smooth muscle. Although this diagnostic term is often used as though it describes a single entity, there seems to be a great deal of variability in the manifestations of this disease, as there is in esophageal spasm. The abnormal physiology that is present in all cases, though, constitutes two problems: the failure of the lower esophageal sphincter to relax in response to a swallow, and the failure of a swallow to make the smooth-muscled part of the esophagus (the distal two-thirds) contract normally. Other features that may be found in some cases include an abnormally increased closure tension in the lower esophageal sphincter, a massively dilated esophageal body, and contractions of the esophageal body that are weak, spontaneous and nonpropulsive. Other variables are consequences of the esophageal obstruction; these include episodes of aspiration pneumonia, malnutrition, and a fermentative esophagitis.

Much more has been written on the pathology of achalasia than on the pathology of esophageal spasm. So many accounts have been published reporting a deficit or absence of ganglion cells in the myenteric plexus that this abnormality must be considered a well-established fact[2, 10, 22, 40, 42, 54, 61, 62]. These reports, all of them together, deal with only a few cases, of course, since autopsy material and adequate surgical specimens are only rarely available from these patients. Those reports do not fully agree as to the distribution and completeness of the deficit in intramural plexus cells. Ganglia are sparse in the esophagus as compared to the rest of the gut, and gross dilation of the esophagus may make distances between ganglia seem greater than normal. Thus, a considerable sampling error is possible. Vagal lesions have also been reported by some investigators[11].

A superior histological technique to examine the myenteric plexus has been introduced by Smith[72] and applied to the study of the myenteric plexuses in achalasia. By this technique, one can distinguish two types of ganglion cells in the myenteric plexus named, on the basis of their affinity for the silver stain, argyrophobe and argyrophil cells. Smith[73] has described the absence of argyrophilic ganglion cells in achalasia. Argyrophobic cells may or may not be deficient.

The smooth muscle of the esophagus is also variably reported to be abnormal. Grossly, hypertrophy at one level or another is reported. Electron microscopy has revealed changes like those seen in denervated striated muscle, detachment or displacement of myofibrils[12].

These changes though, are either less notable or less noted than those of the ganglion cells.

The pathology reviewed briefly above suggests strongly that there is a neuropathic basis for achalasia. That idea is supported by physiological studies as well. The muscle of the esophageal body can be made to contract artificially in these patients, even if it does not do so physiologically. The hypersensitivity of the esophageal smooth muscle to the muscarinic cholinergic agonist, acetyl-β-methacholine (methacholine chloride), was described long ago and has been used as a diagnostic test[48]. This hypersensitivity is attributed to denervation, this being taken as an example of Cannon's famous principle to the effect that denervated structures become hyperreactive to substances to which they normally respond. There is nothing specific about denervation supersensitivity, and so it is not surprising that supersensitivity to gastrin exists as well[21]. Supersensitivity ought to be demonstrable to a variety of other agents that can normally excite esophageal smooth muscle.

Recent studies on the physiology of esophageal function allow one to understand the coexistence of the two invariable features of the achalasia, the failure of swallowing to induce normal contractions of the esophageal body and the failure of swallowing to induce full relaxation of the lower esophageal sphincter. This would be easily understood if it were true that both these functions represent the consequence of the operation of one class of nerves. Evidence exists to establish that this is indeed the case.

Earlier in this chapter it was pointed out that the peristaltic contraction that sweeps that smooth-muscled segment of the esophagus after a swallow is really the consequence of the action of inhibitory nerves, a rebound contraction that follows a period of inhibition. The inhibitory nerves that are responsible for this have been studied extensively in the opossum, to a lesser degree in the cat. The inhibitory nerves that are responsible for relaxation of the lower esophageal sphincter have also been studied in these species. The inhibitory nerves that serve these two functions seem to be physiologically identical.

They may also be identical anatomically, but there have been no sufficiently detailed studies of the morphology of the intramural plexuses of the esophagus in experimental animals. Such studies as have been done do not reveal any marked distinction in the morphology or the innervation between sphincteric and nonsphincteric regions.

These inhibitory nerves that cause contraction of the circular muscle layer of the esophageal body and relaxation of that of the lower esophageal sphincter, influence the muscle by a mechanism that is unknown. A long search to identify the inhibitory neurotransmitter has not been fruitful. In other autonomically innervated tissues, both purine compounds and various peptides have been proposed as inhibitory transmitters for such nonadrenergic inhibitory nerves, but none have been convincingly established.

It seems quite reasonable to propose that achalasia is a consequence of death or dysfunction of this particular class of nerves. Much evidence exists to support this. Neuropathic changes have commonly been described, and they seem especially to affect one class of ganglion cells, the argyrophils. The nonadrenergic inhibitory nerves that pass through vagal tracts seem to be chiefly important in regulation of esophageal muscle, so that the major manifestations of disease of these nerves might be expected to be mainly esophageal. The close resemblance of achalasia to the esophageal lesion of Chagas's disease is also significant since the latter is clearly a neuropathic disease.

In view of this hypothesis, then, there is a need to know more about the structure and function of these nerves, for something about them makes them particularly susceptible to whatever toxic or infective process it is that initiates their destruction or disorder. The selectivity of the process is emphasized by the fact that patients with achalasia do not give evidence of dysfunction of cholinergic or adrenergic nerves. Although no other such disorder is grossly apparent in patients with achalasia, it is possible that a subtle degree of autonomic neuropathy could exist without being apparent.

These nonadrenergic inhibitory nerves are connected with the brain stem through the vagi and so must have representation among the cells of the vagal nuclei. This is consistent with the observation that destruction of the vagal nuclei can produce an achalasia-like syndrome in animals. These nerves, however, cannot be selectively identified by morphologic means in the nuclei, in the vagi, or in the intramural plexuses.

The nonadrenergic inhibitory nerves appear to be distinct physiologically from other known autonomic motor nerves. Their action is unaffected by the selective antagonists to neurochemical transmission at adrenergic and cholinergic synapses. They seem to be especially resistant to the removal of calcium from the extracellular environment[24.] They appear to be more resistant to the actions of local anesthetics than are the cholinergic nerves, and they have a much shorter chronaxie than do cholinergic nerves (unpublished data). All this would suggest that these nerves, at least those in the esophageal intramural plexus, are of larger average diameter than are cholinergic cells. Smith[72, 73] has said, from morphologic studies, that the processes of the argyrophil cells of the myenteric plexus tend to be thicker than those of the argyrophobe cells. Furthermore, the ratio of the number of argyrophil cells to argyrophobe cells in the esophagus is greater than it is elsewhere in the gut[72, 73]. Thus, it seems reasonable to propose that the argyrophil cells of the plexus are the ganglion cells of the nonadrenergic inhibitory system.

Gastroesophageal reflux

Gastroesophageal reflux and its complications are, of course, extremely common and troublesome afflictions. Esophagitis, esophageal ulcer, and stricture are usually thought of as inflammatory rather than motor disorders, but it is now clear that, except for those cases associated with the ingestion of corrosive agents, these problems represent a consequence of the return of gastric content into the esophagus. The forces that normally operate to prevent this occurrence are forces generated by smooth muscle, and so these clinical entities should properly be considered among the motor disorders of the alimentary canal. Two motor abnormalities that contribute to gastroesophageal reflux, occurring either singly or together, have been proposed: the failure of the esophagus to clear itself of refluxed gastric content and failure of the lower esophagus sphincter to prevent such reflux from occurring.

Of course, several secondary factors, too, have been proposed that may normally act to minimize the reflux or to mitigate its effects. These include the esophageal mucosal resistance to the corrosive action of gastric contents, the pinchcock action of the diaphragm at the level of the gastroesophageal sphincter, the nature of the gastric content, the quantity of saliva, and factors that are hydrostatic in nature, like posture and intra-abdominal pressure. These secondary factors will not be discussed here.

The first of the two motor mechanisms, the abnormality of which can contribute to gastroesophageal reflux, is failure of the esophagus to clear itself of refluxed gastric content. The fact that such reflux is a normal event is well-established. Healthy (or at least asymptomatic) people will have several such episodes of reflux day and night. These episodes are asymptomatic and brief. Their occurrence has been demonstrated chiefly at night during sleep, by continuous monitoring of intraesophageal pH through the use of a pH probe, a small pH electrode attached to a wire that is positioned in the distal esophagus. Several times during a period of nocturnal recumbency, the pH will fall abruptly from the normal, near neutrality, to a much lower value and the pH will rise over a matter of minutes to the normal value[41]. The reversal of the transient acidification of the esophageal lumen is thought to be accomplished in part by peristaltic sweeps that clear the esophageal lumen of the acidic material that has entered it from the stomach. Patients with reflux symptoms may show either more such episodes or retardation in the rate at which the abnormal pH is reversed, or both.

Several abnormalities can be proposed that could account for these observations. First, the sphincter itself could be abnormal, a possibility that will be dealt with later. Also, the peristaltic sweeps could be reduced in frequency. Third, peristaltic contractions of normal frequency could be reduced in force. Finally, esophageal contractions could be nonperistaltic. Not all of these were clearly established to occur in the few studies reported[8, 75]. It is possible, of course, that the peristaltic contractions occurring as a consequence of an episode of gastroesophageal reflux are initiated voluntarily by swallowing. That is, they could constitute primary peristalsis. Swallowing can be initiated reflexly, and normal people must swallow salivary secretions during sleep. But esophageal clearance could also be accomplished by secondary peristalsis, a mechanism that involves the ability of esophageal distension to excite reflexly a peristaltic contraction. This reflex is usually considered to be excited by mechanoreceptors whose location and appearance are unknown.

From these considerations, a variety of possibilities are evident that could be proposed to account for poor esophageal clearance of refluxed gastric content. Reflex swallowing during sleep could be depressed, or the mechanism of secondary peristalsis could be defective. Neither of these possibilities has been sought. But evidence exists to support two other possible mechanisms, peristaltic contractions of diminished force and nonperistaltic contractions. This evidence is inferential, arising from studies of patients with esophageal aperistalsis.

Reflux esophagitis is a well-known presenting complaint in those disorders characterized by absence of peristalsis in the smooth-muscled segment. This is most commonly seen in those patients who have the various forms of disorders collectively called scleroderma or diffuse systemic sclerosis. It is true, though, that such patients also usually have a weak lower esophageal sphincter, and so in such cases it is not usually possible to attribute the difficulty mainly to one or the other abnormality. Weak contractions may be detected in some patients with diabetes and alcoholism, but these patients may also have a weak sphincter at the gastroesophageal junction. Patients with achalasia who have had the sphincter breached by pneumatic dilation or operative section are notoriously prone to esophagitis, in part because of the breach but also because of the atony of the distal esophagus. Many patients with achalasia are found to have esophagitis before breach of the sphincter, but this is usually attributed to bacterial fermentation of the retained food and secretions.

Nonperistaltic contractions likewise have not been firmly established as causative of reflux esophagitis, but it is not uncommon to find these two abnormalities coexisting. Unfortunately, both esophagitis and nonperistaltic contractions are independently very common, and so their coexistence must not be rare. It is possible that long-standing esophagitis is causative of nonperistaltic contractions, of course, but no evidence exists to establish that point further.

The greater part of the investigation in the pathogenesis of esophagitis has been directed to the study of strength of the lower esophageal sphincter. A great mass of literature exists that has engendered a good deal of controversy. These controversies have been mostly methodological, dealing with the successive refinements in the technique of esophageal manometry, in which sphincter pressure is measured by the use of a tube that lies in the esophageal lumen. It should be pointed out that the pressure actually measured by all such methods is that pressure that is required to force the mucosa away from a hole (usually 1 mm in diameter) in the side of a plastic tube through which fluid is being pumped. Obviously, several factors can contribute to this pressure. Many of these are technical matters, related to such things as rate of perfusion, the compliance of the tube, the diameter of the tube, the size of the hole, and so on. These problems are circumvented by the use of a tube that contains miniature pressure transducers, but other physiological variables present problems. The tone of the sphincter muscle itself is the only contributor to sphincter pressure that is usually considered. But such other possible factors as the tone in the muscularis mucosae, tissue turgor, and pressure in the intramural blood vessels could also contribute. Also, the sphincter seems not to have a uniform tone throughout its length, 3–4 cm, so that tube placement is an important variable. As well, it is not established that the tone of the sphincter muscle is constant even over rather short intervals of time. It is not surprising, then, that 'normal' values for sphincter pressure (which reflects sphincter closure tension) vary widely. Nevertheless, the preponderance of the evidence indicates that defective tone in the sphincteric muscle is a major cause of gastroesophageal reflux. It is important, then, to learn by what means this tone is maintained.

The very existence of a special kind of smooth muscle in the circular layer at the gastroesophageal junction was a matter of controversy until recent times, and there are even yet claims that such muscle does not exist in man. In fact, no studies have been made of human muscle to attempt to confirm what has been found in muscle from this region in opossum and, to a limited degree, in cat and monkey. The North American opossum, not at all an exotic or unusual laboratory animal, has been studied extensively because it has smooth muscle throughout the distal half of the esophagus, as do man and many other primates. There is abundant evidence that the circular layer of smooth muscle at the level of the lower esophageal sphincter differs from that of immediately adjacent regions in that it has a high degree of tone, a sustained contraction[18].

The source of this tone is not well understood. It is accompanied by continuously generated spike potentials[6]. It is not neurogenic, for little or no reduction in tone is produced by the selective neurotoxin, tetrodotoxin, both *in vitro* and *in vivo*[17, 36]. Also, *in vitro*, this tone is not affected by nerve-blocking concentrations of local anesthetics (unpublished data). It is unaffected by selective antagonists of autonomic neurohormonal transmitters[16]. It is maintained *in vitro* for very low periods. From all this evidence, it is concluded that this tone is myogenic. The special properties of this muscle that cause it to maintain a contraction remain unknown. It is known, however, that this tone is wholly dependent upon oxidative phosphorylation, for it promptly disappears under conditions of hypoxia and promptly returns when oxygen is restored to the tissue[77]. This raises the possibility that sphincter tone could be influenced by abnormalities that would lead to muscle hypoxia, like chronic hypoxemia or a reduced blood flow.

The variability of sphincter closure tension over relatively short intervals of time is a matter not often considered. Yet, such variability exists[13, 60] and it is of obvious relevance to the occurrence of reflux esophagitis. The source of the variability is not understood. Although sphincter closure tension, at least in the opossum, is not reduced by the neurotoxin, tetrodotoxin, this does not establish that the tone of the sphincter muscle *in vivo* is wholly myogenic. The claim that the hormone gastrin is the major determinant of lower esophageal sphincter pressure has now been abandoned, but it remains possible that small changes in sphincter muscle tone could be hormonally mediated. The number of candidate hormones is enormous and the possibilities are still not exhausted. There is one established hormonal influence. Sphincter closure tension *in vivo* is reduced by estrogen together with progesterone, and this is evidence for an action of steroid hormones on the sphincter muscle, directly or indirectly[67, 82, 83].

Nerves, too, could influence tone, and they have long been thought to do so, though on little real evidence. Studies with autonomic neurohormonal agents and selective antagonists establish that the lower esophageal sphincter muscle responds to cholinergic agents by contracting and to norepinephrine, the usual transmitter of adrenergic nerves, by contracting as well. That is, the adrenergic α-receptor is excitatory, but the adrenergic α-receptor is inhibitory. Thus, nerves liberating acetylcholine should cause contraction and those liberating norepinephrine could be either excitatory or inhibitory, depending upon which adrenergic receptor is activated. The α-receptor response is reduced by atropine, potentiated by physostigmine and opposed by hemicholinium, suggesting that α-receptor excitation of the muscle is accomplished through release of acetylcholine from cholinergic stores, presumably cholinergic nerves. This is consistent with the morphologic observation that adrenergic nerves, in the gastrointestinal musculature in general, terminate in a synaptic relationship with ganglion cells, presumably secondary parasympathetic neurons. The few studies that have been made of the morphology of the nerves of esophageal and esophagogastric sphincteric smooth muscle suggest no departure from the general pattern[7, 59], but adequately detailed studies remain to be done.

Nerve–muscle preparations, in which nerves can be selectively excited and muscle responses observed *in vitro*, should help to clarify the situation. Such preparations have been examined extensively. In sphincteric muscle, electrical excitation of the intramural plexus yields only one response, a relaxation that cannot be attributed to the release of norepinephrine. A great number of other established and candidate inhibitory neurotransmitters have been examined as possible agents responsible for this neural inhibition[16]. These include dopamine, γ-amino butyric acid, adenosine triphosphate, and many other less likely candidates. For none of them has evidence been fully supportive. Thus, these nerves can still be classified only as nonadrenergic inhibitory nerves.

On the present evidence, therefore, the lower esophageal sphincter muscle seems to have only one kind of innervation, a nonadrenergic inhibitory innervation. Variations in sphincter tone caused by nerves, therefore, could only be attributed to this set of nerves. It is quite conceivable that such variations could be caused by variations in the tonic level of activity of these nerves alone, but this possibility has not been examined, largely because methods have not been applied to measure tonic activity in such nerves directly in sphincter muscle.

Sphincter closure tension *in vivo* can be made to fall physiologically from time to time. The best-established stimuli that reduce it are smoking[26] and the ingestion of fats[58] and of alcohol[39]. The effect of smoking can be attributed to the action of nicotine, for nicotinic receptors are present on the nonadrenergic inhibitory nerves and can excite them to relax the sphincteric muscle. The way in which alcohol weakens the sphincter is not known. The means by which fat ingestion relaxes the sphincter is also not established. It has been known for a long time that fat ingestion delays gastric emptying as well, and this effect is attributed to excitation of duodenal mucosal receptors to fats. Whether this action on gastric emptying is a consequence of the release of cholecystokinin or some other hormone, or to excitation of inhibitory nerves is still controversial. Whatever the mechanism, it seems reasonable to suppose that the same process brings about the weakening of sphincter closure tension that is seen after the ingestion of fats.

In summary then, the present evidence indicates that the tone of the lower esophageal sphincter muscle is the major variable among the various motor factors that could affect the development of reflux esophagitis. A major component of this tone arises within the muscle itself but the special properties of these muscle cells that lead to this tone are undefined. This tone depends wholly upon oxidative phosphorylation. Both nerves and hormones could modulate the degree of this tone physiologically, but convincing evidence to establish such an influence is yet lacking. The female sex hormones do affect tone *in vivo*. Gastrin seems to have no role; cholecystokinin may have. The only nerves that can be implicated in modulation of tone are the nonadrenergic inhibitory nerves. A great deal remains to be learned of their mechanism of action, morphology, and means of activation, including connections to other autonomic nerves and to the central nervous system.

Surgeons are well aware of the fact that operations designed to compress the esophagogastric junction or to shorten the fibers of the sphincteric muscle will abate gastroesophageal reflux. Because such operations present a variety of familiar and sometimes serious problems, a nonoperative means to minimize the degree of gastroesophageal reflux remains an important goal. On the present evidence, several maneuvers seem logical, though none has been fully subjected to controlled therapeutic trial. Abstinence from tobacco should be beneficial because nicotine can excite the nonadrenergic inhibitory nerves. A reduction in dietary fats is appropriate because of the influence of fat ingestion on tone, though the mechanism is unknown. Chronic ingestion of long-acting cholinomimetics, like bethanecol, seems to be effective, but this practice is limited by the expense and by the other undesirable cholinergic effects of such agents. Chronic ingestion of anticholinergic agents should at least be avoided in view of the evidence (which is not wholly convincing) to indicate that cholinergic nerves tend to raise sphincter muscle tone physiologically. Metoclopramide raises the pressure in the lower esophageal sphincter, and that agent is widely used to treat reflux esophagitis outside the United States. Other practices designed to oppose the hydrostatic differences that exist etween the stomach and esophagus, such as elevation of the torso in recumbency, weight reduction and the avoidance of garments that compress the abdomen are, of course, familiar. The combined use of all these nonoperative practices can do much for victims of gastroesophageal reflux.

Stomach

Gastric retention

The failure of the mechanism that empties the stomach is a problem that is common. An occlusion of some sort at the gastroduodenal junction is usually suspected in patients with gastric retention, but when one is not found one must suspect a defect in the motor mechanisms that empty the stomach. These disorders are still so poorly understood that they are best described under the general heading above. A fuller appreciation of the varieties of dysfunctions that can lead to gastric retention may later give rise to more specific terms.

The view that the fundus is a reservoir and the antrum a pump must now be dismissed as too simplistic, for the fundus also has a major effect on emptying. Still, it is best to consider the stomach to have two distinct divisions whose motor functions are quite different. The line that separates these divisions does not correspond to those separating the stomach into its usual components, fundus, body, antrum, and pylorus. These latter terms are derived from differences in mucosal anatomy and these differences do not correspond to regions defined by anatomic or physiologic distinctions in the gastric musculature. The two regions are distinguished by how they move[45, 46]: in the antrum, there is peristalsis, a term that refers to ring-contractions that sweep toward the pylorus, while the fundus, exhibiting no peristalsis, shows only slow sustained contractions, like tonus changes, that involve all or most of the fundus simultaneously.

The smooth muscle of the fundus is organized into three layers that have long been known. It has been forgotten, however, that there is great species variation in the extent and thickness of the inner muscle layer, the oblique layer[79]. Nevertheless, it is this oblique layer that is the distinctive feature of the musclature of the gastric fundus. It seems reasonable to suppose that the movements that seem to define the fundus could be assigned rather specifically to this oblique layer, but that association has not been established. The study of the muscle physiology of the fundus, to the extent that it has been undertaken at all, has not been specifically directed to the oblique layer.

The smooth muscle cells of the proximal stomach exhibit a stable resting membrane potential that is rather low, about 50 mV. Only small slow depolarizations of the membrane accompany contraction: spike potentials are not detected[55, 56]. Extracellular recordings usually record the same kind of thing, although rather few studies have been done[38, 43].

The contractions of the proximal stomach are often very slow and sustained in character, like tonus changes, but more rapid transients, called phasic contractions, have also been described. The former, lasting 1–3 minutes, can raise intragastric pressure up to 40 or 50 cm H_2O. Phasic contractions, in contrast, last 10–15 seconds and raise intragastric pressure only 5–15 cm H_2O. Both types of contractions seem to involve the whole of the fundus at the same time rather than showing migration from one region to another.

The sources of fundic contractions have been mainly described in terms of control systems external to the muscle and nerve. Fundic muscle strips, however, exhibit a tone *in vitro* that is resistant to tetrodotoxin, and it seems likely that this property can be attributed to the oblique muscle layer alone[20]. Possession by fundic muscle of a myogenic tone like that of the lower esophageal sphincter would be consistent with the fact that the sphincter muscle and the oblique muscle layer of the fundus are continuous. In the fundus, however, this tone seems to be variable, the modulation being mediated, probably, by nerves. Both excitatory and inhibitory pathways have been found in the vagi[1]; the former are cholinergic and the latter are nonadrenergic inhibitory nerves. The recent enthusiasm for proposing new neurotransmitters in the gut has not been applied much to nerves of the proximal stomach. Adequate experiments to establish the nature of neuromuscular transmission in autonomic nerves to the fundus muscle remain to be done.

There is evidence that these nerves are excited by vagovagal reflexes, the afferent pathways of which arise in the distal stomach or small intestine. Here also, precise experimental studies are lacking. It is conceivable that vagal pathways are the effectors for the important receptor-modulated inhibition of gastric emptying that has been so well described for fats, acids, and osmotically active substances.

The enthusiasm for finding hormones and seeking actions for them in physiology has not yet much influenced our thinking about the motions of the proximal stomach. It is sufficient to summarize this active area of research by pointing out that no hormones can be fully accepted as normally active physiological regulators of fundic motility, though cholecystokinin is effective in doses in the physiological range[23, 87].

The effects of fundic contractions are related to both gastric filling and emptying. It is clear that, during eating, gastric volume increases many times over with little change in intragastric pressure. This requires an increase in gastric diameter through relaxation of the muscle, a process that takes place mainly in the fundus. The process, called receptive relaxation, is neurogenic, vagal, and nonadrenergic[1].

Eating is not required, however, for the stomach to show its ability to relax in order to receive a large volume. Filling of the stomach through a tube or inflation of a balloon in the stomach will also demonstrate the capacity of the stomach to accommodate a great increase in volume with a trivial increase in pressure. Such accommodation, also a property mainly of the proximal stomach, seems to be very similar to receptive relaxation in the gastric fundus in response to eating.

The contractions that occur in the fundus of the filled stomach seem to have little mixing effect, but serve rather to deliver gastric content steadily to the distal stomach. The fundus serves to set the level for the head of pressure of luminal content that perfuses the antrum. As a result, the fundus seems to be of major importance in the emptying of liquids: resection of the fundus accelerates the emptying of liquids but has little effect on that of solids[85].

In the distal stomach the oblique layer is either absent, indistinguishable, or thin, except for two broad bands that lie along the lesser curvature. The longitudinal and circular muscle layers are credited mainly with the operation of this region. The circular muscle gradually thickens toward the pylorus. The smooth muscle of the distal stomach shows a resting membrane potential that is higher than that of the proximal stomach. It is unstable, fluctuations in resting membrane potential occurring at quite regular intervals with a uniform configuration. Extracellular electrodes show these depolarizations as signals that appear to progress from a point midway along the greater curvature toward the pylorus with a consistent frequency, velocity and pattern of spread[44,66]. These signals have variously been called pacesetter potentials, slow waves, the basic electrical rhythm and electrical control activity, but the preferred term, pacesetter potentials, indicates their function. It is now well accepted that these myogenic signals, moving as a ring along the distal stomach, establish the time and location of the progressive ring-contractions of the distal stomach, antral peristalsis. That is, they are pacesetters for contractions. These signals are not always accompanied by contractions. The muscle may or may not respond to any single electrical signal by contracting.

It used to be thought the pacesetter potentials *in vivo* were maintained in a quite constant state as to frequency, velocity and pattern of migration. They are not quite so constant as once thought, however, and they are influenced by both nerves and hormones. The physiological importance of neural or hormonal influences on pacesetter potentials remain to be detailed.

The nonmyogenic controls of antral contractions are usually said to include both neural and hormonal mechanisms. It is likely that such controls do operate *in vivo*, for the general level of contractions in the stomach varies greatly. If one examines rather short-time intervals, of the order of 10 minutes, the antrum may respond to all pacesetter potentials generated in that time, to none, or to some proportion between these extremes. The greatest variations seem to occur after a prolonged fast (4–6 hours) when the proportion of pacesetter potentials inducing peristaltic contractions varies cyclically between 0 percent and 100 percent as a part of the migrating motor complex of fasting, a phenomenon much better known in the small intestine where it has been better studied. In the stomach, as in the small intestine, after a prolonged fast, antral peristaltic contractions fluctuate in incidence cyclically, the cycles being the same as those of the small intestine, 70–100 minutes or more. In a single cycle, a long period of inactivity gives way to a long crescendo of contractions culminating in a period of maximal activity lasting 5–7 minutes that is followed again by inactivity.

If this cycling of the incidence of peristaltic contractions in fasting is neurogenic, it could involve either of the generally accepted motor pathways, vagal cholinergic or vagal nonadrenergic inhibitory pathways. Adrenergic mechanisms have not been wholly ruled-out. The phenomenon could, obviously, represent slow cyclic changes in nerve tone such that there is either progressive excitation to a climax or progressive disinhibition to a climax.

Again, those who seek and find other neurotransmitters and hormones have considered the stomach in suggesting physiological significance for the actions of such substances[78, 80, 81], but no physiological significance has been fully established for such substances in antral contraction.

The consequences of antral contractions are familiar. Each contraction is visualized as sweeping before it a bolus of the gastric content. Since antral contractions are shallow when they begin, deepen as they progress, and occlude the lumen only just above the pylorus, a fraction of the propelled bolus squirts back through the core of the contraction ring, the quantity diminishing as the contraction moves through the antrum. In this way, antral contractions push gastric content to and through the pylorus, and they also do a good deal of stirring or grinding of solid material. The ability of the distal stomach to allow the escape only of solid particles of a very small size is called the sieving function of the antrum[53]. Antral resection accelerates the gastric emptying of solids because it destroys this sieving function.

Although quite a lot can be said about the physiology of motor activity of the stomach, much less is known as to the cause of gastric atony. This is because it is much easier to study what needs to be studied in animals than it is in ill patients. Nevertheless, sufficient studies have been done to allow reasonable speculation as to some mechanisms.

The most exciting theory for the mechanism of gastric atony currently discussed is dysrhythmia of the gastric slow waves. It has been clear for a long time, from studies both in animals and in man, that vagotomy disturbs the frequency, velocity, and patterns of spread in the pacesetter potentials. The duration of this disruption is variable, but it can be very prolonged. That such disruption may severely affect gastric emptying of food is without question. A particular kind of dysrhythmia has been induced by electrical pacing of the stomach in animals to produce pacesetter potentials (and accompanying contractions) that begin at the pylorus and migrate retrograde[46, 65]. Such a procedure greatly retards gastric emptying. Also, cases have been described recently in which patients with greatly delayed emptying of the stomach were found to have a spontaneous tachyarrhythmia[76].

A second mechanism for gastric atony, fibrosis of the gastric muscle, is less discussed, probably because it seems so obvious. Degeneration of smooth muscle and replacement with collagen has long been known to occur in those disorders encompassed by the term scleroderma, but the stomach has had much less attention than the esophagus in this condition. It is usually thought that the mechanism is simply a loss of contractile force because of the loss of muscle cells, but other possibilities seem evident. First, since the pacesetter potentials themselves are myogenic and since a period (perhaps prolonged) of dysfunction of the muscle may well precede muscle-cell death and fibrosis, it would be reasonable to think that a dysrhythmia in scleroderma could underlie gastric retention as well. This possibility can be based, also, on the consideration that spread of the myogenic pacesetter potentials requires cell-to-cell communication throughout the muscle, and the fibrosis may interfere with the spread of pacesetter potentials. These possibilities remain to be investigated.

A third theory for a basis for gastric atony, autonomic neuropathy, is much discussed because it is blamed for a very common form of gastric atony, the gastric retention that is associated with diabetes. That the problem is, indeed, neuropathic is certainly possible but it is not well-established in the absence of sufficiently thorough investigation.

An idea recently advanced suggests that there may be a metabolic basis for the gastric atony that is often seen in patients with acidosis, notably diabetic acidosis[69]. This is the observation that the frequency of gastric pacesetter potentials is slowed greatly when the extracellular pH is reduced to 7.0, certainly within the pH that can be achieved in metabolic acidosis of various causes.

Small intestine

Megaduodenum

It seems artificial to distinguish the foregut from the midgut in respect to motor disorders, for the foregut region (the duodenum) does not appear to exhibit motor patterns different from those of the portions of the intestine beyond the ligament of Treitz. Nevertheless, one disorder, megaduodenum, is named as though it spares the midgut, even though it probably does not.

Dilatation of the duodenum has been recognized as a clinical entity for a long time. It is often considered to be a consequence of obstruction of the intestine by compression from the base of the superior mesenteric artery, and operative treatment in some cases is designed to bypass such obstruction.

It is now clear that at least some of these cases of duodenal dilatation are not due to external compression at the ligament of Treitz but to a primary failure of the musculature of the duodenum. Thus, this term megaduodenum may constitute the clinical presentation of a more generalized disorder, a general disorder of gastrointestinal smooth muscle. The generalized disorder may cause acute attacks that resemble bowel obstruction, so that such cases may present themselves in a clinical syndrome that has been called intestinal pseudo-obstruction[4, 32]. The best-described such entities are familial ones, hence they have been called familial or hereditary visceral myopathies[44]. There is a semantic proliferation that only reflects the pathogenetic confusion and the protean manifestations of this class of disorders. Since most of them may exhibit megaduodenum, this term seems an appropriate way to introduce the recent thinking on the topic. The term megaduodenum should be used to exclude all those cases in which an actual obstruction, extrinsic or intrinsic to the intestinal wall, can be demonstrated to be occlusive to the flow of luminal content. The term should be reserved to those conditions in which the primary problem seems to be a loss of the motive power of the duodenal musculature itself.

The factors that establish the motive power of the duodenum have been studied for a long time and may now be considered to be, at least in general, well understood[14, 52]. The situation is very much like that in the gastric antrum as described above.

The muscularis propria of the duodenal wall contains two layers of smooth muscle, longitudinal and circular in orientation. The functions of these two layers are quite different. Contractions of the longitudinal layer produce mainly mixing of the intestinal content and circulation of the content across the absorptive mucosal surface, at least as indicated by extensive studies in an analytical model[52]. Contractions of the circular muscle layer have very little influence on mixing or transmucosal flux, but they are mainly propulsive in function, serving to move the intestinal content from one level to the next along the cylindrical conduit of the intestine.

Contractions of the circular muscle layer are always propulsive. That is, they are always peristaltic in nature. The contraction always begins at one level of the intestine and sweeps caudad, the distance of migration or spread being highly variable. When the contraction front moves only a matter of a few centimeters or less, the ring-contraction may appear, on gross inspection, to be a 'segmentation', a standing contraction. That is, its caudad bias may not be apparent. A caudad bias is, however, always present, so that contractions of the circular muscle layer are always propulsive caudad.

The occurrence of such contractions both in time and location is seemingly random along the duodenal segment for most of the time, except after a prolonged fast[86]. After a fast of 4–12 hours (the time varying among species and among individuals) the contraction pattern alters to one in which, at a single point along the duodenum, the incidence of contractions passes through cycles. A single cycle lasts 1–3 hours, varying among species and among individuals. During a single cycle, there is, at first, no contraction activity for a period of perhaps 10–40 minutes. Then contractions begin to occur, increasing in incidence progressively until they occur as a maximum incidence for 5–10 minutes when the cycle begins over again as a prolonged period of inactivity. The reasons for this cycling are not known.

The distribution of duodenal contractions is determined by an electrical phenomenon like the pacesetter potentials of the gastric antrum. These are usually called the slow waves in the duodenum. Occurring constantly at a frequency of 10–12 cycles per minute, they appear to begin at a pacemaker near the duodenal bulb and to sweep caudad. Frequency, velocity and direction seem to be very constant physiologically (except in vomiting, where these briefly change). As in the gastric antrum, these myogenic electrical signals are pacemaking signals, establishing the time and place at which contractions will occur.

The likelihood that the muscle at any given level of the duodenum will respond to a slow wave by contracting is determined by nonmuscular factors that may be classified as neural and hormonal. As in the stomach, none of the numerous and growing number of hormones and candidate hormones that are studied by gastrointestinal physiologists can yet be given any physiological role in regulation of duodenal motility. The chief controls appear to be neural, but a detailed knowledge of these controls is also lacking. Those nerves that have been best demonstrated include both cholinergic excitatory nerves and nonadrenergic inhibitory nerves, but little more can be said. It is clear that the two muscle layers differ greatly from one another, both in their innervation and in their responses to a variety of drugs and hormones. No complete concept, though, can yet be presented as to the nature of the physiological controls that establish the incidence of duodenal contractions.

A list has been published of the reported conditions thought to be causative of the syndrome of chronic intestinal pseudo-obstruction, in which megaduodenum is a common feature[32]. For no entries on this list can the full explanation of failure of contractions of the duodenal muscle be advanced.

Theoretically, megaduodenum could come about through failure of any of the three kinds of controls that are thought to exist on duodenal contractions, myogenic, neurogenic, and hormonal controls. Myogenic disease seems to be the best established. At least one group of these disorders, exemplified by the kindred described as a 'familial visceral myopathy', is characterized by pathological degeneration and fibrosis of the circular muscle layer of the duodenum[33]. Since many patients operated upon for megaduodenum by bypass of the superior mesenteric artery may have no intestinal wall resected for histological examination, it is not excluded that at least some of these patients may have, in fact, a visceral myopathy.

The failure of myogenic controls could also take the form of functional deficits not reflected in anatomical changes. These would include alterations in frequency, velocity or direction of spread of electrical slow waves like those dysrhythmias demonstrated in some cases to be causative of gastric retention. Only one duodenal dysrhythmia has been demonstrated. Abnormal frequencies of duodenal slow waves were long ago described in association with thyroid disease[19]. The very slow frequency found in myxedema could be a major factor in myxedema ileus, though it would undoubtedly be contributed to by such other abnormalities as reduced mucous secretion and perhaps swelling of the muscular wall or the gut itself.

This new knowledge about megaduodenum can greatly affect the approach to patients. Some cases of megaduodenum are due to neuromuscular disease of the duodenum itself and not to extrinsic compression. In some such cases, the muscular disease will be revealed also in the fact that there will be found a coexistent esophageal atony, gastric dilatation or megacystis. The finding of one of these abnormalities in association with megaduodenum would suggest the true cause of the duodenal dilatation.

Significant morbidity may result from the alteration of food in the dilated duodenum through bacterial proliferation and fermentation. Indeed, the latter process may lead to much more trouble than the 'obstruction'. The content of the dilated duodenal segment is almost invariably septic in character, and appropriate antibiotic preparation before operation will greatly reduce the likelihood of peritoneal soilage.

References

1 ABRAHAMSSON, H. Studies on the inhibitory nervous control of gastric motility. *Acta Physiologica Scandinavica (Stockholm)*, Supplement 390, 1–38 (1973)

2 ADAMS, H. D. Amyenteric achalasia of the esophagus. *Surgery, Gynecology and Obstetrics*, **119**, 251–256 (1964)

3 ANDREW, B. L. The respiratory displacement of the larynx: a study of the innervation of accessory respiratory muscles. *Journal of Physiology*, **130**, 474–487 (1955)

4 ANURAS, S. and CHRISTENSEN, J. Recurrent or chronic intestinal pseudo-obstruction. *Clinics in Gastroenterology*, **10**, 177–190 (1981)

5 ASOH, R. and GOYAL, R. K. Manometry and electromyography of the upper esophageal sphincter in the opossum. *Gastroenterology*, **74**, 514–520 (1978)

6 ASOH, R. and GOYAL, R. K. Electrical activity of the opossum lower esophageal sphincter in vivo. Its role in the basal sphincter pressure. *Gastroenterology*, **74**, 835–840 (1978)

7 BAUMGARTEN, H. G. and LANGE, W. Adrenergic innervation of the oesophagus in the cat (*Felis domestica*) and rhesus monkey (*Macacus rhesus*). *Zeitschrift für Zellforschung und Mikroskopische Anatomie (Berlin)*, **95**, 529–545 (1969)

8 BOOTH, D. J., KEMMERER, W. T. and SKINNER, D. B. Acid clearing from the distal esophagus. *Archives of Surgery*, **96** 731–734 (1968)

9 CAR, A. and ROMAN, C. L'activité spontanée du sphincter oesophagien supérieur chez le mouton. Ses variations au cours de la déglutition et de la rumination. *Journal de Physiologie (Paris)*, **62**, 505–511 (1970)

10 CASSELLA, R. R., BROWN, A. L., JR., SAYRE, G. P. and ELLIS, F. H., JR. Achalasia of the esophagus: Pathologic and etiologic considerations. *Annals of Surgery*, **160**, 474–487 (1964)

11 CASSELLA, R. R., ELLIS, F. H., JR. and BROWN, A. L., JR. Fine-structure changes in achalasia of the esophagus. I. Vagus nerves. *American Journal of Pathology*, **46**, 279–288 (1965)

12 CASSELLA, R. R., ELLIS, F. H., JR. and BROWN, A. L., JR. Fine-structure changes in achalasia of the esophagus. II. Esophageal smooth muscle. *American Journal of Pathology*, **46**, 467–475 (1965)

13 CASTELL, D. O. The lower esophageal sphincter. Physiologic and clinical aspects. *Annals of Internal Medicine*, **83**, 390–401 (1975)

14 CHRISTENSEN, J. The physiology of gastrointestinal transit. *Medical Clinics of North America*, **58**, 1165–1180 (1974)

15 CHRISTENSEN, J. The controls of oesophageal movement. In *Clinics in Gastroenterology*, edited by M. Atkinson, **5**, 15–27. London, W. B. Saunders Co., Ltd (1976)

16 CHRISTENSEN, J. The innervation and motility of the esophagus. In *Frontiers of Gastrointestinal Research: The Esophagus*, edited by L. van der Reis, **3**, 18–32. Basel, S. Karger AG (1978)

17 CHRISTENSEN, J. and CONKLIN, J. L. Studies on the origin of the distinctive mechanics of smooth muscle at the esophagogastric junction. In *Proceedings of the Fourth International Symposium on Gastrointestinal Motility*, edited by E. E. Daniel *et al.*, Session I, 63–71. Vancouver, Mitchell press (1974)

18 CHRISTENSEN, J. CONKLIN, J. L. and FREEMAN, B. W. Physiologic specialization at esophagogastric junction in three species. *American Journal of Physiology*, **225**, 1265–1270 (1973)

19 CHRISTENSEN, J., SCHEDL, H. P. and CLIFTON, J. A. The basic electrical rhythm of the duodenum in normal human subjects and in patients with thyroid disease. *Journal of Clinical Investigation*, **43**, 1659–1667 (1964)

20 CHRISTENSEN, J. and TORRES, E. I. Three layers of the opossum stomach: responses to nerve stimulation. *Gastroenterology*, **69**, 641–648 (1975)

21 COHEN, S., LIPSHUTZ, W. and HUGHES, W. Role of gastrin supersensitivity in the pathogenesis of lower esophageal sphincter hypertension in achalasia. *Journal of Clinical Investigation*, **50**, 1241–1247 (1971)

22 CROSS, F. S. Pathologic changes in megaesophagus (esophageal dystonia). *Surgery*, **31**, 647–653 (1952)

23 DEBAS, H. T., FAROOQ, O. and GROSSMAN, M. I. Inhibition of gastric emptying is a physiological action of cholecystokinin. *Gastroenterology*, **68**, 1211–1217 (1975)

24 DE CARLE, D. J., CHRISTENSEN, J., SZABO, A. C., TEMPLEMAN, D. C. and MCKINLEY, D. R. Calcium dependence of neuromuscular events in esophageal smooth muscle of the opossum. *American Journal of Physiology*, **232**, E547–E552 (1977)

25 DECKTOR, D. L. and RYAN, J. P. Intracellular analysis of esophageal membrane response to electrical stimulation. In *Gastrointestinal Motility*, edited by J. Christensen, 45–50. New York, Raven Press (1980)

26 DENNISH, G. W. and CASTELL, D. O. Inhibitory effect of smoking on the lower esophageal sphincter. *New England Journal of Medicine*, **284**, 1136–1137 (1971)

27 DIAMANT, N. E. and EL-SHARKAWAY, T. Y. Neural control of esophageal peristalsis. A conceptual analysis. *Gastroenterology*, **72**, 546–556 (1977)

28 DODDS, W. J., STEF, J. J., STEWART, E. T., HOGAN, W. J., ARNDORFER, R. C. and COHEN, E. B. Responses of the feline esophagus to cervical vagal stimulation. *American Journal of Physiology*, **235**, E63–E73 (1978)

29 DOTY, R. W. Neural organization of deglutition. In *Handbook of Physiology*, edited by C. F. Code, **4**, 1861–1902. Washington DC, American Physiological Society (1968)

30 ELLIS, F. H., JR., OLSEN, A. M., SCHLEGEL, J. F. and CODE, C. F. Surgical treatment of esophageal hypermotility disturbances. *Journal of the American Medical Association*, **188**, 862–866 (1964)

31 ELLIS, F. H., JR., SCHLEGEL, J. F., LYNCH, V. P. and PAYNE, W. S. Cricopharyngeal myotomy for pharyngo-esophageal diverticulum. *Annals of Surgery*, **170**, 340–350 (1969)

32 FAULK, D. L., ANURAS, S. and CHRISTENSEN, J. Chronic intestinal pseudoobstruction. *Gastroenterology*, **74**, 922–931 (1978)

33 FAULK, D. L., ANNURAS, S., GARDNER, G. D., MITROS, F. A., SUMMERS, R. W. and CHRISTENSEN, J. A familial visceral myopathy. *Annals of Internal Medicine*, **89**, 600–606 (1978)

34 FERGUSON, T. B., WOODBURY, J. D., ROPER, C. L. and BURFORD, T. H. Giant muscular hypertrophy of the esophagus. *Annals of Thoracic Surgery*, **8**, 209–218 (1969)

35 GILLIES, M., NICKS, R. and SKYRING, A. Clinical, manometric, and pathological studies in diffuse oesophageal spasm. *British Medical Journal*, **2**, 527–530 (1967)

36 GOYAL, R. K. and RATTAN, S. Genesis of basal sphincter pressure: effect of tetrodotoxin on lower esophageal sphincter pressure in opossum in vivo. *Gastroenterology*, **71**, 62–67 (1976)

37 HELLEMANS, J., VANTRAPPEN, G., VANDENBROUCKE, J. The electrical activity of the human esophagus. *Gastroenterology*, **58**, 959 (1970)

38 HINDER, R. A. and KELLY, K. A. Human gastric pacesetter potential. Site of origin, spread, and response to gastric transection and proximal gastric vagotomy. *American Journal of Surgery*, **133**, 29–33 (1977)

39 HOGAN, W. J., VIEGAS DE ANDRADE, S. R. and WINSHIP, D. H. Ethanol-induced acute esophageal motor dysfunction. *Journal of Applied Physiology*, **32**, 755–760 (1972)

40 HURST, A. F. and RAKE, G. W. Achalasia of the cardia (so-called cardiospasm). *Quarterly Journal of Medicine*, **23**, 491–508 (1930)

41 JOHNSON, L. F. and DEMEESTER, T. R. Twenty-four-hour pH monitoring of the distal esophagus. A quantitative measure of gastroesophageal reflux. *American Journal of Gastroenterology*, **62**, 325–332 (1974)

42 KAY, E. B. Observations as to the etiology and treatment of achalasia of the esophagus. *Journal of Thoracic Surgery*, **22**, 254–270 (1951)

43 KELLY, K. A. Gastric motility in health and after gastric surgery. *Viewpoints on Digestive Diseases*, **8**, No. 2, (1976)

44 KELLY, K. A. and CODE, C. F. Canine gastric pacemaker. *American Journal of Physiology* **220**, 112–118 (1971)

45 KELLY, K. A., CODE, C. F. and ELVEBACK, L. R. Patterns of canine gastric electrical activity. *American Journal of Physiology*, **217**, 461–470 (1969)

46 KELLY, K. A. and LAFORCE, R. C. Pacing the canine stomach with electric stimulation. *American Journal of Physiology*, **222**, 588–594 (1972)

47 KOPALD, H. H., ROTH, H. P., FLESHLER, B. and PRITCHARD, W. H. Vasovagal syncope: report of a case associated with diffuse esophageal spasm. *New England Journal of Medicine*, **271**, 1238–1241 (1964)

48 KRAMER, P. and INGELFINGER, F. J. Esophageal sensitivity to mecholyl in cardiospasm. *Gastroenterology*, **19**, 242–253 (1951)

49 KRAVITZ, J. J., SNAPE, W. J., JR. and COHEN, S. Effect of thoracic vagotomy and vagal stimulation on esophageal function. *American Journal of Physiology*, **234**, E359–E364 (1978)

50 LEVITT, M. N., DEDO, H. H. and OGURA, J. H. The cricopharyngeus muscle, an electromyographic study in the dog. *Laryngoscope*, **75**, 122–136 (1965)

51 LUND, W. S. The cricopharyngeal sphincter: its relationship to the relief of pharyngeal paralysis and the surgical treatment of the early pharyngeal pouch. *Journal of Laryngology and Otology*, **82**, 353–367 (1968)

52 MACAGNO, E. O and CHRISTENSEN, J. Fluid mechanics of the duodenum. *Annual Review of Fluid Mechanics*, **12**, 139–158 (1980)

53 MEYER, J. H., THOMSON, J. B., COHEN, M. B., SHADCHEHR, A. and MANDIOLA, S. A. Sieving of solid food by the canine stomach and sieving after gastric surgery. *Gastroenterology*, **76**, 804–813 (1979)

54 MISIEWICZ, J. J., WALLER, S. L., ANTHONY, P. P. and GUMMER, J. W. P. Achalasia of the cardia: pharmacology and histopathology of isolated cardiac sphincteric muscle from patients with and without achalasia. *Quarterly Journal of Medicine*, **38**, 17–30 (1969)

55 MORGAN, K. G., GO, V. L. W. and SZURSZEWSKI, J. H. Motilin increases the influence of excitatory myenteric plexus neurons on gastric smooth muscle in vitro. In *Gastrointestinal Motility*, edited by J. Christensen, 129. New York, Raven Press (1980)

56 MORGAN, K. G., SCHMALZ, P. F. and SZURSZEWSKI, J. H. Action of pentagastrin on nonadrenergic inhibitory intramural nerves of the canine orad stomach. *Gastroenterology*, **76**, 1206 (1979)

57 MUKHOPADHYAY, A. K. and WEISBRODT, N. W. Neural organization of esophageal peristalsis: role of vagus nerve. *Gastroenterology*, **68**, 444–447 (1975)

58 NEBEL, O. T. and CASTELL, D. O. Inhibition of the lower oesophageal sphincter by fat – a mechanism for fatty food intolerance. *Gut*, **14**, 270–274 (1973)

59 NISHIMURA, T. and TAKASU, T. The adrenergic innervation in the esophagus and respiratory tract of the rabbit. *Acta Oto-Laryngologica (Stockholm)*, **67**, 444–452 (1969)

60 POPE, C. E., II. Pathophysiology and diagnosis of reflux esophagitis. *Gastroenterology*, **70**, 445–454 (1976)

61 RAKE, G. W. A case of annular muscular hypertrophy of the oesophagus (achalasia of the cardia without oesophageal dilatation). *Guy's Hospital Reports*, **76**, 145–152 (1926)

62 RAKE, G. W. On the pathology of achalasia of the cardia. *Guy's Hospital Reports*, **77**, 141–150 (1927)

63 ROMAN, C. Contrôle nerveux du péristaltisme oesophagien. *Journal de Physiologie (Paris)*, **58**, 79–108 (1966)

64 RYAN, J. P., SNAPE, W. J., JR. and COHEN, S. Influence of vagal cooling on esophageal function. *American Journal of Physiology*, **232**, E159–E164 (1977)

65 SARNA, S. K. and DANIEL, E. E. Electrical stimulation of gastric electrical control activity. *American Journal of Physiology*, **225**, 125–131 (1973)

66 SARNA, S. K., DANIEL, E. E. and KINGMA, Y. J. Simulation of the electric-control activity of the stomach by an array of relaxation oscillators. *American Journal of Digestive Diseases*, **17**, 299–310 (1972)

67 SCHULZE, K. and CHRISTENSEN, J. Lower sphincter of the opossum in pseudopregnancy. *Gastroenterology*, **73**, 1082–1085 (1977)

68 SCHULZE, K., CONKLIN, J. L. and CHRISTENSEN, J. A potassium gradient in smooth muscle segment of the opossum esophagus. *American Journal of Physiology*, **232**, E270–E273 (1977)

69 SCHULZE-DELRIEU, K. and REUBER, M. Frequency decline of gastric pacesetter potential during acidosis. *Clinical Research*, **27**, 635 (1979)

70 SCHULZE, K., HAJJAR, J. J. and CHRISTENSEN, J. Regional differences in potassium content of smooth muscle from opossum esophagus. *American Journal of Physiology*, **235**, E709–E713 (1978)

71 SHIPP, T., DEATSCH, W. W. and ROBERTSON, K. Pharyngoesophageal muscle activity during swallowing in man. *Laryngoscope*, **80**, 1–16 (1970)

72 SMITH, B. The myenteric plexus in man. In *The Neuropathology of the Alimentary Tract*, edited by B. Smith, 12–16. London, Edward Arnold (1972)

73 SMITH, B. Achalasia of the cardia. In *The Neuropathology of the Alimentary Tract*, edited by B. Smith, 25–34. London, Edward Arnold (1972)

74 SOERGEL, K. H., ZBORALSKE, F. F. and AMBERG, J. R. Presbyesophagus: esophageal motility in nonagenarians. *Journal of Clinical Investigation*, **43**, 1472–1479 (1964)

75 STANCIU, C. and BENNETT, J. R. Oesophageal acid clearing: one factor in the production of reflux oesophagitis. *Gut*, **15**, 852–857 (1974)

76 TELANDER, R. L., MORGAN, K. G., KREULEN, D. L., SCHMALZ, P. F., KELLY, K. A. and SZURSZEWSKI, J. H. Human gastric atony with tachygastria and gastric retention. *Gastroenterology*, **75**, 497–501 (1978)

77 TEMPLEMAN, D. C. (sponsored by J. Christensen). The myogenic active tension that defines lower esophageal sphincter muscle is aerobic. *Gastroenterology*, **72**, 1189 (1977)

78 THOMAS, P. A. and KELLY, K. A. Hormonal control of interdigestive motor cycles of canine proximal stomach. *American Journal of Physiology*, **237**, E192–E197 (1979)

79 TORGERSEN, J. The muscular build and movements of the stomach and duodenal bulb. *Acta Radiologica Scandinavica*, Supplementum 45, 1–191 (1945)

80 VALENZUELA, J. E. Effect of intestinal hormones and peptides on intragastric pressure in dogs. *Gastroenterology*, **71**, 766–769 (1976)

81 VALENZUELA, J. E. Dopamine as a possible neurotransmitter in gastric relaxation. *Gastroenterology*, **71**, 1019–1022 (1976)

82 VAN THIEL, D. H., GAVALER, J. S., JOSHI, S. N., SARA, R. K. and STREMPLE, J. Heartburn of pregnancy. *Gastroenterology*, **72**, 666–668 (1977)

83 VAN THIEL, D. H., GAVALER, J. S. and STREMPLE, J. Lower esophageal sphincter pressure in women using sequential oral contraceptives. *Gastroenterology*, **71**, 232–234 (1976)

84 WEISBRODT, N. W. and CHRISTENSEN, J. Gradients of contractions in the opossum esophagus. *Gastroenterology*, **62**, 1159–1166 (1972)

85 WILBUR, B. G., KELLY, K. A. and CODE, C. F. Effect of gastric fundectomy on canine gastric electrical and motor activity. *American Journal of Physiology*, **226**, 1445–1449 (1974)

86 WINGATE, D. L. Backwards and forwards with the migrating complex. *Gastroenterology*. (In press)

87 YAMAGISHI, T. and DEBAS, H. T. Cholecystokinin inhibits gastric emptying by acting on both proximal stomach and pylorus. *American Journal of Physiology*, **234**, E375–E378 (1978)

9
Carcinogenesis in the foregut

M. Siurala, K. Varis and P. Sipponen

Part 1 Oesophageal carcinoma

Epidemiology

General considerations

The death rate of oesophageal carcinoma (OC) is considerably lower than those of gastric and colonic carcinomas. Its geographical distribution is also very different, indicating a different aetiopathogenetic background.

Males are significantly more frequently affected than females. OC seems to be most common in France: the age-adjusted death rate among French males in 1966–7 was 14.00 per 100 000 inhabitants[9]. Next in order are non-Caucasian males in the United States (9.85) and Chilean males (9.40).

In OC the differences between high- and low-risk areas within the same country may be very high. Thus, in Iran there is within a few hundred miles a 20-fold variation in the death rate[4], and in North China the death rate of OC is, in the Linhsien area, 100 times higher than in the lowest risk area[14]. Small areas with high death rates are also Singapore, Curaçao, some Caribbean islands, the Turkmenian and Kazakhstan SSR, southern shore of the Caspian Sea, and others[9].

Some differences in death rate have been noted in different populations living in the same area. Thus, Jews have a lower death rate than other ethnic populations in the same country[18]. Little is known about the genetics of OC. Familial accumulation of the disease is rare; however, 24 cases have been reported in two English families[3]. OC shows interesting genetic associations to tylosis, which is known to be inherited in a dominant Mendelian way. The risk of getting OC is 95 per cent in tylosis, suggesting a close genetic association. It is probable that a single mutant gene is responsible for the development of both diseases[3].

Risk factors

It has generally been assumed, and there is indeed some evidence supporting the assumption, that abuse of alcohol and tobacco increases the risk of OC[12, 16]. Similarly, it has been known for a long time that the Paterson-Brown Kelly-Plummer-Vinson syndrome accompanying iron deficiency is associated with OC[17]. The high death rate of OC among Turkomans of North Iran is thought to be due to deficient diet[15] or to the habit of chewing tar from opium pipes[7]. Likewise, a deficiency of molybdenum is suspected of increasing the risk of OC among Bantus living in the Transkei district of South Africa[1]. Hot tea, betel nuts and nitrosoamines, and deficiency of riboflavin have been considered additional risk factors of OC. Because of the high tannin content of tea, it is interesting to note that there is some epidemiological evidence for an association between the use of tannin-containing extracts and OC[10].

In addition to external environmental factors, some aberrations and alterations in the oesophagus might be considered risk factors of OC. Thus, it is generally assumed that Barrett's syndrome, i.e. the presence of gastric mucosa at an abnormally high level in the oesophagus predisposes to the development of OC[5]. The recent interesting epidemiological study by Crespi et al.[4] of a large population sample from a high-risk area in North Iran, suggests that chronic oesophagitis could be related to OC. Two experienced endoscopists in the team performed oesophagoscopy and oesophageal biopsy on more than 400 subjects. They reported oesophagitis in 86 per cent of the subjects (males and females). It was severe in 11 per cent of the males. Distinct epithelial dysplasia was found in 16 and invasive carcinoma in 11 out of 430 subjects. Thus this high-risk population was characterized by the occurrence of epithelial dysplasia and a high prevalence of oesophagitis. The authors point out that the morphology in their oesophagitis cases was similar to the early changes induced in rats by administration of nitroso-compounds. They also refer to a study in China where oesophageal carcinomas were detected in a high percentage during a follow-up of cases with oesophageal dysplasia. On the other hand, no relation could be demonstrated between the occurrence and severity of oesophagitis and reflux, nor were the epithelial changes considered to be due to deficiency of riboflavin. The study of Crespi *et al.* seems to link oesophagitis and epithelial dysplasia with the development of oesophageal carcinoma, and similar results have been obtained in an extensive epidemiologic study in North China[14]. However, the results of the study cannot be considered conclusive because of its principles of selection and lack of adequate controls.

Mechanism of action of the presumed risk factors

The environmental carcinogens are in contact with the oesophageal mucosa for a short time only. It is possible, however, that alcohol may fix some substances and attach them to the oesophageal mucosa for a longer time[8]. In addition, alcoholic beverages sometimes contain nitroso-compounds, but their amount is probably too small to be of any significance. It is generally believed that the alcohol itself and its amount are of importance, rather than its quality[2, 15].

In connection with smoking, nitroso-compounds may be solubilized in the saliva and so come in contact with oesophageal mucosa[6]. Moreover, both alcohol abuse and smoking decrease the pressure in the lower oesophagus and predispose to reflux. Reflux with or without concomitant oesophagitis has been claimed to be of pathogenetic significance, although conflicting results have also been reported. On the other hand, the simultaneous use of alcohol and tobacco may have a multiplicative effect[15].

Theoretically, deficiency states may predispose to OC. Thus, iron and riboflavin act as coenzymes for some respiratory enzymes, and their deficiency is associated with epithelial alterations of the upper gastrointestinal tract. This mechanism could explain the increased risk of OC assumed to be associated with alcoholism and Paterson-Brown Kelly-Plummer-Vinson syndrome[17, 18], and a stomach operated for benign gastroduodenal disease[13]. However, the epidemiological study of Crespi *et al.*[4] cited above does not support the significance of riboflavin deficiency as a risk-increasing factor in OC.

Possibilities to improve the prognosis of OC

Elimination of alcohol and tobacco is a theoretically possible but practically overwhelming task. Moreover, it will hardly be achieved for the sake of such a rare disease as oesophageal carcinoma. The correction of deficiency states is simple on an individual level, but on a population level it is a large economic and sociopolitical problem.

Tea-drinking has attracted some interest because of the high tannin content of tea. There has not been a question of abandoning it, but the British habit of adding milk to it has been advocated, since milk proteins are capable of binding tannin. Indeed, Morton states in a recent article[11]: 'Thanks to early warnings from the British Medical Association, the British have traditionally added milk to their tea to bind tannin'.

References

1 BURRELL, R. J., ROACH, W. A. and SHADWELL, A. Esophageal cancer in the Bantu of the Transkei associated with mineral deficiency in garden plants. *Journal of the National Cancer Institute*, **36**, 201–204 (1966)

2 CHILVERS, C., FRASER, P. and BERAL, V. Alcohol and oesophageal cancer: An assessment of the evidence from routine collected data. *Journal of Epidemiology and Community Health*, **33**, 127–133 (1979)

3 MCCONNELL, R. B. Epidemiology of gastrointestinal tumours: a review. *Journal of the Royal Society of Medicine*, **71**, 278–281 (1978)

4 CRESPI, M., MUÑOZ, N., GRASSI, A., ARAMESH, B., AMIRI, G., MOJTABAI, A. and CASALE, V. Oesophageal lesions in northern Iran: a premalignant condition? *Lancet*, **2**, 217–220 (1979)

5 HAGGITT, R. C., TRYZELAAR, J., ELLIS, F. H. and COLCHER, H. Adenocarcinoma complicating columnar epithelium-lined (Barrett's) esophagus. *American Journal of Clinical Pathology*, **70**, 1–5 (1978)

6 HECHT, S. S., CHEN, C. B., HIROTA, N., ORNAF, R. M., TSO, T. C. and HOFFMANN, D. Tobacco-specific nitrosamines: Formation from micotine in vitro and during tobacco curing and carcinogenicity in strain A mice. *Journal of the National Cancer Institute*, **60**, 819–824 (1978)

7 HEWER, T. F. Opium and oesophageal cancer in Iran. *Lancet*, **1**, 45 (1979)

8 HORIE, A., KOCHI, S. and KURATSUNE, M. Carcinogenesis in the esophagus. II. Experimental production of esophageal cancer by administration of ethanolic solution of carcinogens. *Gann*, **56**, 429–441 (1965)

9 LOGAN, W. P. D. Cancers of the alimentary tract: international mortality trends. *WHO Chronicle*, **30**, 413–419 (1976)

10 MORTON, J. F. Plant products and occupational materials ingested by oesophageal cancer victims in South Carolina. *Quarterly Journal of Drug Research*, **13**, 2005–2022 (1973)

11 MORTON, J. F. Tea with milk. *Science*, **204**, 909 (1979)

12 SCHWARTZ, D., LELLOUCH, J., FLAMANT, R. and DENOIX, P. F. Alcohol et cancer. Résultats d'une enquête retrospective. *Revue Française d'Etudes Cliniques et Biologiques*, **7**, 590–604 (1962)

13 SHEARMAN, D. J. C., FINLAYSON, N. D. C., ARNOTT, S. J. and PEARSON, J. G. Carcinoma of the oesophagus after gastric surgery. *Lancet*, **1,** 581–582 (1970)

14 The Coordinating Group for Research on Etiology of Esophageal Cancer in North China. The epidemiology and etiology of esophageal carcinoma in North China. *Chinese Medical Journal*, **1,** 167–183 (1975)

15 TUYNS, A. J., PÉQUIGNOT, G. and JENSEN, D. M. Role of diet, alcohol and tobacco in oesophageal cancer, as illustrated by two contrasting high-incidence areas in the north of Iran and west of France. *Frontiers in Gastro-intestinal Research*, **4,** 101–110 (1979)

16 WYNDER, E. L. and BROSS, I. J. A study of etiological factors in cancer of the oesophagus. *Cancer*, **14,** 389–413 (1961)

17 WYNDER, E. L., HULTBERG, S., JACOBSSON, F. and BROSS, I. J. Environmental factors in cancer of the upper alimentary tract. A Swedish study with special reference to Plummer-Vinson (Paterson-Kelly) syndrome. *Cancer*, **10,** 470–487 (1957)

18 WYNDER, E. L., REDDY, B. S., McCOY, G. D., WEISBURGER, J. H. and WILLIAMS, G. M. Diet and gastrointestinal cancer. *Clinical Gastroenterology*, **5,** 463–482 (1976)

9
Carcinogenesis in the foregut

M. Siurala, K. Varis and P. Sipponen

Part 2 Gastric carcinoma

Epidemiology

General considerations

Malignancies are a major cause of death throughout the world. However, in spite of countless time and money-consuming studies the final problem is still unsolved: we do not know what makes the cell behave like a cancer cell. It has therefore not been possible to develop methods which would permit a specific treatment of the disease. Indeed, no substantial progress has been achieved in the treatment of carcinomas of most organs. This failure has prompted anew an intensive search for environmental carcinogenic factors by epidemiological methods, with some success, as is exemplified by recent progress in the field of skin and lung cancer.

Epidemiological studies have shown that geographical factors are of significance in the development of carcinomas of organs directly exposed to the action of environmental carcinogens, as in carcinomas of the stomach and colon[48]. On the other hand, a geographical dependence cannot be demonstrated as distinctly for carcinomas of prostate, pancreas, brain and breast, which are less subject to direct effects of environmental carcinogens.

An intensive search for carcinogens has disclosed in our environment many substances that have strong carcinogenic properties under experimental conditions. However, it has not been possible to show that any of these carcinogens would alone be responsible for the development of gastric carcinoma (GCA) in man[77, 110]. In addition, there is some evidence indicating that pathological conditions of the gastric mucosa, such as atrophic gastritis, the gastric lesion of pernicious anaemia and the operated stomach and gastric polyps increase the risk of GCA. Accordingly, both internal and external factors are operating in the development of this malignancy. Thus achlorhydria accompanying atrophic gastritis may facilitate the formation of carcinogenic nitroso-compounds in the gastric lumen[78], and there is evidence indicating that an altered gastric mucosa may be more susceptible to the action of carcinogens than is a normal one[11]. Epidemiological research in GCA must, therefore, take into account both the environmental carcinogens and the alterations in the morphology, function and immunology of the gastric mucosa, and in addition to these the effects of genetic factors. The problem is further complicated by the probability that not all the above factors are always necessary for the development of GCA. Therefore, various combinations of these factors may be operating on an individual level. It should also be noted that the histologically different types of GCA, the intestinal and the diffuse[50, 56], (*see* p. 283), seem to have different aetiopathogenetic backgrounds and different biological behaviours[8, 9, 10, 56, 67, 68, 69, 70], (*see* page 279 and *Table 9.1*).

Mortality rate

The death rate of GCA has decreased during the last decades in many western countries. The reason for the decrease is not known; it is not due to any active preventive, diagnostic or therapeutic attempts. The simultaneous increase in the death rate of colonic carcinoma would indicate the effects of changed environmental conditions such as dietary habits. There is, however, one significant exception from this trend: the 'stump carcinoma' which occurs as a late complication after surgery for benign gastroduodenal ulcer[12].

High- and low-risk areas

The death rate of GCA in immigrants from a high- to a low-risk area may give a clue as to the significance of environmental factors. Thus the death rate among Japanese who have emigrated to the United States has been lower than that of Japanese living in Japan. The death rate decreased further in the second generation but still remained higher than in the United States[96]. This indicates that there must be acting in Japan some factors typical for this area which exert their influence already in childhood and are able to increase the risk of GCA in immigrants who have lived in a low-risk country for a long time before the appearance of GCA.

Table 9.1 Characteristics of histologically different types of gastric carcinoma (classification of Lauren)

	Intestinal type	*Diffuse type*
Prevalence	Higher than that of the diffuse type. High prevalence in high-risk areas: 'epidemic' cancer type	Lower than that of the intestinal type. Probably unaffected by the environment: 'endemic' cancer type
Age	More common in old age groups. Infrequent in young people	Not uncommon in young age groups
Sex	Male/female ratio about 2	Male/female ratio about 1
Site of predilection	Antrum and cardia	Body of the stomach
Macromorphology	Tumour-forming	Ulcerating
Metastases	Usually in the liver	Usually in the lymph nodes and the serosa
Blood-group distribution	The expected one	Blood group A more common than expected
Heredity	No evidence	Family accumulation and association with genetic markers
Relation to chronic gastritis	Severe atrophic gastritis present around the cancer area	Atrophic gastritis uncommon in early stages of the cancer
Relation to intestinal metaplasia	Possibly direct pathogenetic relationship	Probably no relationship in the majority of patients
Relation to dysplasia	Relationship to dysplasia of 'intestinal' type	Relationship to dysplasia of 'foveolar' type

'Epidemic' and 'endemic' types

The proportion of intestinal type of all GCAs is high in high-risk areas and among high-risk populations[8, 10, 14, 69]. The decrease in the incidence of GCA is mainly due to a decrease in the intestinal type, while the incidence of the diffuse type remains virtually unchanged[14, 68, 69]. Similarly, the decrease in the death rate of GCA among immigrants from high- to low-risk areas is mainly due to the decrease in the intestinal type[8, 10]. It also should be noted that intestinal carcinoma mainly affects elderly persons while the diffuse is often found in patients below 50 years of age. Therefore, the intestinal type has been designated as the 'epidemic' and the diffuse the 'endemic' type of GCA[20].

Environmental factors

Because the stomach is directly exposed to environmental factors one could expect that such factors would easily be identified. However, despite world-wide extensive epidemiological research work it has been possible to show only slight correlations between living habits and risk of GCA. It is obvious that the finding of a correlation does not imply the existence of causal relationship. Thus, it has been claimed that a diet rich in fish would contribute to the high incidence of GCA in Japan. However, fish is the main source of protein in many low-risk areas. Similarly it has been suggested that the use of talc rice would increase the GCA risk in the Japanese. However, careful dietary analyses among the different populations living in Hawaii disclosed that Philippinos consumed more talc rice than the Japanese, but had a very low incidence of GCA[97]. On the other hand, epidemiological studies concerned with the relationship of environmental nitrates and nitrites to GCA have brought out data that have opened an exciting explanation route for the existence of high- and low-risk areas of GCA.

Nitroso-compounds

In 1970 it was observed in Chile that the incidence of GCA was highest in areas with a high content of nitrate in the water and soil[112]. Likewise the high incidence of GCA in Japan has been related to the mutagenic effects of food treated with nitrites[62]. Nitrates are readily reduced in the gastric lumen to nitrites which in the presence of amines may form nitroso-compounds[105]. Small amounts of such nitroso-compounds are potent carcinogens in animals. The formation of nitroso-compounds is markedly facilitated at the higher pH levels of the gastric contents[78]. Thus, the nitrite-nitrate ratio at above pH 5 is more than 20-fold as compared with that below pH 5[100]. The high nitrite content of gastric juice at higher pHs may be due to the presence of nitrite-producing bacteria[79, 85], and *in vitro* addition of such bacteria to the gastric juice of healthy subjects has resulted in increased formation of nitrosamines[79]. Nitrite and consequently nitrosamine formation are inhibited by vitamin C[65] and freezing[107].

The possibility of drugs being a source of nitroso-compounds has been discussed recently in connection with the treatment of peptic ulcer with cimetidine. Three cases of gastric cancer diagnosed during cimetidine treatment have been published and the relation of GCA to cimetidine has been discussed[15]. Cimetidine is a guanide derivative and is *in vitro* in the presence of nitrites readily transformed to mono-nitroso-cimetidine, the structure of which is analogous to N-methyl-N'-nitro-N-nitrosoguanidine. The latter causes in the rat the development of adenocarcinoma when administered as one large dose[37] or when repeatedly present in small amounts in the drinking water[89]. However, despite the experimental evidence, it is probable that when making the diagnosis in the three described cases of GCA the possibility of malignant ulcers was overlooked.

The discussion presented above has been mainly focused on the effects of environmental carcinogens. However, many other environmental factors in addition to carcinogens, such as occupation, dietary habits and deficiency-states[25, 110] may be of equal or even greater significance in the development of GCA.

Genetics

Associations with genetic markers

It has been known for a long time that the prevalence of blood group A in GCA is greater than expected. This finding indicates the effect of a hereditary component in the development of the disease. However, the increase in risk related to blood group A is only about 20 per cent. Later on it was found that blood group A was mainly associated with the diffuse type of GCA[10]. Likewise, blood group A is associated with an increased risk of pernicious anaemia[61], a disease with a higher-than-expected risk of GCA. Moreover, the ABO blood-group distribution in GCA associated with pernicious anaemia was similar to its overall distribution in GCA[7]. The association of pernicious anaemia with GCA demonstrates the presence of one distinct biological model: a genetic marker (blood group A) is associated with an unknown genetic factor which, independent of its carcinogenic properties, contributes to the development of pernicious anaemia.

In spite of intensive research it has not been possible to show any relationship between HLA antigens and GCA.

Family studies

When dealing with family associations one has to take into account that members of the same family share not only a similar genetic background but also a family environment in common. It should also be noted that GCA is not a rare disease and may therefore occur in more than one member of a family by chance. However, earlier family studies seem to indicate that near relatives of gastric carcinoma patients have an increased risk of developing this disease[61]. Recently Lehtola[57] studied the mortality from gastric carcinoma in 2243 first-degree relatives of 341 GCA probands. Control probands were matched by age, sex and birthplace and the death rate in GCA was evaluated in their first-degree relatives. It appeared that the risk of developing GCA was significantly higher (1.50, $P = 0.05$) in GCA relatives than in control relatives. In relatives of probands with diffuse GCA the risk was sevenfold ($P = 0.005$), but in relatives of those with intestinal carcinoma it was slightly and insignificantly higher than in controls. No case of GCA was found in the spouses of the GCA probands. It was noted in addition that the familial factors appeared to be most significant in the young female probands with diffuse type of GCA. These results suggest that the higher risk in diffuse carcinoma families is due to genetic variation rather than to a common family environment.

Lehtola's results are well in line with the results of earlier authors and with the recent studies of Ihamäki, Varis and Siurala[45] and Ihamäki and Sipponen[44] who found that conditions commonly considered precancerous, such as atrophic gastritis, intestinal metaplasia, epithelial dysplasia and achlorhydria, were significantly more common and occurred at a younger age in first-degree relatives of GCA probands than in controls, the probands of whom were computer-matched from the general population by age, sex, places of birth and residence, and occupation. The differences were most pronounced between diffuse carcinoma relatives and their controls, while no differences were seen between relatives of intestinal GCA patients and their controls. These results could explain the increased risk for gastric carcinoma in near relatives of persons with this disease.

Geographical and racial approach

One possibility of evaluating the significance of genetic factors is by comparing the prevalence of a disease in different races living in the same area. Although the living habits may differ in different races, the most important environmental factors such as the quality of air, water and soil are similar. Using this approach it was found that in Wales the GCA risk was 70 per cent higher in the Welsh population than in people of other origins[2]. Indians living in Arizona had significantly more GCA and pernicious anaemia than Caucasians[88]. The Ainu people of North Japan have significantly less GCA than Japanese of the same area[73]. Moreover, in the United States the intestinal/diffuse carcinoma ratio was higher in Negroes than in Caucasians, and the ratio has rapidly decreased during recent years in the Caucasian population[14]. These results emphasize the significance of genetic factors. However, the intestinal/diffuse GCA ratio may also reflect environmental differences. Thus, the lower death rate of the mainly environmentally influenced intestinal type of GCA in Caucasians may be due in part to their higher living standard.

Pathogenesis and dynamics

General considerations

To explain the pathogenesis of malignant tumours, two main hypotheses have been proposed and both have been applied to the pathogenesis of gastric carcinoma as well. One, the random multiple-hit hypothesis, implies that multiple single-occasional events lead to mutation-like changes in single cells or cell populations and by this pathway to malignant transformation. The second, the altered differentiation hypothesis, presupposes a programmed process which stepwise follows a pathway that resembles the embryogenic development of the target organ. The latter theory explains easily the association of carcinoma with a more primitive kind of epithelium, such as intestinal metaplasia and epithelial dysplasia, as well as the production of embryogenic antigens by the diseased mucosa.

Recently Farber *et al.*[17], basing upon experiences with experimental liver carcinoma[87], have proposed a theory which combines the two alternatives. Carcinogen-induced hits lead to the development of a carcinogen-resistant cell population which begins to proliferate (initiation of the carcinogenic process) and grow over the normal cell population, which remains inhibited by the carcinogen. Some of the initiated cells are capable of following the normal process of maturation but others do not. The latter remain immature (promotion of the carcinogenic process) and eventually undergo malignant transformation. Whether this theory can be applied to human gastric carcinoma remains to be proved.

Pathogenesis of the morphologically different types

Several trials have been made to classify GCA, but only during the last few years have there been presented classifications which show some fit with aetiopathogenetic and clinical aspects of the disease. The classifications are those of Mulligan[67], Lauren[56] and that suggested by a subcommittee of WHO[108]. Morphologically these classifications are similar in that they separate into a major group the gastric carcinomas with characteristics of intestinal epithelium (intestinal or adenomatous type, *Figure 9.1*). In addition, all three classifications distinguish a type of carcinoma which is formed of signet-ring cell type, (*Figure 9.1*). The differentiation of GCAs into intestinal and diffuse is most clearly put forward by Lauren[56], who in addition to these two main types accepts an intermediate form.

The characteristics of the two types of GCA are shown in *Table 9.1*. The differences are most pronounced in the epidemiology and genetics of the disease.

Gastric carcinoma in young people

Quite recent data published by Japanese authors and by the authors' own team seem to lend further support to the different natures of the

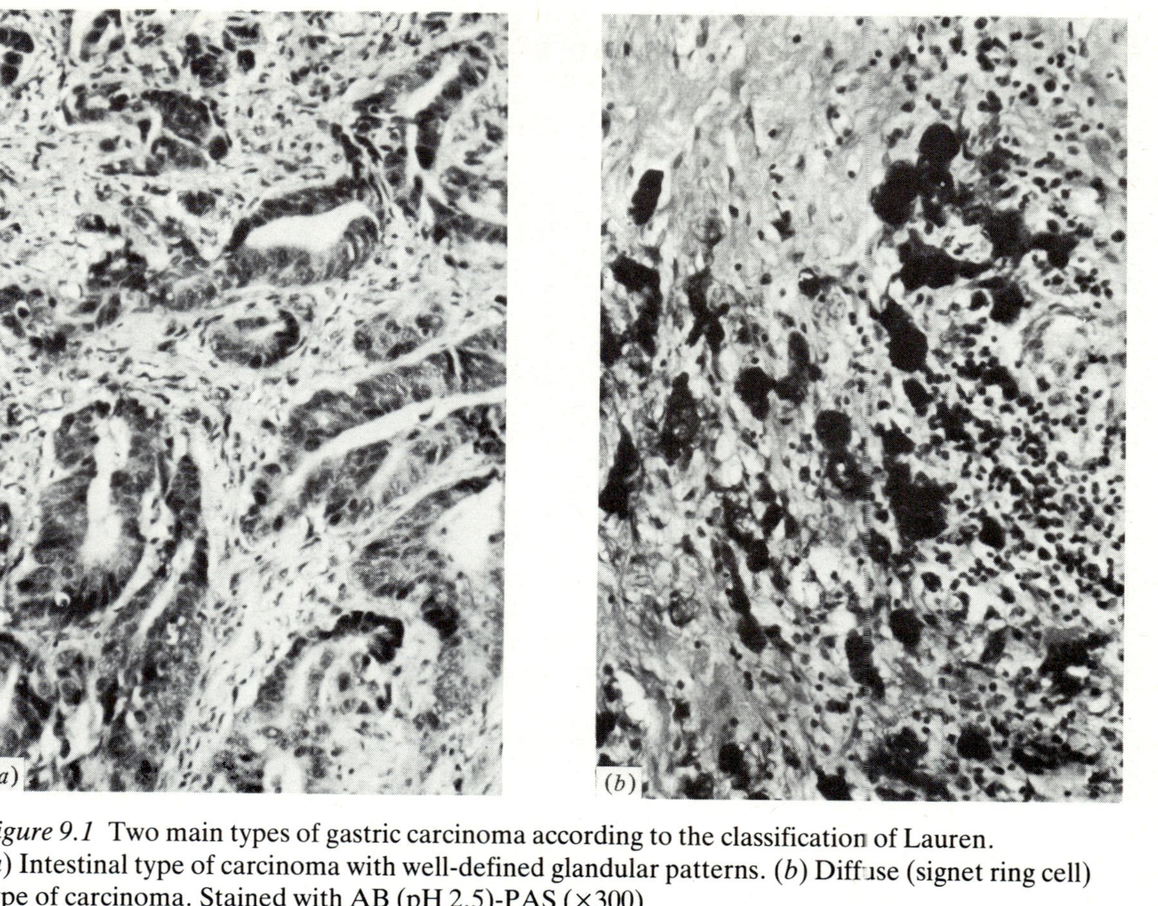

Figure 9.1 Two main types of gastric carcinoma according to the classification of Lauren.
(*a*) Intestinal type of carcinoma with well-defined glandular patterns. (*b*) Diffuse (signet ring cell) type of carcinoma. Stained with AB (pH 2.5)-PAS (×300)

two morphological types of GCA. The Japanese authors[98, 111] have studied the behaviour of GCA in a notably large series consisting of patients below 30 years of age. Most of these carcinomas were of the diffuse type. Endoscopically they were, like diffuse GCAs in general, found mainly in the body or around the antrofundal border and appeared as a rule as ulcerating lesions. In addition, the male/female ratio was similar to that of diffuse carcinomas in general. In these respects the carcinomas differed substantially from GCAs in aged persons, most of which are of the intestinal type.

Relation of different types to gastritis

Gastritis is in some way genetically associated with diffuse GCA. Kekki *et al.*[52] subjected first-degree relatives of GCA patients and appropriately matched control relatives from a general population to mathematical analysis based on stochastic principles. It appeared that the mean family age-adjusted score of gastritis showed in intestinal carcinoma families a distribution similar to that in control families, while in diffuse carcinoma the score decreased with increasing age of the proband. In other words, the occurrence of diffuse GCA at a young age, i.e. a high predisposition to diffuse GCA, is associated with a high predisposition to gastritis in relatives, and vice versa, a low predisposition of the proband to diffuse GCA with a low predisposition to gastritis in the relatives. This points to a genetic relationship between gastritis and diffuse GCA. This opinion seems valid in view of the findings that genetic factors are of importance in the development of both gastritis[93, 102] and diffuse GCA[57]. In addition, diffuse gastric carcinoma, particularly in its early stages, is rarely associated with marked atrophic changes and accompanying intestinal metaplasia[80], which does not support the concept of direct aetiopathogenetic relationship between the two conditions. The authors' own experience is in accordance with these findings. *Figure 9.2* on p. 295 shows that the age-dependent prevalence curve of intestinal metaplasia around the tumour in diffuse GCA is almost identical with that of a representative sample of a Finnish population, indicating that the occurrence of intestinal metaplasia in diffuse GCA is the expected one and without aetiopathogenetic significance. On the other hand, the more environmentally determined intestinal type of GCA is assumed to be aetiopathogenetically directly related to atrophic gastritis and intestinal metaplasia[18, 19, 20, 26, 29].

Natural course

Assuming that at least a considerable proportion of GCAs develop as a programmed process, the natural course of GCA from normal state to death must certainly take a long time. The development of the premalignant stages such as atrophic gastritis with metaplasia and pernicious anaemia is a very slow process, as clearly indicated by long-term follow-up examinations and dynamic evaluation of epidemiologically valid cross-sectional data[39, 43]. Thereafter the progression of the process from initiation up to the critical point of Hutchinson is still a slow process, and further time is needed before the appearance of macroscopical tumour. Thus, in an operated stomach in which atrophic changes with metaplasia and dysplasia develop already within one year after operation[21, 83], carcinoma does not appear until 10 to 30 years later.

Progression of the disease from the establishment of a macroscopical tumour onwards may still be rather slow in many cases. However, data on the natural course of the tumour in its early stages are regrettably scarce. Gutman[27] followed up radiologically for more than 20 years ulcerating lesions which later proved to be malignant. Recently Yamaha (for reference *see*[18]) described three cases of early GCA followed up for 17–31 years. Kawai, Miyaoka and Kohli[51] observed 14 patients with ulcerating lesions up to 3 years, and other Japanese authors (for references *see*[18]) two similar cases for about 8 years. All authors noted the very slow progression of these early lesions. The observations seem to be in line with cross-sectional data obtained in Japan by the screening of large populations. Most of the carcinomas found by screening belonged to the advanced Borrman types or early ulcerating GCAs. According to basic dynamic laws the speed of the progression is inversely proportionate to the prevalence of early and intermediate forms of the disease in the population at large. If these laws are applicable to the present data on GCA, the high prevalence of early ulcerating GCAs in screening series would indicate a very slow progression of such lesions[75].

Dynamic aspects

Recent developments in endoscopy and autoradiography have yielded some additional interesting data on the dynamics of GCA. Measurements of the growth of malignancy[18] have shown that the doubling time of the lesion[18, 51] in the early stages is very long (555–3076 days) as compared with metastatic lesions (17–90 days). Thus growth of the GCA is about 30 times more rapid in the late than in the early stages. Indeed, the progression of the diseases in the premalignant stages can be measured in decades, in the early stages in years, but in the end stages merely in months. Thus a marked acceleration of the progression of the disease towards the end is characteristic of the dynamics of GCA. However, there is an apparent discrepancy between the doubling time and the generation time of the early lesions. The generation time for normal epithelial cells has been estimated to be one day[59], for intestinal metaplasia 1.5 days[19], and for the early carcinomatous lesions 4–15 days[18]. The contrast between the rapid generation time and the macroscopically slow growth of the early lesions has been explained by their growth pattern[18]. They grow along the surface and are therefore more exposed to the peptic action of the gastric juice. However, the discrepancy can as well be explained by difference in host-response in early and late stages of the disease. It is regrettable that the facilities for measuring the capability of the body to cope with growing malignancy are very limited.

Significance of the host response

The capability of the body to protect and restore a normal DNA synthesis after exposure to mutagens must be very high, otherwise it would be impossible to understand why the species have remained unchanged in spite of exposure to mutagenic factors during millions of years. Knowledge of these protective mechanisms is certainly limited but their existence is generally acknowledged, and it is assumed that there exists some kind of alarm system that primarily is called into service to cope with the mutagenic affects of a carcinogen. Several methods have been proposed for measurement of the susceptibility of the body to the effects of carcinogens, such as estimation of the rapidity of DNA exchange and determination of ornithine decarboxylase. However, the application of such systems to clinical use is still questionable and outside the scope of this paper.

Studies of the immunoresponse of the body to malignant transformation and growth have yielded conflicting results[95], but there is some evidence indicating that the local response of macrophages and immunocompetent round cells may affect the prognosis of GCA[47, 84]. Moreover, there is some evidence indicating a lowered immunoresponse in later stages of the malignant process[13, 66], which could explain the differences in the rapidity of growth at different stages of the disease.

It is important to note that the data given above on the natural course of GCA are based upon examination of small series only; in view of the varying behaviour of different types of gastric carcinoma this is very unsatisfactory. All in all, it must be concluded that our overall knowledge of the natural course of GCA is greatly deficient. Long-term follow-up examinations would give substantial information, but large series have been collected only in Japan, and only a few cases been followed up and in general for a rather short time so far. On the other hand, the long time necessary for the development of tumour provides an opportunity to interfere with the natural course of the disease, an aspect which will be discussed below.

Possibilities of improving the prognosis

Prevention

The ideal solution of the problem would be prevention of the disease. This, on the other hand, presupposes knowledge of the factors that have been found to act as carcinogens or cocarcinogens under experimental conditions. Most potent of these have been shown to be some nitroso-compounds. Although they occur in the diet and water in very small concentrations, it is possible that under certain conditions they may be formed in the gastric lumen and accumulate in the mucosa in concentrations high enough to induce malignant transformation[64]. However, we still do not know whether they play any significant part in the development of gastric carcinoma in man, and even if we could prove it, their elimination from the environment would be an overwhelming task.

Nitrates are present in water and soil and their complete removal is hardly possible. On the other hand, the transformation of nitrates to nitrites can be inhibited by storage of food in the refrigerator or by vitamin C, which will be more closely discussed below. Refraining from the use of vegetables grown in nitrogen fertilized soil and from canned meat and fish to which nitrates have been added could be justified theoretically, but there is no proof of the benefit of such measures. These measures seem of particular importance in risk groups such as achlorhydrics and patients with various degrees of atrophic gastritis, but this concerns mainly elderly people who in view of the long natural history of GCA hardly need any preventive measures. The role of nitroso-compound-forming drugs as carcinogens in man is still uncertain; however, the authors would like to refer to the statement of a WHO team: 'Any orally administered readily nitrosable drug that generates demonstrable carcinogenic derivates should be withdrawn provided a suitable replacement is available'[109].

To be successful, the elimination of deleterious factors should not interfere with sound dietary and living habits and it should be managed easily and at reasonable expense. Accordingly, even the identification of carcinogenic factors may not make an effective prevention possible. Moreover, in the case of gastric carcinoma, which is caused by many genetic and environmental factors, the elimination of one factor might not substantially affect its prognosis at a population level. In fact, the decline in the death rate of gastric carcinoma noted during the last decades is not due to any active measures but has occurred spontaneously concomitantly with an increase in the living standard.

Technically the addition of anticarcinogenic substances to the diet might be an easier procedure than the elimination of carcinogens. Developments in the field of chemical carcinogenesis has indeed focused anew the interest upon the anticarcinogenic action of some compounds, such as vitamins E and C. Earlier epidemiological studies have indicated an inverse correlation between the supply of vitamins E and C and the gastric carcinoma death rate[106], and recent experimental and *in vitro* studies have shown that vitamin C can inhibit the formation of carcinogenic nitroso-compounds in the gastric lumen[65]. Accordingly, there is a theoretical basis for a recommendation to add vitamin C to the diet for the prophylaxis against GCA.

Diagnosis and treatment

Another alternative which could affect the prognosis of the disease is improved diagnosis and treatment. However, the effectiveness of the present diagnostic methods is already very high. Thus gastroscopy combined with direct vision gastric biopsy and/or brush cytology yields a diagnostic reliability of about 100 per cent. Nevertheless, the prognosis of the disease is still poor. It is true that in recent years some centres have reported 5-year survival rates markedly exceeding the earlier ones[46] and have usually attributed the good results to employment of more radical surgical procedures. However, the better results can as well be ascribed to improved diagnosis, advances in anaesthesia, improved early and late postoperative care, and particularly to more rigid criteria for operative intervention. Thus Bennigshoff and Tsien[4] have clearly demonstrated the effect of the principles of selection upon the 5-year survival rate of carcinoma of the breast. Indeed, critical evaluation of data in the literature suggest that no substantial change has occurred during the recent decades in the 5-year survival rate of carcinoma of the breast[55]. It also can be shown that operations and radiotherapy have not affected the overall long-term survival in bronchial carcinoma[3, 74]. Likewise the overall 5-year and 10-year survival rates of gastric carcinoma have not, according to Pichlmayr[76], changed during the last 2–3 decades. On the other hand, the epidemiological evaluation of Humphrey et al.[40] indicates that gastric carcinoma differs from other visceral carcinomas with respect to survival. The authors calculated standardized mortality ratios for lung, colon and gastric carcinomas treated by 'curative' surgery, and found in gastric carcinoma only a subgroup (26 per cent of cases) which could be identified as cured, i.e. which showed a return to the expected survival rate for age, sex and race. It is certainly not an easy task to evaluate the many reported 5-year survival rates in GCA. Many factors seem to affect it. Thus, in addition to therapeutic measures, the general condition of the patient and the stage of the tumour, such factors as sex, age, macroscopical and histological type of the tumour, and quality and quantity of the tissue stomal reaction should be considered[86].

Developments in chemotherapy and immunotherapy seem not to have affected the natural course of gastric carcinoma. Some healing effect has been described[113], but from the curative point of view the results have been rather disappointing. Nor is it probable that recent exciting advances in operative endoscopy, which permit endoscopic removal of small, early nonulcerating carcinomas[34], will affect the overall prognosis of the disease.

Screening

While the overall prognosis of gastric carcinoma has shown little change during the last decades, high survival rates have been reported in a subgroup of gastric carcinoma diagnosed by chance, i.e. by screening of large populations, and called 'early' gastric carcinoma. Japanese authors have reported a 5-year survival rate of about 95 per cent in the 'early' cases found by endoscopical or fluoroscopical mass screening. Because of this the authors consider it necessary to review the problem more closely.

From a time aspect the term 'early' is not quite appropriate[31] because a circumscribed small lesion does not necessarily imply that it is an early one: it might have existed for a long time. The Japanese classification of early cancers in more than 10 subtypes can also be criticized. The complicated classification is based upon morphological and endoscopical criteria. Such criteria are justified if they correlate with certain other parameters: aetiopathogenetic, epidemiological and clinical. Accordingly, one is tempted to ask whether there exist such correlations: what for instance are the clinical features that distinguish type IIc+III from III+IIc? Hermanek and Roesch[35] have suggested a simpler classification of the early types into ulcerating and non-ulcerating. On the other hand, there is some evidence indicating that the Japanese type IIc differs epidemiologically from type III: Nagayo[72] has shown that during the last 10 years the prevalence of type IIc has significantly increased and that of III decreased, indicating the existence of differently behaving subgroups of the early gastric carcinoma. Therefore, the Japanese subclassification can be considered justified as a starting point for a closer identification of this probably rather heterogeneous group.

It was already noted above that epidemiological and follow-up considerations and the results of long-term follow-up studies emphasize that at least a part, if not most, early ulcerating types grow slowly. Accordingly, the 5-year survival rate in such cases is probably *a priori* high without any operative interventions. However, the data on the natural course of different types of gastric carcinoma are very scanty, which makes it impossible to judge the true benefit of large screening projects. Indeed, there is not yet *definite proof* that a surgical intervention improves the prognosis of GCA: it may only fit in the natural course of the carcinoma without altering it. Furthermore, one must also reckon with various psychologically adverse effects of mass screening in addition to the direct risks due to radiation or invasive diagnostic procedures[53]. The cost/benefit aspect is, moreover, of particular importance when whole populations are screened for a rather rare disease such as gastric carcinoma.

The difficulties involved in judging the benefit of mass-screening are further emphasized by the fact that a considerable proportion of patients with the disease die from causes other than GCA. Thus Kobori *et al.*[54] followed up for 15 years a large series of early gastric carcinoma patients who underwent two-thirds gastrectomy, and found that only 20 per cent of the deaths could be clearly attributed to GCA.

Immunology in diagnosis and screening

The good results obtained in Japan with mass screening have encouraged the search for simpler and less expensive methods than those employed by the Japanese authors. Demonstration of specific carcinoma markers in body fluids would be the ideal solution[36]. Most of these markers are glycoproteins with antigenic properties. They are often found in the fluids and tissues of fetuses but disappear later on and reappear in connection with malignancy: hence they are termed carcinofetal antigens. The best known are the carcinoembryogenic antigen (CEA) of Gold and Friedman[23], the α-fetoprotein of Abelev (AFP)[1], and the fetal sulphoglycoprotein antigen (FSA) of Häkkinen[41], but the list of these antigens is long because of the ability of tumours to produce a great variety of 'strange' proteins[24]. In addition to antigens, abnormal enzymes and isoenzymes have been demonstrated in the blood and tissues of patients with carcinoma[63, 99].

CEA has been used mainly for the diagnosis of colonic carcinoma and as an early sign of relapse after surgery. CEA cross-reacts with the normal cross-reacting antigen (NCA) and the normal cross-reacting antigen 2 (NCA 2) of Burtin, Chavanel and Hirsch-Marie[5, 6]. In addition, it is immunologically indistinguishable from an antigen normally present in gastric juice, the CEA-like or Celia antigen[104] which is closely related or identical with NCA 2[5, 6]. Moreover, radioimmunological quantification of tissue extracts of the stomach did not reveal any significant differences between malignant and benign gastric lesions[58]. Purification of CEA has resulted in further loss of sensitivity in the diagnosis of colonic and gastric malignancy.

The FSA of Häkkinen is the only antigen which has been used for mass screening. Earlier studies indicate a sensitivity of 95 per cent in gastric carcinoma[42]. Häkkinen[41] examined a population of about 30 000 persons for the presence of FSA. Twenty-two of about 2300 FSA-positive subjects proved to have gastric carcinoma and eight of the negative subjects were later found to suffer from gastric carcinoma. This gives a sensitivity of 73 per cent and a specificity of 92 per cent. However, the usefulness of the method is limited because the examination is carried out on gastric juice. Moreover, attempts to quantify FSA immunologically have so far failed.

It seems that despite the early encouraging results the use of these markers for the diagnosis and screening of GCA has proved to be of limited value, as could be expected because the different types of gastric carcinoma at different stages of differentiation and progression most probably produce a variety of different strange elements with antigenic properties. Moreover, the methodological difficulties inherent in immunological methods are considerable: cruder antibody preparations lead to low specificity and their purification to loss of sensitivity. If, on the other hand, the presence of oncofetal antigens is considered a sign of differentiation with a return to embryonal conditions, it is possible that these antigens could be produced by all poorly differentiated tissues, such as epithelial dysplasia and colonic type of intestinal metaplasia[41, 94]. Accordingly, the appearance of oncofetal antigens could also be a sign of an early premalignant alteration.

The considerations presented above do not encourage a wider employment of mass screening for GCA although high prevalence of the disease in Japan and the excellent results obtained by Japanese investigators make their enthusiasm understandable. It also should be noted that some evidence[28] indicates that the prognosis of the rapidly growing Borrman type of GCAs is markedly better when they are diagnosed by chance or by screening than at routine outpatient examination. This is an important point in favour of mass screening and should be further evaluated. Moreover, according to Hara[30], annually performed mass screenings of smaller populations have reduced the death rate by about 50 per cent. However, comparable reductions have been noted lately in some countries without any preventive or mass-screening attempts. Moreover, in Japan the decrease in the mortality rate was found to be associated with a distinct decrease in the incidence of the disease[38].

Follow-up of risk groups

General considerations

A further possibility of improving prognosis of GCA is by screening and following up high-risk groups. The advantages of such an approach are obvious: the group to examine is smaller and accordingly its handling is simpler and less expensive. There is evidence that pernicious anaemia, adenomatous polyps, a stomach operated for peptic ulcer, and Menetrier's disease can be considered risk groups of GCA. However, only a few subjects with these diseases develop malignancy, and all together they can explain the occurrence of GCA in only a small proportion of cases. Similar conclusions can be drawn with respect to atrophic gastritis where there is evidence of a higher than expected risk of gastric carcinoma, but only a very small proportion of these subjects will ever develop GCA. Atrophic gastritis is a very common condition, the prevalence of atrophic gastritis of the body mucosa being, in two Finnish and one Estonian population samples, 26, 16 and 20 per cent respectively[45, 92, 103]. On the other hand, the death rate of GCA in Finland is only 24 per 100 000 of population. Accordingly, there is an urgent need of closer identification of the characteristics of high-risk groups.

Assuming that the four conditions mentioned above (atrophic gastritis, pernicious anaemia, polyps and operated stomach) are precancerous, the question arises: what signs have they in common? An answer to this question may give hints as to the characteristics responsible for their possible precancerous properties.

The four conditions in question have in common atrophic gastritis and the following signs associated with it: intestinal metaplasia, epithelial dysplasia, hyperplasia, cyst formation, and achlorhydria.

The significance of achlorhydria has already been discussed (*see* p. 280). A high pH of gastric contents and bacterial invasion accompanying it may assist in the intraluminal formation of water-soluble nitroso-compounds (*see* p. 280). In addition, achlorhydria, which is commonly accompanied by duodenal regurgitation, may facilitate the solubilization and uptake of fat-soluble environmental carcinogens such as dimethylbenzanthracene and methylchloranthrene. Concerning cyst formation it has been assumed that cysts permit sporadic cancer cells to avoid shedding in the course of renewal of the gastric mucosa and thus permit the cells to live long enough to form a tumour. Such a hypothesis has been put forward by Fujita and Hattori[19], but as yet there is no convincing evidence to support it.

Intestinal metaplasia

Intestinal metaplasia (IM) is virtually always found in the close vicinity of an intestinal-type GCA[16, 56], but less frequently around GCA of the diffuse type[16]. Similarly, in early GCA the tumours of intestinal type are as a rule associated with IM, but those of diffuse-type more rarely[16]. It is also known that in both types of GCA the tumour itself shows morphological, histochemical and immunological[90] characteristics of IM. In addition, there can be found in the same stomach

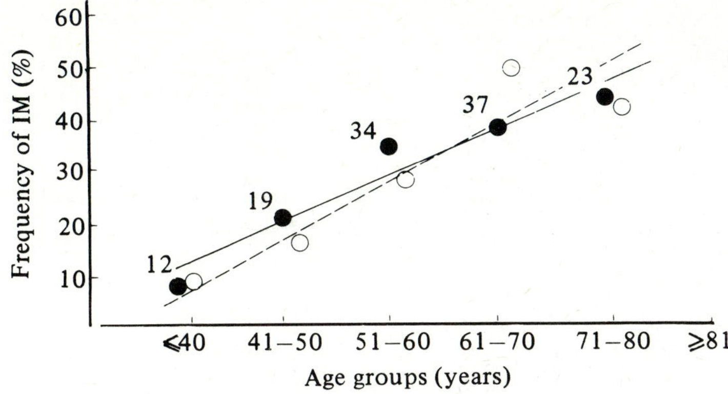

Figure 9.2 Age-behaviour of intestinal metaplasia (IM) in
the mucosa surrounding carcinoma (GCA) of diffuse type
(●) and in a sample of a Finnish population (358 subjects) (○)

transitional forms between IM and GCA[71, 72]. The prevalence of IM is,
moreover, significantly higher in high than in low-GCA-risk areas[8]. It
should be noted, however, that the prevalence of IM in a representative population increases significantly with age (*Figure 9.2*), so that its
prevalence in elderly age groups approaches almost 50 per cent[45].
Thus the expected prevalence of IM among GCA patients is already
very high.

The common occurrence of IM in the general population and its
rapid increase with age, limits its usefulness for screening purposes.
Moreover, the lack of distinct association with the diffuse type of
GCA, which more often affects young people than does the intestinal
type, specially decreases the value of IM as a screening criterion.
Figure 9.2 clearly demonstrates that the age-behaviour of IM in the
close vicinity of diffuse GCA is similar to that of IM in a general
population. These considerations strongly indicate the need for a
closer identification of those properties of IM which might have a
nearer relationship to GCA.

Relationship of different types of intestinal metaplasia to gastric carcinoma

Recent histochemical studies have succeeded in identifying subtypes of
IM which seem to behave differently with respect to GCA.

The morphological heterogeneity of the mucin-staining properties
of IM has been known for a long time. Most metaplastic glands found

in the gastric mucosa share the main characteristics of the epithelium of the *small intestinal* mucosa: they stain like true small-bowel goblet and absorptive cells by reactions typical of sialylated or neutral mucosubstances[33, 49, 91], they reveal similar antigenic determinants[6, 41], and their overall morphology is similar. However, a small proportion of intestinal metaplasias lack these characteristics and show instead the staining properties of *colonic* epithelium (*Figure 9.3*), i.e. they are stained by reactions typical of acidic sulphated glycoproteins[32, 33, 49, 101] and contain antigens found in a normal colonic mucosa[5, 6].

The synthesis of glycoproteins up to the final residues is determined by deligated, gene-linked internal enzyme systems. Accordingly the appearance of metaplasia with different kinds of glycoproteins may reflect the level of differentiation or dedifferentiation. Sipponen *et al.*[91] found in representative samples of patients that the occurrence of staining characteristics of the colonic type (staining with high-iron-diamine and Alcian blue at pH 1.0) increases with age, so that the mean age of subjects with the colonic type of IM is significantly higher than of those with the small-intestinal type. The staining types correlated also with the extension of IM in the stomach: when large areas were affected by IM the glands often stained strongly with high-iron-diamine, while in less extensive IM the reaction generally was faint[91]. These results suggest that the two types of IM represent different stages of the same process. It is probable that this process, because of the simpler morphology and function of the colonic mucosa, is a dedifferentiation process which might terminate in neoplasia. Indeed, the colonic type of IM seems to be more closely related to malignancy than does the small-intestinal type.

Heilman and Höpker[33] found IM with sulphated glycoproteins (colonic type of IM) in most gastric specimens removed for GCA, but only rarely in specimens from patients with benign gastrointestinal disease. Similar reports have been published by others[33, 49, 101]. Furthermore, Teglbjaerg and Nielsen[101] observed that IM of colonic type was associated particularly with the intestinal type of GCA. Moreover, Sipponen *et al.*[91] found that the colonic type of IM was more common in patients with pernicious anaemia and in patients with GCA and their first-degree relatives than in controls considered to represent a general population. These studies suggest some relationship between colonic-type IM and subpopulations commonly considered GCA risk-groups. However, the data discussed do not prove that the colonic type of IM is directly aetiopathogenetically related to GCA; more conclusive evidence can be obtained only by

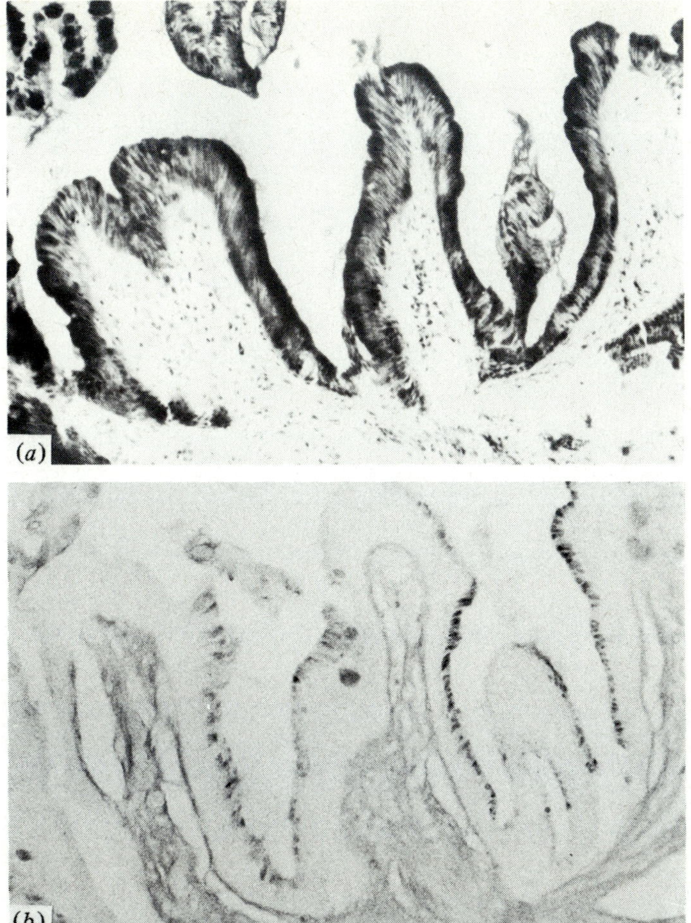

Figure 9.3 Intestinal metaplasia with characteristics of colonic epithelium (enterocolic metaplasia). (*a*) Epithelium stained with AB (pH 2.5)-PAS. (*b*) An adjacent section stained with high-iron diamine (HID) for sulphated mucosubstances. Note the staining of mucosubstances throughout the epithelium (×300)

long-term follow-up studies. The results can as well be interpreted as the occurrence of the colonic type of IM being only of the markers associated with the dedifferentiation phenomena characteristic of a cancerous stomach. Indeed, experimental evidence indicates that GCA induced by administration of nitroso-compounds may develop concomitantly with or before the occurrence of intestinal metaplasia[81, 82].

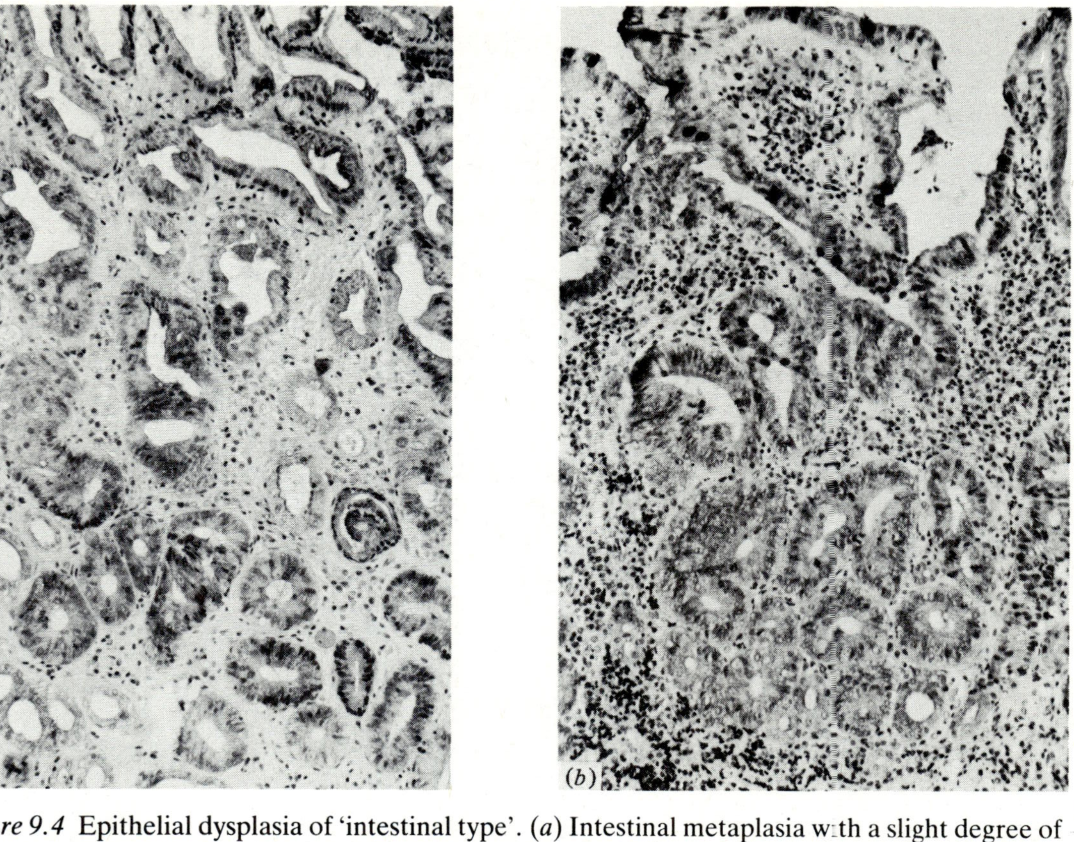

Figure 9.4 Epithelial dysplasia of 'intestinal type'. (*a*) Intestinal metaplasia with a slight degree of atypia: some irregularity in the contour of glands but well-defined brush border in the epithelium. (*b*) Intestinal metaplasia with moderate atypia: the number of goblet cells is reduced and the contour of tubules is irregular and disturbed

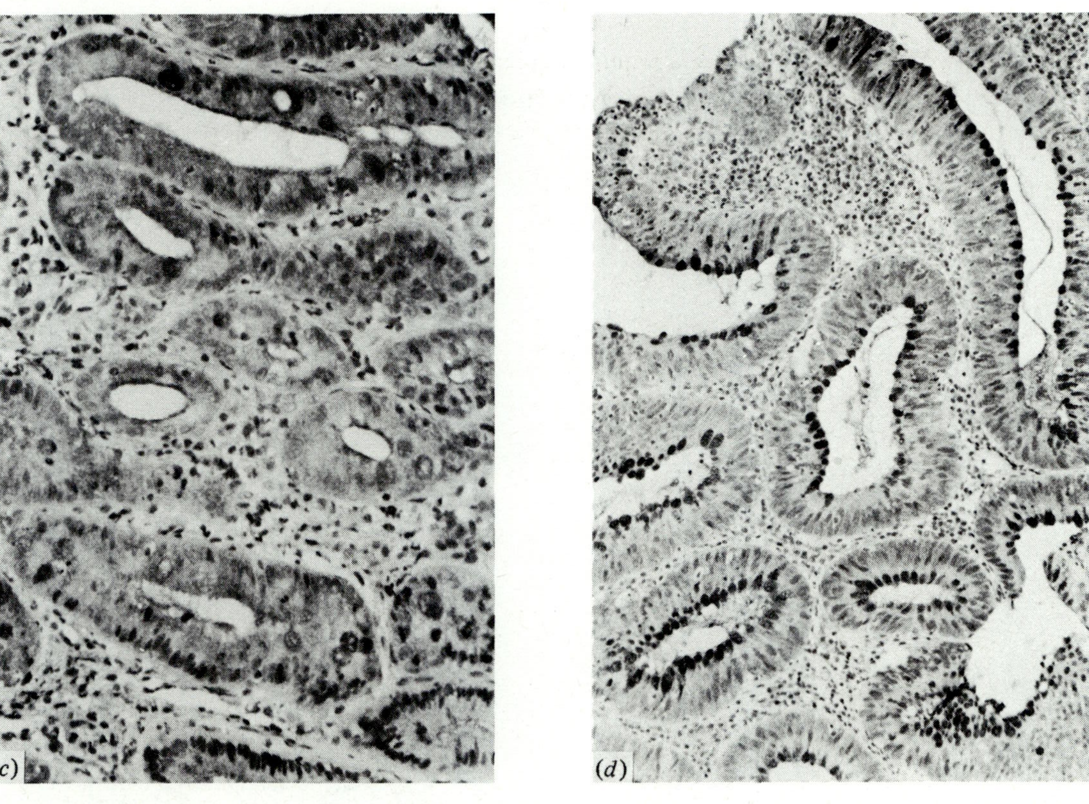

Figure 9.4(c) Intestinal metaplasia with moderate atypia:there is nearly complete loss of goblet cells, anaplasia and stratification of the epithelium and epithelial cells. (*d*) Intestinalized gastric mucosa with dysplasia of severe degree: the epithelium is hyperplastic, pleomorphic and stratified, with only slight mucus secretion in the apical parts of the epithelium. The number of mitoses is high throughout the tubules. Note also the marked resemblance to neoplastic adenomas of colon. AB (pH 2.5)-PAS (×300)

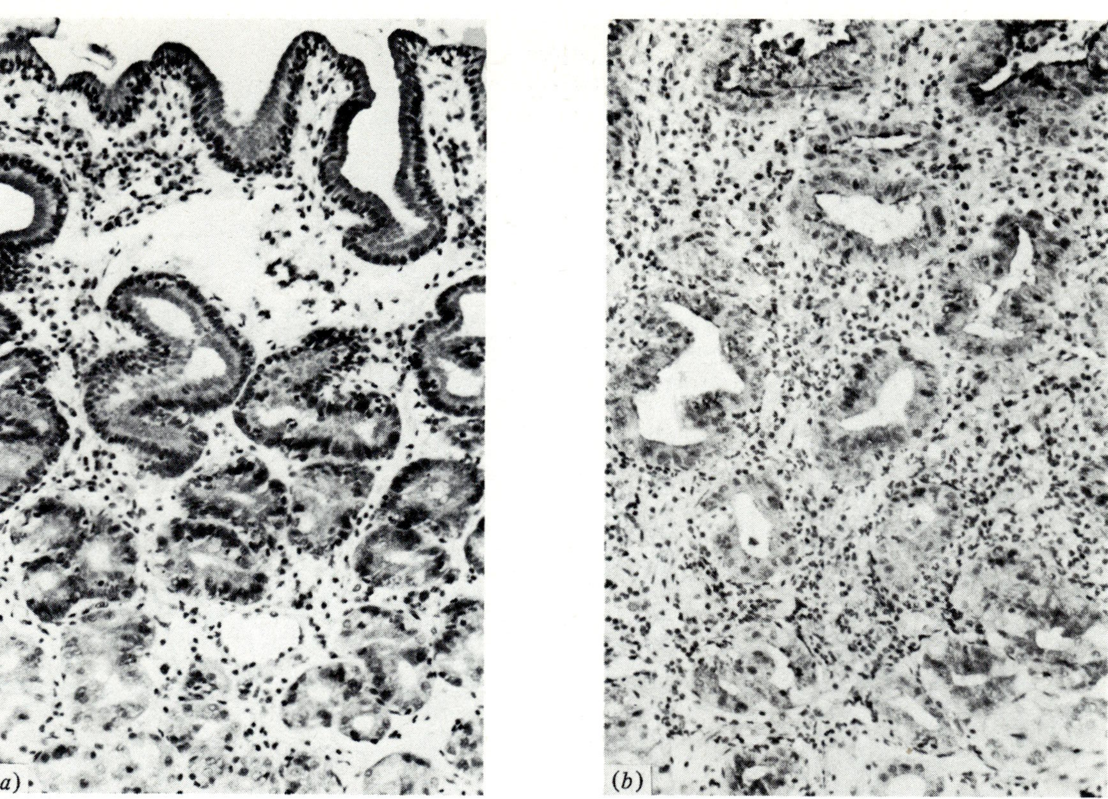

Figure 9.5 Epithelial dysplasia of 'foveolar type'. (*a*) Normal foveoles. (*b*) Slight dysplasia with reduced mucus synthesis and secretion, and with slight irregularities and cell pleomorphism in the epithelium of foveoles

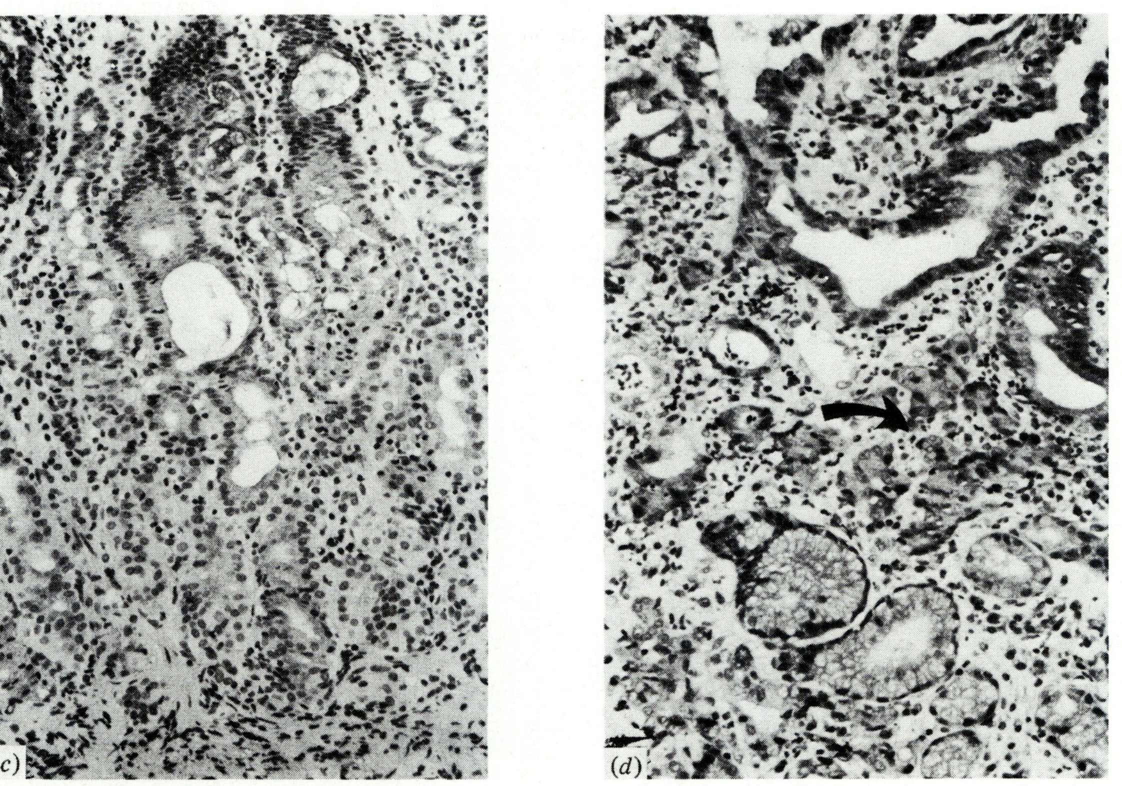

Figure 9.5(*c*) Severe dysplasia with severe irregularity in the contour of glands and with marked cellular pleomorphism in the epithelium. (*d*) Foveolar dysplasia with signs (arrow) of early intramucosal diffuse type carcinoma. AB (pH 2.5)-PAS (×300)

Different types of intestinal metaplasia can also be identified immunologically. Thus, some intestinal glands may reveal a marked carcinoembryogenic antigen-like activity[94], that has been demonstrated in the colonic mucosa[94] and in a cancerous tissue as well[90].

The results discussed above indicate that there exist intestinal metaplasias which histochemically, morphologically and immunologically resemble normal colonic mucosa and which are more closely related to GCA than is the small-intestinal type.

Epithelial dysplasia

The relation of the two types of IM to s.c. epithelial dysplasia (ED) of the gastric mucosa is not clear. Nor is there any distinct and generally accepted definition of epithelial dysplasia. Morphologically there seem to exist at least two main types. One of them can most properly be defined as poorly differentiated and intestinal, here called the intestinal type of ED (*Figure 9.4*). It reveals characteristics of absorptive epithelium, but goblet cells are few or lacking, and the brush border and cytoplasm are less well stained than in the normal small-intestinal mucosa. ED of intestinal type shows further peculiar cell kinetics[22, 29, 60]. Using incorporation with radioactive thymidine[22, 60] it has been shown that in well-differentiated IM there are mitoses at the bottom of the glands around the germinative area, as in the normal small intestine. On the other hand, in ED of intestinal type the mitoses occur throughout the gland[29]. Thus in this type of ED the whole gland continues to synthesize DNA and undergo mitosis, resulting in poor maturation of the gland. If the life-span of such poorly matured epithelium is prolonged, dysplasia invariably develops and possibly also neoplasia. This is the probable mode of development of adenomatous polyps of the stomach, which are composed of poorly differentiated intestinalized glands and which are usually considered precancerous. The distinctly precancerous colonic adenomas also reveal morphological and cell-kinetic features similar to those of gastric ED of intestinal type[60]. However, this sequence of events cannot be considered proven, nor do we know whether the intestinal type of ED is identical with or related to the histochemically identified colonic type of IM.

Another type of ED is characterized by increased numbers of mitotic figures in the pits and nonmetaplastic surface epithelium, where the cells appear poorly differentiated and show a rather high degree of anaplasia (*Figure 9.5*). The authors designate it *the foveolar type of ED*; however, it is less distinctly defined than the intestinal type of ED. The rather high degree of cellular anaplasia may link it with poorly differentiated types of GCA: the diffuse (*Figure 9.5d*) and anaplastic.

Conclusions

(1) Gastric carcinoma (GCA) is a multifactorial disease caused by many genetic and environmental factors.

(2) Living habits and diet show slight and only statistically demonstrable correlations with GCA.

(3) The incidence of GCA correlates with the nitrate content of water and soil. Nitrates may be transformed to nitrites, and these in the presence of amines to nitroso-compounds, which are potent experimental carcinogens. Under *in vitro* conditions the process is facilitated at high pH of gastric juice, and it seems that an altered gastric mucosa is more suspectible to the action of carcinogens than a normal one. The formation of nitrites from nitrates is inhibited by cooling and by vitamin C.

(4) Extensive family studies have demonstrated an increased risk of GCA in near relatives of probands with this disease. This risk is manyfold in relatives of diffuse GCA, but not significantly different from controls in relatives of intestinal GCA. Some evidence suggests that the differences found are mainly due to genetic variation rather than to a common family environment. Alterations of the gastric mucosa commonly considered pre-cancerous tend to occur in these high-risk conditions more often and at a younger age than expected.

(5) The pathogenesis and the natural course of GCA are largely unknown. This limits our possibilities to improve the prognosis of the disease. In spite of many encouraging reports the overall prognosis of the disease has not substantially changed in western countries during the last few decades, and the decreased death rate of GCA in recent decades is not due to any preventive measures. The better results reported to have been obtained by improved diagnostic and surgical methods can probably be ascribed to other reasons.

(6) The excellent results obtained by Japanese authors by radiological and gastrocamera mass screening may in part be due to the very slow rate of growth of some types of 'early' GCA. A fairly long survival time has been reported in a few nonoperated cases followed up so far. The effect of mass screening upon the overall death rate of the disease has not yet been demonstrated.

(7) Attempts to diagnose and screen GCA by means of non-radiological and noninvasive methods, e.g. by immunological methods, have not been succesful. Numerous substances with antigenic properties produced by malignant tissue have been identified immunologically, but none having sufficient usefulness.

(8) Methods of finding and following up conditions considered precancerous have not been very encouraging. Some evidence indicates that atrophic gastritis, pernicious anaemia, the operated stomach and adenomatous polyps are precancerous or cancer-preceding conditions. However, only a small proportion of these patients will ever get GCA. This has prompted a search for those factors that are responsible for the precancerous properties of the above-mentioned conditions. Intestinal metaplasia, particularly its colonic type, and epithelial dysplasia are thought to be such conditions, but no conclusive evidence has been brought up as yet and research work in this field is still in progress.

(9) The lack of success in the treatment of GCA is due to the poor knowledge at present of its aetiopathogenesis. The reason for the difficulty in solving this problem is mainly the multifactorial and greatly variable nature of the disease, as evidenced by the dissimilar pathogenetic backgrounds and biological behaviours of the two histologically different types: the diffuse and the intestinal GCA.

(10) The limited knowledge of the natural course of GCA owing to lack of appropriate long-term follow-up studies of nonoperated cases and of precancerous conditions, makes it difficult to judge the benefit of mass-screening procedures and methods of treatment.

References

1 ABELEV, G. I., PEROVA, S. D., KHRAMKOVA, N. I., POSTNIKOVA, Z. A. and IRLIN, I. S. Production of embryonal alpha-globulin by transplantable mouse hepatomas. *Transplantation*, **1**, 174–180 (1963)

2 ASHLEY, D. J. B. Gastric cancer in Wales. *Journal of Medical Genetics*, **6**, 76–79 (1969)

3 BECKER, H., BROST, H. G., BRIELER, H. S., DAHM, P., DALICHAU, H., DONHÖFER, A., HEGEMANN, G., JUNGINGER, TH., KESSLER, E., KÜMMERLE, F., MÜHE, E., PICHLMAIER, H., REIDEMEISTER, J. CHR., REUSCH, G., SATTER, P., SAVIC, B., SOMMERWERCK, D., SCHOTTE, J. F., SCHWAIGER, R., STÖHR, U., STROTHMANN, A., TÄGER, B., TIMM, D., UNGEHEUER, E., VIERECK, R., WACHE, H., WASSNER, U. J. and ZIEROTT, G. Ergebnisse der operativen Behandlung des Bronchial-karzinoms. *Deutsche Medizinische Wochenschrift*, **101**, 1553–1557 (1976)

4 BENNINGHOFF, D. R. and TSIEN, K. C. Treatment and survival in breast cancer. *British Journal of Radiology*, **32**, 450–454 (1959)

5 BURTIN, P. V. The carcinoembryonic antigen of the digestive system (CEA) and cross-reacting antigens. In *Pathophysiology of Carcinogenesis in Digestive Organs*, edited by E. Farber, *et al.* 259–267. Tokyo, University Press/Baltimore, University Park Press (1977)

6 BURTIN, P., CHAVANEL, G. and HIRSCH-MARIE. H. Characterization of a second normal antigen that cross reacts with CEA. *Journal of Immunology*, **111**, 1926–1928 (1973)

7 CALLENDER, S., LANGMAN, M. J. S., MACLEOD, I. N., MOSBECH, J. and RATHKENS-NIELSEN, K. ABO blood group in patients with gastric carcinoma associated with pernicious anemia. *Gut*, **12**, 465–467 (1971)

8 CORREA, P. CUELLO, C. and DUQUE, E. Carcinoma and intestinal metaplasia of the stomach in Colombian migrants. *Journal of the National Cancer Institute*, **44**, 297–306 (1970)

9 CORREA, P., CUELLO, C., DUQUE, E., BURBANO, L. C., CARCIA, F. T., BOLANOS, O., BROWN, C. and HAENSZEL, W. Gastric cancer in Colombia. III. Natural history of precursor lesions. *Journal of the National Cancer Institute*, **57**, 1027–1033 (1976)

10 CORREA, P., SASANO, N., STEMMERMANN, G. N. and HAENSZEL, W. Pathology of gastric carcinoma in Japanese populations: comparison between Miyagi prefecture, Japan and Hawaii. *Journal of the National Cancer Institute*, **51**, 1449–1459 (1973)

11 DAHM, K. and WERNER, B. Experimentelles Anastomosencarcinom. *Langenbecks Archiv für Chirurgie*, **333**, 211–236 (1973)

12 DOMELLÖF, L. Gastric carcinoma promoted by alkaline reflux gastritis with special reference to bile and other surfactants as promotor of postoperative gastric cancer. *Medical Hypotheses*, **5**, 463–470 (1979)

13 DOUGLASS, H. O. and ZAMCHECK, N. Delayed hypersensitivity skin testing (DHS), total lymphocyte count (TLC) and CEA levels in patients with gastric and pancreatic cancer (meeting abstr.) *Proceedings of the American Association for Cancer Research*, **20**, 197 (1979)

14 DUTZ, W., KOHOUT, E. and VESSAL, K. Epidemiologic studies of gastric carcinoma: comparison between Iranians and two racial groups in the USA. *Israel Journal of Medical Sciences*, **15**, 410–413 (1979)

15 ELDER, J. B., GANGULI, P. C. and GILLESPIE, I. E. Cimetidine and gastric cancer. *Lancet*, **1**, 1005–1006 (1979)

16 ELSTER, K., CARSON, W., WILD, A. and THOMASKO, A. Evaluation of histological classification in early gastric cancer. *Endoscopy*, **3**, 203–206 (1979)

17 FARBER, E., SELT, D., CAMERON, R., LAISHES, B. and MEDLINE, A. Chemical carcinogenesis: An emerging new perspective. *Pathophysiology of Carcinogenesis in Digestive Organs*, edited by E. Faber *et al*. 429–441. Tokyo, University Press/Baltimore, University Park Press (1977)

18 FUJITA, S. Biology of early gastric carcinoma. *Pathology, Research and Practice*, **163**, 297–309 (1978)

19 FUJITA, S. and HATTORI, T. Cell proliferation, differentation and migration in the gastric mucosa: a study in the background of carcinogenesis. In *Pathophysiology of Carcinogenesis in Digestive Organs*, edited by E. Farber *et al*. 21–36. Tokyo, University Press/Baltimore, University Park Press (1977)

20 GEDIGK, P., BECHTELSHEIMER, H. and MUELLER-WALLRAF, R. Premalignant lesions of the stomach. *Israel Journal of Medical Sciences*, **15**, 405–409 (1979)

21 GJERULDSEN, S. T., MYREN, J. and FRETHEIM, B. C. Alteration of gastric mucosa following graded partial gastrectomy for duodenal ulcer. *Scandinavian Journal of Gastroenterology*, **3**, 465–470 (1968)

22 GLASS, G. B. J. and PITCHUMONI, C. S. Atrophic gastritis. *Human Pathology*, **6**, 219–250 (1975)

23 GOLD, P. and FRIEDMAN, S. O. Specific carcinoembryonic antigens of the human digestive system. *Journal of Experimental Medicine*, **122**, 417–481 (1965)

24 GOLDENBERG, D. M. Oncofetal and tumor-associated antigens of the human digestive system. In *Pathology of the Gastro-Intestinal Tract*, edited by B. C. Morson. *Current Topics in Pathology*, **63**, 289–342. Berlin, Springer Verlag (1976)

25 GOLDSMITH, J. R., STEINITZ, R. and WRONKOWSKI, Z. Gastric cancer incidence. *Frontiers in Gastro-intestinal Research*, **4**, 111–121 (1979)

26 GRUNDMANN, E. Histologic types and possible initial stages in early gastric carcinoma. *Beiträge zur Pathologie*, **154**, 256–280 (1975)

27 GUTMAN, R. A. Près de 50 ans de diagnostique précaire du cancer gastrique. *Abstract of papers of the VI World Congress of Gastroenterology*, Madrid. 72 (1978)

28 HAKKILUOTO, A. and LEMPINEN, M. Ulcer stimulating gastric carcinoma. *Annales Chirurgiae et Gynaecologiae Fenniae*, **64**, 5–9 (1975)

29 HANAWA, T., KORBOLA, K. and NAGAYO, T. Growth state from mitotic index in metaplastic intestinal epithelium, atypical epithelium of intestinal epithelium and well-differentiated adenocarcinoma of the stomach. Meeting abstract (Japanese text). Quoted by *Cancergram*, **80**, 7 (1980)

30 HARA, Y. Current procedures for the early detection of cancer. Endoscopical and roentgenological screening. In *Current Views in Gastroenterology*, edited by Varro and Balint, 497–510. Budapest (1977)

31 HAUBRICH, W., SHANNON, E. and SCHUMAN, B. 'Early' gastric cancer. *Gastrointestinal Endoscopy*, **25**, 77–78 (1979)

32 HEILMAN, K. *Gastritis, Intestinale Metaplasie, Carcinom.* Stuttgart, Georg Thieme Verlag (1978)

33 HEILMAN, K. and HÖPKER, W. W. Loss of differentiation in intestinal metaplasia in cancerous stomach. A comparative morphologic study. *Pathology, Research and Practice,* **164,** 249–258 (1979)

34 HERMANEK, P. Local excision – a therapeutic procedure in early gastric carcinoma. In *Gastric Cancer,* edited by Ch. Herfarth and P. Schlag, 215–216. Berlin, Heidelberg, New York, Springer Verlag (1979)

35 HERMANEK, P. and ROESCH, W. Critical evaluation of the Japanese 'early gastric cancer' classification. *Endoscopy,* **5,** 220–223 (1973)

36 HEYMER, B. and QUENTMEIER, A. Biological markers for staging of gastric cancer. In *Gastric Cancer,* edited by Ch. Herfarth and P. Schlag, 157–162. Berlin, Heidelberg, New York, Springer Verlag (1979)

37 HIRONO, I. and SHIBUYA, C. Proceedings of the 2nd International Symposium of the Princess Takamatsu Cancer Research Foundation. *Topics in Chemical Carcinogenesis,* 121, Tokyo (1974)

38 HISAMICHI, S., SASAKI, R., SUGAWARA, N., YANBO, T. and YAMAGATA, S. Stomach cancer in various age groups as detected by gastric mass survey. *Journal of the American Geriatrics Society,* **27,** 439–443 (1979)

39 HOVINEN, E., KEKKI, M. and KUIKKA, S. A theory to the stochastic dynamic model building for chronic progressive disease processes with an application to chronic gastritis. *Journal of Theoretical Biology,* **57,** 131–152 (1976)

40 HUMPHREY, E. W., KEEHN, R. J., HIGGINS, G. A. and SHIELDS, T. W. The long-term survival of patients with visceral carcinoma. *Surgery, Gynecology and Obstetrics,* **149,** 385–394 (1979)

41 HÄKKINEN, I. P. T. Reappearance of fetal sulfoglycoprotein antigen in carcinogenesis of the stomach. In *Pathophysiology of Carcinogenesis in Digestive Organs,* edited by E. Farber *et al.,* 75–88. Tokyo, University Press/Baltimore, University Park Press (1977)

42 HÄKKINEN, I. and VIIKARI, S. Occurrence of fetal sulphoglycoprotein antigen in the gastric juice of patients with gastric disease. *American Journal of Surgery,* **169,** 277–281 (1969)

43 IHAMÄKI, T., SAUKKONEN, M. and SIURALA, M. Long-term observations of subjects with normal mucosa and with superficial gastritis: Results of 23–27 years follow-up examinations. *Scandinavian Journal of Gastroenterology,* **13,** 771–776 (1978)

44 IHAMÄKI, T. and SIPPONEN, P. Morphology and function of the gastric mucosa in first-degree relatives of probands with histologically different types of gastric carcinoma. *Acta Pathologica et Microbiologica Scandinavica, Section A,* **87,** 437–462 (1979)

45 IHAMÄKI, T., VARIS, K. and SIURALA, M. Morphological, functional and immunological state of the gastric mucosa in gastric carcinoma families. Comparison with a computer-matched family sample. *Scandinavian Journal of Gastroenterology,* **14,** 801–812 (1979)

46 INBERG, M. V., HEINONEN, R., RANTAKOKKO, V. and VIIKARI, J. Surgical treatment of gastric carcinoma. A regional study of 2590 patients over a 27-year period. *Archives of Surgery,* **110,** 703–710 (1975)

47 INBERG, M. V., LAUREN, P., VUORI, J. and VIIKARI, S. J. Prognosis in intestinal-type and diffuse gastric carcinoma with special reference to the effect of the stomal reaction. *Acta Chirurgica Scandinavica*, **139**, 273–278 (1973)

48 JANSSON, B., SEIBERT, B. and SPEER, J. F. Gastrointestinal cancer. Its geographic distribution and correlation to breast cancer. *Cancer*, **36**, 2373–2384 (1975)

49 JASS, R. J. and FILIPE, M. I. A variant of intestinal metaplasia associated with gastric carcinoma: A histochemical study. *Histopathology*, **3**, 191–199 (1979)

50 JÄRVI, O. and LAUREN, P. On the role of heterotopias of the intestinal epithelium in the pathogenesis of gastric cancer. *Acta Pathologica et Microbiologica Scandinavica*, **29**, 26–44 (1951)

51 KAWAI, K., MIYAOKA, T. and KOHLI, U. Evaluation of early gastric cancer from the clinical point of view. In *Early Gastric Cancer*, edited by H. Grundmann, H. Grunge, and S. Witte, 63–66. Berlin, Springer Verlag (1974)

52 KEKKI, M., VARIS, K., IHAMÄKI, T., SIPPONEN, P. and SIURALA, M. (Unpublished observations)

53 KITABAKE, T., YOKOYAMA, M., SAKKA, M. and KOGA, S. Estimation of benefits and radiation risks from mass x-ray survey in Japan. *Strahlentherapie*, **146**, 352–358 (1973)

54 KODORI, O., MACHIDA, T., HOSAKA, S., KUSAMA, S., SHOJI, M. and SCHIKAWA, K. Kritische Untersuchung des Todesfalle bei rezidiwierten Magenfrühkarzinomen. *Langenbecks Archiv für Chirurgie*, **348**, 167–175 (1979)

55 KROKOWSKI, E. Verändertes Konzept der Krebsbehandlung. In *Neue Aspekte der Krebsbekämpfung*, edited by E. Krokowski, 93. Stuttgart, Georg Thieme Verlag (1978)

56 LAUREN, P. The two histological main types of gastric carcinoma, diffuse and so-called intestinal type carcinoma. *Acta Pathologica et Microbiologica Scandinavica*, **64**, 31–49 (1965)

57 LEHTOLA, J. Family study of gastric carcinoma; with special reference to histological types. *Scandinavian Journal of Gastroenterology*, **13** (Supplement 50) (1978).

58 LINDGREN, J., SIPPONEN, P., SEPPÄLÄ, K., TARPILA, S., NORDLING, S., WAHLSTRÖM, T. and SEPPÄLÄ, M. Carcinoembryonic antigen in endoscopical brush specimens from benign and malignant gastric lesions. *British Journal of Cancer*, **40**, 848–856 (1979)

59 LIPKIN, M., SHERLOCK, P. and BELL, B. Cell proliferation kinetics in the gastrointestinal tract of man. *Gastroenterology*, **45**, 721–729 (1963)

60 LIPKIN, M. Neoplastic transformation of cells in the gastrointestinal tract. In *Pathophysiology of Carcinogenesis in Digestive Organs*, edited by E. Farber *et al.*, 413–428. Tokyo, University Press/Baltimore, University Park Press, (1977)

61 MCCONNELL, R. B. *The Genetics of Gastro-intestinal Disorders*. 46–75. London, Oxford University Press (1966)

62 MARQUARDT, H., RUFINO, F. and WEISBURGER, J. H. Mutagenic activity of nitrite: Human stomach cancer may be related to dietary factors. *Science*, **196**, 1000–1001 (1977)

63 MIKI, K., ODA, T., SUZUKI, H., IINO, S. and NIWA, H. Alkaline phosphatase isoenzymes in carcinoma tissues of gastrointestinal tract. *Scandinavian Journal of Immunology*, **8**, 536–570 (1978)

64 MIRVISH, S. S. Formation of N-Nitroso compounds: Chemistry, kinetics and *in vivo* occurrence. *Toxicology and Applied Pharmacology*, **31**, 325–351 (1975)

65 MIRVISH, S. S. and SHUBIK, P. Ascorbic acid and nitrosamines. *Nature*, **250**, 684–689 (1974)

66 MOERTEL, C. G., RITTS, R. E., O'CONNELL, M. J. and SILVERS, A. Non-specific immune determinants in patients with unresectable gastrointestinal carcinoma. *Cancer*, **43**, 1483–1492 (1979)

67 MULLIGAN, R. M. Histogenesis and biologic behavior of gastric carcinoma. *Annals of Pathology*, **7**, 349–415 (1972)

68 MUÑOZ, N. and ASVALL, J. Time trends of intestinal and diffuse types of gastric cancer in Norway. *International Journal of Cancer*, **8**, 144–157 (1971)

69 MUÑOZ, N. and CONNELLY, R. Time trends of intestinal and diffuse types of gastric cancer in the United States. *International Journal of Cancer*, **8**, 158–164 (1971)

70 MUÑOZ, N., CORREA, P., CUELLO, C. and DUQUE, E. Histologic types of gastric carcinoma in high- and low-risk areas. *International Journal of Cancer*, **3**, 809–818 (1968)

71 NAGAYO, T. Histological diagnosis of biopsied gastric mucosa with special reference to the borderline cases. *Gann Monograph on Cancer Research*, **11**, 245–256 (1971)

72 NAGAYO, T. Precursors of human gastric cancer. Their frequences and histological characteristics. In *Pathophysiology of Carcinogenesis in Digestive Organs,* edited by E. Farber *et al.*, 151–160. Tokyo, University Press/Baltimore University Park Press (1977)

73 NAMIKI, M., SEKIYA, C., YAZAKI, Y., MUTO, E. and HARADA, K. Disease specificity in the Ainos with special reference to gastrointestinal disease. In *10th International Congress of Gastroenterology*, 750, Budapest (1976)

74 OESER, H. *Strahlenbehandlung der Geschwülste.* München, Urban and Schwarzenberg (1954)

75 OKABE, H. Growth of early gastric cancer. *Gann Monograph on Cancer Research*, **11**, 67–79 (1971)

76 PICHLMAYR, R., BÜTTNER, D. and MEYER, H.-J. Das Magenkarzinom. *Deutsche Ärzteblatt*, **74**, 2505–2509 (1977)

77 RUBIN, P. MACDONALD, E. J., MING, S. C., NAGAYO, T., YOKOYAMA, H., SCHADE, R. O. K., COLCHER, H. and JANOWER, M. L. Cancer of the gastrointestinal tract. Gastric cancer. *Journal of the American Medical Association*, **288**, 883–896 (1974)

78 RUDDELL, W. S. J., BONE, E. S., HILL, M. J., BLENDIS, L. M. and WALTERS, C. L. Gastric-juice nitrite. A risk factor for cancer in the hypochlorhydric stomach? *Lancet*, **2**, 1037–1039 (1976)

79 RUDDELL, W. S. J., BONE, E. S., HILL, M. J. and WALTERS, C. L. Pathogenesis of gastric cancer in pernicious anaemia. *Lancet*, **1**, 521–523 (1978)

80 RÖSCH, W., HERMANEK, P. and ELSTER, K. Gastritis und Frühkarzinom. *Fortschritte der Endoskopie*, **5,** 23 (1973)

81 SAITO, T., INOKUCHI, K., TAKAYAMA, S. and SUGIMURA. T. Sequential morphological changes in N-methyl-N-nitro-N-nitrosoguanidine carcinogenesis in the glandular stomach of rats. *Journal of the National Cancer Institute*, **44,** 769–783 (1970)

82 SAITO, T., SASAKI, O., TAMAKA, R., IWAMATSU, M., MATSUKUCHI, T. and INOKUCHI, K. Follow-up studies of experimental stomach. Experimental cancer in dogs. In *Pathophysiology of Carcinogenesis in Digestive Organs*, edited by E. Farber *et al.*, 107–120. Tokyo, University Press/Baltimore, University Park Press (1977)

83 SAUKKONEN, M., SIPPONEN, P., VARIS, K. and SIURALA, M. Morphological and dynamic behavior of the gastric mucosa after partial gastrectomy with special reference to the gastroenterostomy area. *Acta Hepato-Gastroenterologica*, **27,** 48–56 (1980)

84 SCHACHENMAYER, W. and HAFERKAMP, O. Prognostic significance of stromal reaction in gastric carcinoma. In *Gastric Cancer*, edited by Ch. Herfarth and P. Schlag, 182–186. Berlin, Heidelberg, New York, Springer Verlag (1979)

85 SCHLAG, P., WONKA, W., MEYER, H., FEYERABEND, G. and MERKLE, P. Bakterielle Besiedlung und Nitritbildung im Magen nach Gastroenterostomie. *Langenbecks Archiv für Chirurgie*, **344,** 109–114 (1977)

86 SCHMITZ-MOORMAN, P. HEIDER, H.-A. and THOMAS, C. Cancer of the stomach – prognosis, independent of therapy. In *Gastric Cancer*, edited by Ch. Herfarth and P. Schlag, 172–181. Berlin, Springer Verlag (1979)

87 SELT, D. and FARBER, E. New principle for the analysis of chemical carcinogenesis. *Nature*, **263,** 701–703 (1976)

88 SIEVERS, M. L. Unusual comparative frequency of gastric carcinoma, pernicious anemia, and peptic ulcer in southwestern American Indians. *Gastroenterology*, **65,** 867–876 (1973)

89 SIGARAN, M. F. and CON-WONG, R. Production of proliferative lesions in gastric mucosa of albino mice by oral administration of N-methyl-N-nitro-N-nitrosoguanidine. *Gann*, **70,** 343–352 (1979)

90 SIPPONEN, P., RUOSLAHTI, E., VUENTO, M., ENGVALL, E., STENMAN, U.-H., IHAMÄKI, T. and SIURALA, M. CEA and CEA-like activity in gastric cancer. *Acta Hepato-Gastroenterologica*, **23,** 276–279 (1976)

91 SIPPONEN, P., SEPPÄLÄ, K., VARIS, K., HJELT, L., IHAMÄKI, T., KEKKI, M. and SIURALA, M. Intestinal metaplasia with colonic type sulphomucins in the gastric mucosa. *Acta Pathologica et Microbiologica Scandinavica*, *Sect. A*, **88,** 217–224 (1980)

92 SIURALA, M., ISOKOSKI, M., VARIS, K. and KEKKI, M. Prevalence of gastritis in a rural population. *Scandinavian Journal of Gastroenterology*, **3,** 211–223 (1968)

93 SIURALA, M. and VARIS, K. Gastritis. In *Scientific Foundations of Gastroenterology*, edited by W. Sircus and A. N. Smith, 357–369. London, William Heinemann Medical Books Ltd (1979)

94 SIURALA, M., VILLAKO, K., IHAMÄKI, T., KEKKI, M., LEHTOLA, J., SIPPONEN, P. and VARIS, K. Atrophic gastritis: Its genetic and dynamic behavior and its relations to gastric carcinoma and pernicious anemia. In *Pathophysiology of Carcinogenesis in Digestive organs*, edited by E. Farber *et al.*, 135–148. Tokyo, University Press/Baltimore, University Park Press (1977)

95 SPECTOR, B. D., PERRY, G. S., GOOD, R. A. and KERSEY, J. Immunodeficiency diseases and malignancy. *Comparative Immunology, Microbiology and Infectious Diseases*, **4,** (1978)

96 STEMMERMANN, G. N. Gastric cancer in the Hawaii Japanese. *Gann*, **6,** 525–535 (1977)

97 STEMMERMAN, G. N. and KOLONEL, L. N. Talc-coated rice as a risk factor for stomach cancer. *American Journal of Clinical Nutrition,,* **31,** 2017–2019 (1978)

98 SUGIYAMA, N. and OHOHASHI, I. Clinico-pathological study on 114 gastric cancers of young men. *Gastroenterologia Japonica*, **13,** 318–319 (1978)

99 TAKEUCHI, T., MIYAYAMA, H., IWAMASA, T. Histochemical demonstration of total phosphorylase activity for diagnosis of carcinoma cells in human stomach and intestines. *Stain Technology*, **53,** 257–260 (1978)

100 TANNENBAUM, S. R., MORAN, D., RAND, W., CUELLO, C. and CORREA, P. Gastric cancer in Colombia. IV. Nitrite and other ions in gastric contents of residents from a high-risk region. *Journal of the National Cancer Institute*, **62,** 9–12 (1979)

101 TEGLBJAERG, P. S. and NIELSEN, H. O. 'Small intestinal type' and 'colonic type' intestinal metaplasia of the human stomach and their relationship to the histogenetic types of gastric adenocarcinoma. *Acta Pathologica et Microbiologica Scandinavica, Section A*, **86,** 351–355 (1978)

102 VARIS, K. A family study of chronic gastritis. *Scandinavian Journal of Gastroenterology*, **6,** Supplement 13 (1971)

103 VILLAKO, K., TAMM, A., SAVISAAR, E. and RUTTAS, M. Prevalence of antral and fundic gastritis in a randomly selected group of an Esthonian rural population. *Scandinavian Journal of Gastroenterology*, **11,** 817–822 (1976)

104 VUENTO, M., RUOSLAHTI, E., PIHKO, H., SVENBERG, T., IHAMÄKI, T. and SIURALA, M. Carcinoembryonic antigen-like substance in gastric juice. *Immunochemistry*, **13,** 313–316 (1976)

105 WALKER, E. A., BOGOVSKI, P. and GRICIUTE, L. Environmental N-nitroso-compounds, analysis and formation. *IARC Scientific Publications*, No. **14,** Lyon (1976)

106 WEISBURGER, J. H. Mechanism of action of diet as a carcinogen. *Cancer*, **43** (5 Supplement) 1987–1995 (1979)

107 WEISBURGER, J. H. and RAINERI, R. Assessment of human exposure and response to N-nitroso compounds: A new view on the etiology of digestive tract cancers. *Toxicology and Applied Pharmacology*, **31,** 396–374 (1975)

108 WORLD HEALTH ORGANIZATION Histological typing of gastric and oesophageal tumours. *International Histological Classification of Tumours* No. **19.** Geneva, WHO (1977)

109 WORLD HEALTH ORGANIZATION Nitrosatable drugs. *Drug Information*, **2,** 4, Geneva, WHO (1978)

110 WYNDER, E. L., REDDY, B. S., McCOY, G. D., WEISBURGER J. H. and WILLIAMS, G. M. Diet and gastrointestinal cancer. *Clinical Gastroenterology*, **5**, 463–482 (1976)

111 YOSHII, Y. and KOBAYASHI, S. Carcinoma of the stomach in the young. Comparative study with that in the aged (meeting abstract). *Gastroenterologia Japonica*, **13**, 318–319 (1978)

112 ZALDIVAR, R. Geographical pathology of oral, oesophageal gastric and intestinal cancer in Chile. *Zeitschrift für Krebsforschung*, **75**, 1–13 (1970)

113 ZEITOUN, P., MARTIN, F. and NASCA, S. Progrès thérapeutiques en cancerologie digestive. *Médecine et Chirurgie Digestives*, **8**, 655–660 (1979)

Index